THE PLANT BASED DIET cookbook

600 QUICK AND EASY HEALTHY RECIPES TO PREPARE FLAVORFUL DISHES FOR ALL THE FAMILY, FROM BREAKFAST TO DESSERT. 4-WEEK WEIGHT LOSS MEAL PLAN

Eva Mirville

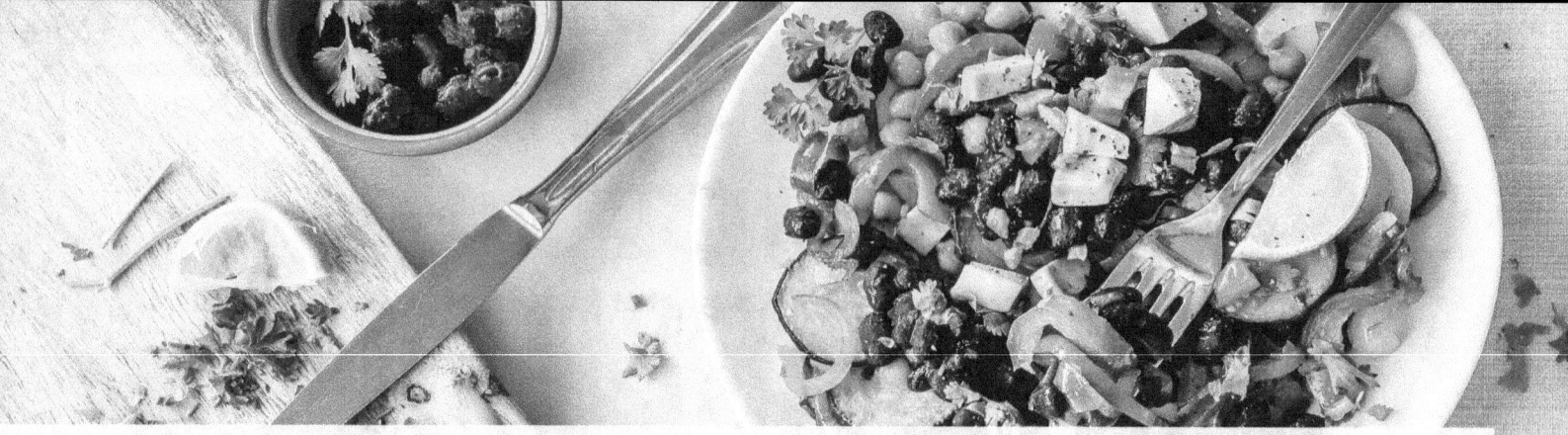

Copyright - 2020 -

All rights reserved.

The content contained within this book may not be reproduced, duplicated or transmitted without direct written permission from the author or the publisher.

Under no circumstances will any blame or legal responsibility be held against the publisher, or author, for any damages, reparation, or monetary loss due to the information contained within this book. Either directly or indirectly.

Legal Notice:

This book is copyright protected. This book is only for personal use. You cannot amend, distribute, sell, use, quote or paraphrase any part, or the content within this book, without the consent of the author or publisher.

Disclaimer Notice:

Please note the information contained within this document is for educational and entertainment purposes only. All effort has been executed to present accurate, up to date, and reliable, complete information. No warranties of any kind are declared or implied. Readers acknowledge that the author is not engaging in the rendering of legal, financial, medical or professional advice. The content within this book has been derived from various sources. Please consult a licensed professional before attempting any techniques outlined in this book.

By reading this document, the reader agrees that under no circumstances is the author responsible for any losses, direct or indirect, which are incurred as a result of the use of information contained within this document, including, but not limited to, - errors, omissions, or inaccuracies.

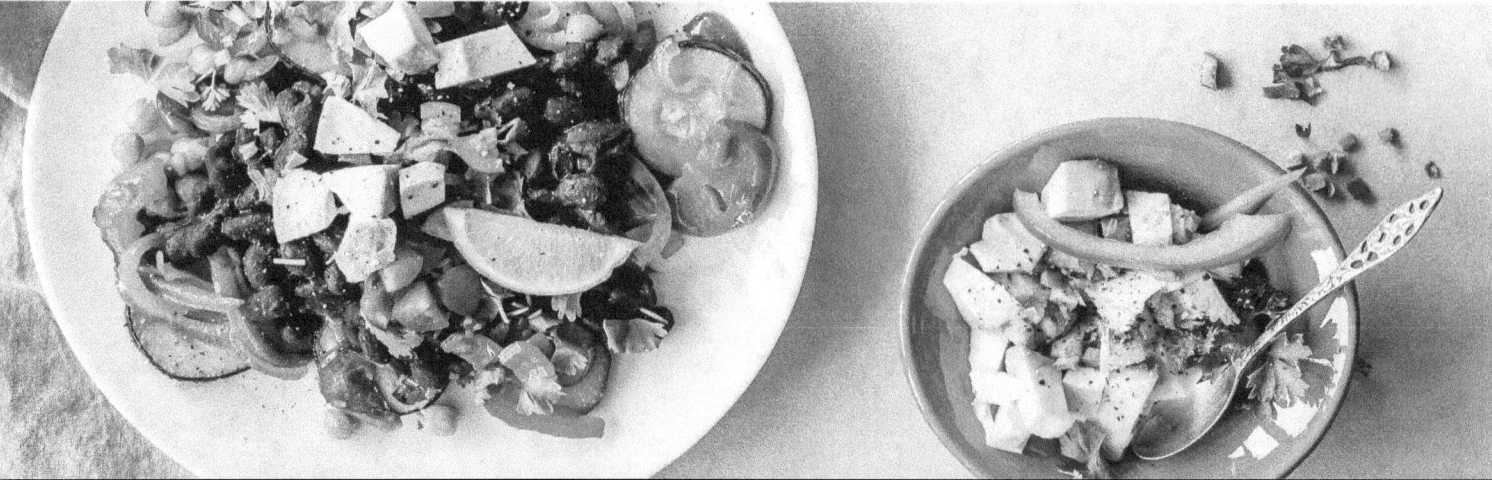

TABLE OF CONTENTS

INTRODUCTION — 4

CHAPTER 1:
WHAT IS A PLANT BASED DIET — 8

CHAPTER 2:
BENEFITS OF A PLANT-BASED DIET — 12

CHAPTER 3:
LOOKING FOR ALTERNATIVES — 14

CHAPTER 4:
SUPERFOODS — 18

CHAPTER 5:
UNDERSTANDING PLANT MICRONUTRIENTS — 22

CHAPTER 6:
4-WEEK WEIGHT LOSS MEAL PLAN — 26

CHAPTER 7:
BREAKFAST — 32

CHAPTER 8:
SMOOTHIES AND FRESH JUICES — 52

CHAPTER 9:
GRAINS — 70

CHAPTER 10:
PASTA & NOODLES — 94

CHAPTER 11:
LEGUMES — 102

CHAPTER 12:
SOUPS AND STEWS — 118

CHAPTER 13:
SALADS AND SIDE DISHES — 140

CHAPTER 14:
SNACK AND SIDES — 166

CHAPTER 15:
WRAPS AND SANDWICHES — 184

CHAPTER 16:
SAUCES, DRESSINGS, AND DIPS — 196

CHAPTER 17:
VEGETABLES RECIPES — 220

CHAPTER 18:
APPETIZER AND SNACK — 248

CHAPTER 19:
DESSERTS — 268

CHAPTER 20:
FRUIT SALAD — 298

CONCLUSION — 302

RECIPES INDEX — 303

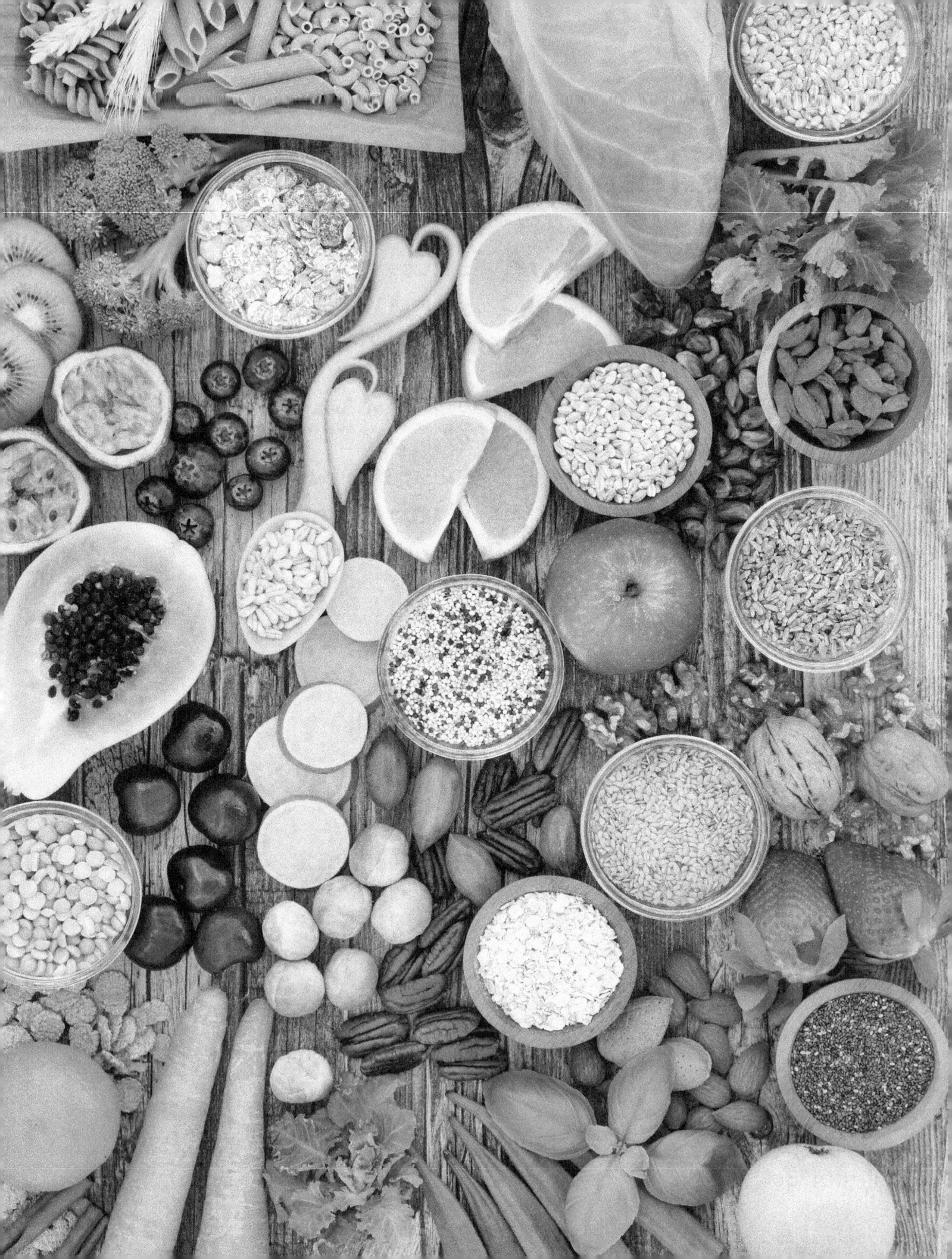

INTRODUCTION

There are a lot of arguments out there about which diet is the best for you. Despite this, a lot of health and wellness communities are going to agree that those diets that emphasize fresh and whole ingredients, while making sure to minimize the foods that are processed are the ones that are the best for your wellness overall. And as you can imagine, the plant-based whole foods diet will be able to do this very well. Let's dive into how this diet works, and what this kind of nutrition is all about, so you can use it for some of your own needs as well.

There isn't a clear definition of what this kind of diet would entail because it is more about eating healthy and ensuring that we provide our bodies with all of the nutrition it needs from plant sources. This is often seen more as a lifestyle change than anything because there are various plant-based diets that you can go on, and each one will vary based on how much a person decides to include or exclude animal products into the diet. For example, some vegetarians include fish in it, and some will be vegan and won't include any animal product.

It is a natural fact that only through watching what we eat we will have the most impact on our weight. Plant-based diet helps you appreciate automatic, easy Fat: burning without all other diets' usual calorie constraints.

Weight loss is an almost certain result you will enjoy once you start the plant-based diet, but this is not the only benefit you will enjoy. Think of all those activities you have always wanted to pursue but shelved because you simply had no energy left after your usual day's work.

Well, it's time to dust off those hobbies and the things you enjoy doing, because on the plant-based you will have more energy for your daily work and play! The accompanying mental clarity and sharpness of thought are also positive effects that you will have due to this diet. A better health report card, by way of optimized cholesterol readings, normalized blood sugar and a corresponding lowered risk of cardiovascular diseases are also just some of the beneficial health effects experienced by most on the diet.

A plant-based diet is a diet based primarily on whole plant foods. It is identical to the regular diet we're used to already, except that it leaves out foods that are not exclusively from plants. Hence, a plant-based diet does away with all types of animal-sourced foods, hydrogenated oils, refined sugars, and processed foods. A whole food plant-based diet comprises not just fruits and vegetables. It also consists of unprocessed or barely-processed oils with healthy monounsaturated fats (like extra-virgin olive oil), whole grains, legumes (essentially lentils and beans), seeds and nuts, as well as herbs and spices.

What makes a plant-based meal (or any meal) fun is how you make them, the seasoning process, and the combination process that contributes to a fantastic flavor and makes every meal unique and enjoyable. There are many delicious recipes (all plant-centered), which will prove helpful when you intend making mouthwatering, healthy plant-based dishes for personal or household consumption. Provided you're eating these plant-based foods regularly, you'll have very few problems with Fat: or diseases that result from bad dietary habits, and there would be no need for excessive calorie tracking.

Plant-based diet can vary from one person to another. However, the foundational idea is that we try to avoid processed food as much as possible and choose to use what we receive from the beautiful planet that we live in. By that, I mean the incredible ingredients derived from the earth. In essence, plant-based diet comes with a few benefits.

Plant-based diet avoids using processed foods as much as possible.

- There are no animal products in the diet.
- The categories included are vegetables, fruits, seeds and nuts, legumes, whole grains, and herbs and spices.
- The diet tries to limit the use of sugar, wheat-flour, and oil as much as possible.
- It focuses on the quality of food, mostly utilizing locally or

farm-produced organic foods

An important thing to remember here is that there are minimally processed foods included in the plant-based diet, such as non-dairy milk, tofu, and whole-wheat paste, to name a few. Overall, we aim to keep processed foods where they belong: on supermarket shelves, not in our refrigerators.

When people look at the list of foods that come in a plant-based diet, they are often focused on how little we have to work on. However, that is probably because many of the meat options have suddenly been removed. It feels as though a major part of the diet has been excluded due to it. How can life be fun without a nice steak? What can we do without chicken wings? Is there anything that can be done without a delicious fish?

In reality, there are numerous ingredients that you can work with. Additionally, the fun is not just in the ingredients but how we prepare them. The growing demand has seen a rise in people trying out new recipes and mashing up ingredients in interesting ways. Have you heard of smoothies that contain cayenne pepper? Sounds pretty exciting, doesn't it? We are going to look at such wonderful and delicious recipes along with so many more dishes that use wholesome and natural ingredients.

Some people are doing it; some people are talking about it, but there is still a lot of confusion about what a whole plant-based diet entails. Since we split food into their macronutrients: sugars, proteins, and fats, most of us are uncertain about nutrition. What if we were able to put these macronutrients back together to free your mind from confusion and stress? The secret here is simplicity.

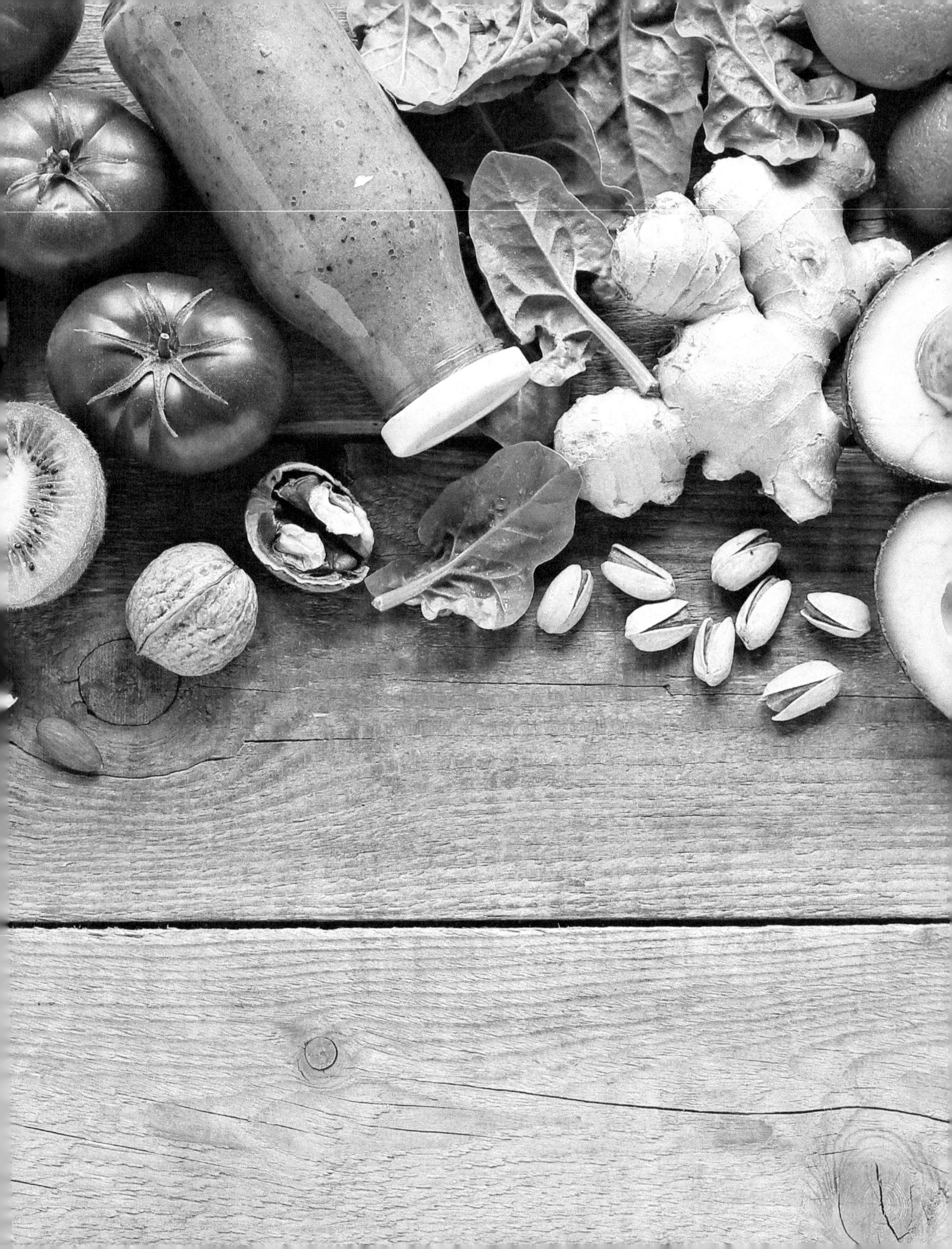

CHAPTER 1:
WHAT IS A PLANT BASED DIET

The first step to following a whole food plant-based diet is understanding what it means. To put it plain and simple, it means filling a majority of your diet with foods that are not processed or refined and come directly from plants. They are foods that are as close as possible to their source and are completely unmodified. It is not a diet restricted solely to fruits and vegetables; there are many delicious alternatives to help you have a satisfying choice of foods to eat.

Many people mistake the plant-based diet for a vegan one. So, let's talk about the difference. There are parallels in both of them, but there are small differences. A vegan diet does not include any products based on animals. This, of course, includes meats and eggs and outcomes of these animals, such as honey. Vegans will carry this perspective into their lives, which is more than a diet to them. A plant-based diet will keep you from eating anything based on animals, but it will not prevent you from using animal products in your life.

Get your Phytochemicals

The only place to get phytochemicals is in whole foods, such as fruits, vegetables, beans and whole grains. These essential nutrients have a direct impact on your health. The latest research determines that a few of the key phytochemicals might help to prevent certain cancers, lower cholesterol, keep the gastrointestinal tract healthy and protect various cells throughout the body. There are thousands of different forms available, but the most commonly known nutrients are terms that might be a little more familiar to you: flavonoids, antioxidants and carotenoids.

How do you fill your diet with these amazing nutrients? Start by creating a rainbow of colors on your plates. The more colorful fruits and vegetables you consume, the higher your body's chances of consuming the nutrients your body needs. There are many beautiful colored fruits and vegetables to choose from, including red tomatoes, blue blueberries, orange carrots, pink watermelon, pink grapefruit, green spinach, green kale, red strawberries and red raspberries. The more colors on your plate, the more benefits you are providing your body.

In addition to fruits and vegetables, phytonutrients can be found in whole-grain bread, whole-grain cereal, walnuts, sunflower seeds, peas, lentils, green tea and black tea. If you consume bread and cereals, it is important to ensure that they are truly made from whole grains, not processed grains that could be stripped of the nutrients you assume you are obtaining by eating it.

Is Organic a Requirement?

Eating whole foods does not mean that they must be locally grown or even organic; that is a completely different topic. This does not mean that your whole foods cannot be organic; it is just not a prerequisite to qualify as whole or natural. Organic or locally grown food could provide you with the added benefit of eliminating harmful toxins and chemicals, which can further benefit eating whole foods.

Maximize Nutrients in Vegetables

The reason why we eat food, besides that it tastes good, is to obtain the vital nutrients necessary for good health. When you consume food that has been modified, processed or refined, the important nutrients are removed. This is even true for those foods that you consider healthy. For example, you might think you are doing your body well by eating spinach or broccoli. But if you do not eat it raw or prepare it properly, you are likely losing some of its nutrients, especially water-soluble elements. Vitamin B and C are two of the water-soluble vitamins found in both vegetables that are lost when these vegetables are cooked in water, whether boiled or steamed. Choosing to eat these vegetables raw is the best way to consume all vital nutrients. If you prefer them cooked, choose methods such as sautéing, stir frying or blanching as each of these methods are considered "quick cooking" methods and avoid the risk of losing many nutrients.

Choosing Whole Grains

In addition to eating fruits and vegetables, a whole foods diet also includes eating various whole grains. Care should be taken when you choose your grains, however. Not all whole grains are as "whole" as they sound. When you choose the right grains, you can reap the benefits of complex Carbs: and vital vitamins and nutrients, adding taste, texture and proper nutrition to your diet.

Grains are found in the seeds of various grasses. They can be found in wheat, oats, rice, cornmeal and barley. When grains start, they are considered whole and their most important ingredients, bran and germ are intact. During the processing of these grains, they are stripped of bran and germ as well as their vital nutrients. This results in refined and enriched grains, which make up the products that have a longer shelf life, such as white bread and white rice. These foods, as you probably know, are less healthy for you. When you read product labels, look for the words refined or enriched grains and steer clear. In refined grains, the lost nutrients are never replaced. In enriched grains, the products are fortified with the stripped nutrients, but it does not provide the same benefits as eating whole foods with the natural nutrients right from the start.

Creating the Perfect Meals

Creating the perfect meals with the right plant-based whole foods does not have to be difficult. It is best to get creative to maximize the nutrients that you consume. Start with the basics including whole grain breads, whole grain pasta, steel cut oats, colorful fruits and raw vegetables. Then you can get creative:

- Add fruits and spices to your oatmeal
- Add flax seed to your whole grain cereal
- Make salad the main course for lunch or dinner and get creative
- Add your favorite vegetables to whole grain pasta or rice
- Make smoothies with as many fruits and vegetables as possible
- Add plant-based, natural nut butters to whole grain bread
- Eat fruit for dessert
- Add beans to lunch and dinner entrées
- Include at least one fruit and vegetable at every meal.

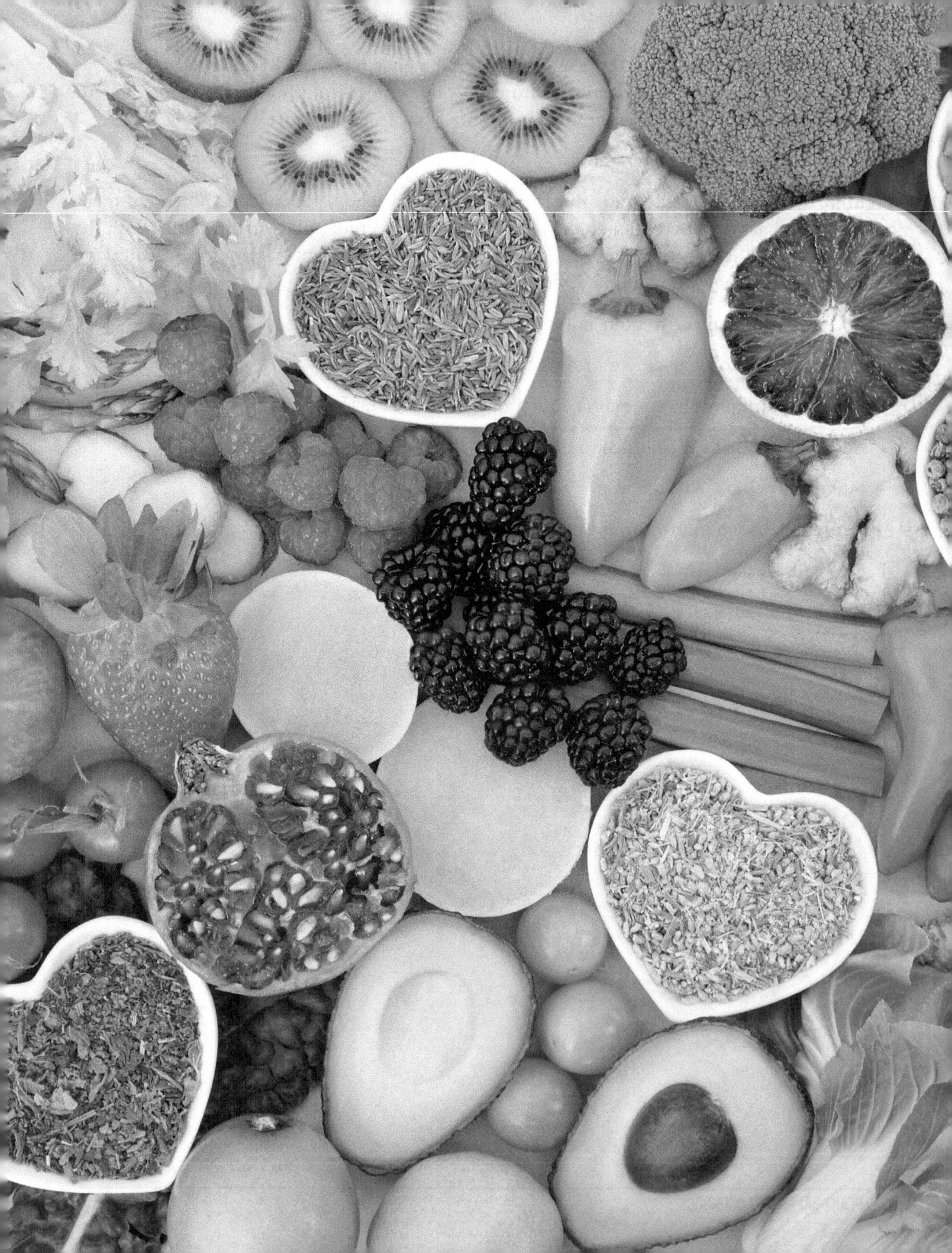

CHAPTER 2: BENEFITS OF A PLANT-BASED DIET

Now that you know what the plant-based diet is, it's essential to look at the host of benefits that it has to offer. It's hard to stick to a diet that makes you drastically change your current way of eating if you don't have a good reason. That's what this chapter is about—giving you that good reason to meet your health and weight loss goals using the plant-based diet.

Better Nutrition

Plants are very healthy foods to eat, and most people fail to eat the appropriate number of veggies and fruits; therefore, following a plant-based diet will boost your productivity. Vegetables and fruits are rich in antioxidants, vitamins, fiber, and minerals. Based on studies, fiber is a nutrient that most people don't get an adequate amount of, and it comes with tons of healthy perks—it is good for the heart, waistline, blood sugar, and the gut.

Weight Loss

When following a plant-based diet, people tend to have a lower body mass index (BMI) than people on an omnivorous diet. However, research shows that you will be more successful at dropping lb. and keeping them off when you follow a plant-based diet to lose weight. In societies that follow a mainly plant-based lifestyle, obesity is also lower. Since you're taking in more vitamins and nutrients and fiber, which your body has to break down, with a plant-based lifestyle, you're also likely to stay fuller for longer, which means you'll eat less overall. To lose weight, you have to burn more calories than you take in, so eating less is an essential part of that.

Healthier Hearts

Following a plant-based diet is likely to reduce the risk of cardiovascular diseases, and enhance other heart disease risk factors. Following a plant-based diet can also help quell inflammation, which increases the risk of heart disease by regulating plaque buildup in the arteries.

Lowers Blood Pressure

A plant-based diet has been proven to lower blood pressure because it has a high potassium content. A plant-based diet reduces blood pressure as well as stress and anxiety. Potassium-rich foods include seeds, whole, almonds, beans, berries, and grain. However, meat contains almost no potassium, which is why the plant-based diet offers a better way to control your blood pressure.

Lowers Cholesterol

Plants don't contain cholesterol, which includes saturated forms such as coffee or chocolate. When you live a plant-based diet lifestyle, you're reducing the amount of cholesterol you take in to next to zero. This plant-based diet will lessen the danger of heart illness and disease since cholesterol is an important cause of stroke and heart attack.

Lowers Diabetes Risk

Irrespective of your body mass index (BMI), following a plant-based diet lowers the risk of diabetes. Another study, published in February 2019, states that you tend to have higher insulin sensitivity when you follow a plant-based diet, which is significant for maintaining a healthy blood sugar level.

Reduces the Risk of Cancer

The consistent consumption of adequate legumes, veggies, fruits, and grains is associated with lower cancer risk. However, disease-fighting phytochemicals, which can be found in plants are known to prevent and halt cancer. Lastly, studies also indicate an association between processed meats' consumption and a rise in cancer risk, especially colorectal cancer. Therefore, there's a benefit from consuming more plants and choosing healthy plant foods rather than unhealthy ones.

More Energy

Within days of this type of eating, you'll feel energized because you'll get the nutrients you need. The foods that you'll be eating will also have higher water content, which can hydrate your skin and leave you feeling better overall. Plant-based foods are easier to digest and lighter, so you'll feel better than ever in just a few days. You'll also get a better sleep when you eat right. When you feed your body the vitamins and minerals it needs, you'll help your body relax and give it a peaceful sleep. Calcium and magnesium, which this diet is packed with, can help relax the body for quiet rest.

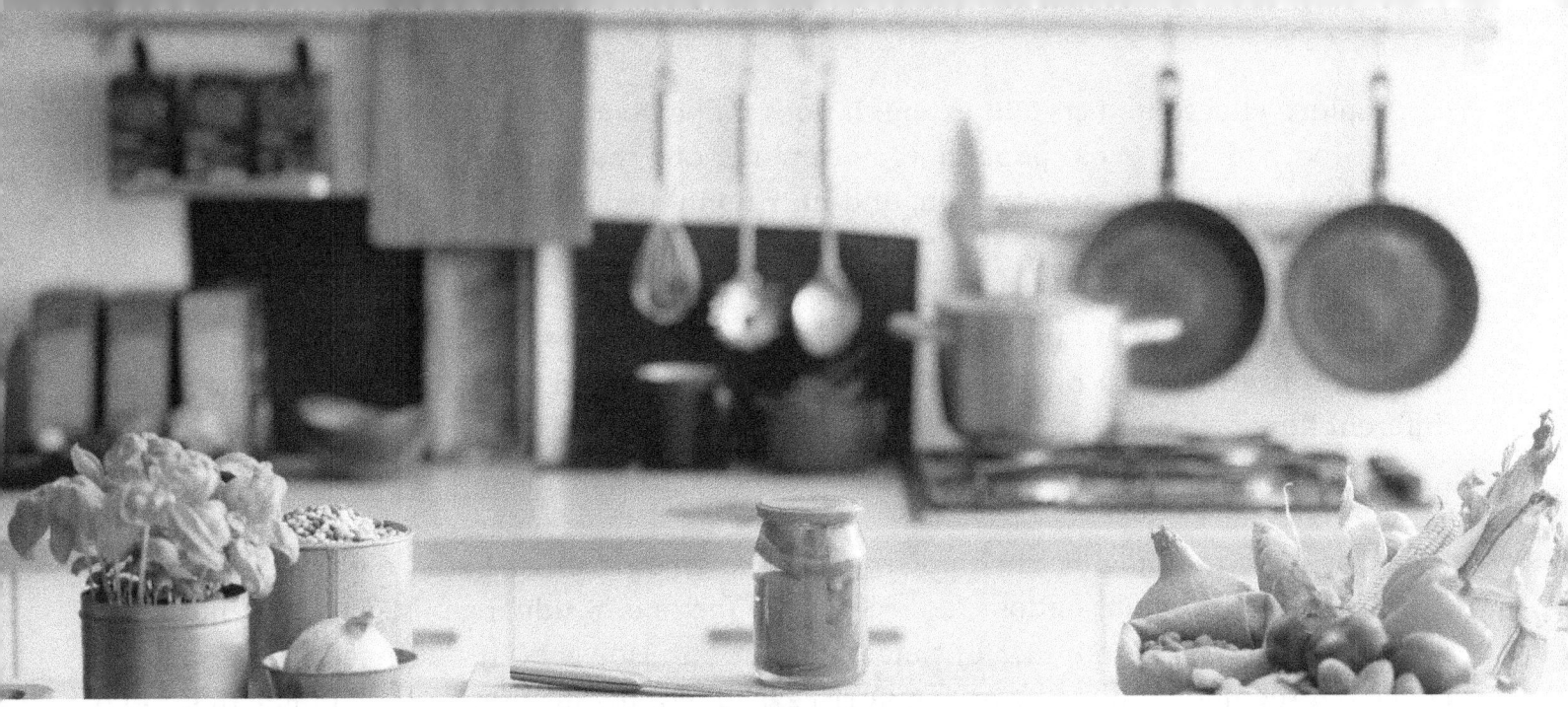

CHAPTER 3:
LOOKING FOR ALTERNATIVES

While a plant-based diet is not a vegan diet, you may want to avoid animal products as much as possible. Here are some tips to get you started so you can stick to this diet with ease and limit your animal product intake.

Look for Milk Alternatives

There are many non-dairy milk alternatives out there. There is coconut, cashew, Brazil nut, rice, almond and even hemp seed milk substitutes. Most can be used in equal measurements, especially in baking. Just make sure you're using their unsweetened versions. The best is that most of these kinds of milk are rich in calcium so you won't be missing out.

Look for Egg Alternatives

You can also replace eggs in recipes. You can use six tablespoons of water with three tablespoons of chia seeds or ground flaxseeds. Just soak them for five to ten minutes so that the mixture becomes gelatinous. You can also use a quarter cup of pureed banana or a quarter cup of applesauce, depending on the recipe. Each one of these is the equivalent of a single egg.

Look for Cheese Alternatives

There isn't a substitute for cheese, but the plant world has soft and creamy textures that can replace cheese to a certain extent. It does make a small change in the dish's taste, but it isn't too bad. The most popular replacements are soaked and blended cashews, sliced avocado, sprouted soft organic tofu, and nutritional yeast.

Look for Meat Alternatives

For a rich, hearty texture that will help fill you up, there are beans, Portobello mushrooms, tempeh, and tofu. Each of these is chewy and hearty, and they can be marinated to get different flavors. You can also use these for chili, stews, and burgers or can be served baked.

Be Careful Eating Out

It can be hard to dine out when you're trying to enjoy a plant-based diet. However, many restaurants offer vegan options, so try to look for one in advance. Just realize that you'll need to minimize the number of times you eat out. However, if you need to go out, then check out the menu online before you arrive. Look for dishes that are low in Fat: and full of vegetables, and then look for grilled, baked and steamed options. Try to avoid any dishes that are fried, rich, creamy or crispy. Just don't be shy about asking for a different salad dressing or side dish either. Make sure sauces and cheeses are left out too. If there's bread, ask for whole wheat. If there is rice, ask for brown rice.

Purge Your Kitchen

You should get rid of any temptation that's in your kitchen and calling your name if you're trying to start a plant-based diet. It's not good to have unhealthy foods in front of you, or you're bound to give in.

Plan Your Meals

Luckily this book comes with a meal plan that will help you stick to your first 4 weeks of your diet. However, you may want to stick to planning your meals for the first few months if you find yourself struggling.

Choose the One for You

You can choose the plant-based diet for you! Here are some of the most common plant-based diets out there.

- **Veganism:** This is a diet that includes legumes, fruits, grains, vegetables, nuts and seeds, but you'll not be able to eat any food that's sourced from animals.

- **Raw Veganism:** This is a diet that includes uncooked and some dehydrated foods.

- **Vegetarianism:** This is a diet that consists of legumes, vegetables, nuts and fruit. You can include eggs and dairy in this diet, but you aren't allowed meat.

- **Fruitarianism:** This is a vegan diet that primarily involves fruit, but you should not use this if you have diabetes.

- Ovo-Lacto Vegetarianism: This encourages that you eat eggs and dairy along with your fruit and vegetables.
- Ovo Vegetarianism: This is where you can eat eggs with your fruits and vegetables, but you still can't have dairy.
- Lacto Vegetarianism: This allows you to have dairy but no eggs with your fruits and vegetables.
- Semi-Vegetarianism: This is a mostly vegetarian diet with the occasional time that you can have meat.
- Pescatarian: This is a semi-vegetarian diet that allows you to have dairy, eggs, shellfish and fish.
- Macrobiotic Diet: This diet highlights whole grains, beans, miso soup, sea vegetables, vegetables, and naturally processed foods. This can be done with or without seafood and other animal products.

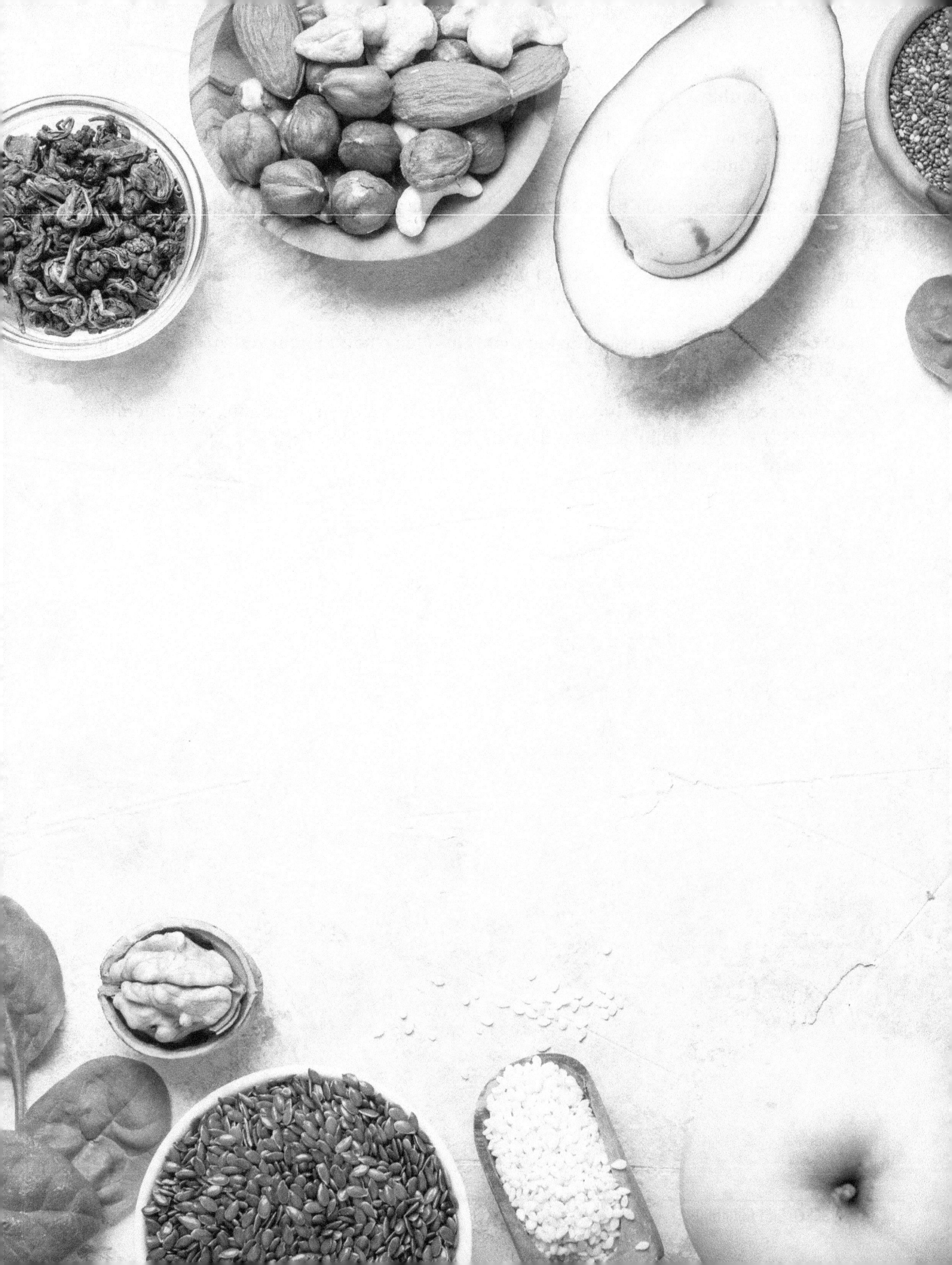

CHAPTER 4: SUPERFOODS

To be clear, most superfoods are already vegan, but some are particularly high in nutrient content. The following are the top vegan superfoods available today. These should be incorporated into your diet every chance you get. The following are twelve of the best superfoods that you will find at your local grocery store.

Dark Leafy Greens

Kale, swiss chard, spinach, and collard greens are all classed as dark leafy greens and these superfoods should be incorporated into your daily meal plan. Not only are they a great digestive aid due to their high fiber content, but they're also dense sources of vitamins C and K, zinc, calcium, magnesium, iron and folate. They have a high antioxidant profile that assists the body in removing harmful free radicals, reducing the risk of cancer, heart disease, and stroke.

Berries

Nature's little antioxidants are also the most delicious and delicate fruits we know. Berries host an array of benefits to the body and each one has its special powers:

Strawberries contain more vitamin C than oranges! They are antioxidant rich and provide us with fiber, potassium, anthocyanins, and folate. Strawberries reduce the risk of cancer, are supportive in the control of diabetes, and are great anti-inflammatories.

Blueberries are one of the most antioxidant-rich foods out there. They contain manganese and vitamins C and K, are supportive of cognitive function and mental health.

Raspberries are rich in vitamin C, selenium and phosphorus. Research shows they are beneficial in controlling blood sugar in people with diabetes. They are a great source of quercetin, known to slow the onset and growth of cancer cells.

Blackberries are incredibly high in antioxidants and fiber and are loaded with phytochemicals that fight cancer. They are also packed with vitamin C and K.

Nuts and Seeds

Nuts and seeds are a vegan's best friend when it comes to texture, variety, healthy fats, and proteins. They are incredibly nutrient dense and contain excellent levels of fats, protein, complex carbs, fiber. They are loaded with vitamins and minerals that are easily absorbed and fun to eat, while at the same time helping to protect our bodies against disease. Every nut and seed have their special traits:

- Pine nuts have an excess amount of manganese.
- Brazil nuts are the leading source of selenium.
- Pistachios are well known for their lutein content that supports eye health
- Almonds and sunflower seeds are great sources of vitamin E.
- Cashews have more iron than any other food in this category.
- Pumpkin seeds are one of the best possible sources of zinc.

Olive Oil

A staple of the Mediterranean diet for a reason, this oil is rich in antioxidants and monounsaturated fats that support cardiovascular health, prevent strokes and feed your hair and skin like nothing else. Despite being fat, it supports healthy weight maintenance.

Mushrooms

The best vegan meat source is low in calories while being high in Protein: and fiber. They're a great source of B vitamins, vitamin D, potassium and selenium. They are high in antioxidants, support healthy gut bacteria and are beneficial in weight loss.

Seaweed

Used in medicine for centuries, seaweed has antiviral properties and has recently tested positively in killing certain cancer cells. Seaweed benefits cholesterol levels and is rich in antioxidants proven to lower the instance of heart disease. Seaweed is incredibly rich in vitamin A, B, C, D, E and K. It's brimming with iron and iodine, which is essential for thyroid function and having decent amounts of calcium, copper, potassium, and magnesium.

Garlic

Garlic is a powerful medicinal ally to have on hand. It is rich in vitamins B6 and C, but most importantly, it boosts immune function, lowers blood pressure, improves cholesterol levels and supports cardiovascular health. Fresh garlic is brimming with antioxidants that have a potent effect on overall health.

Avocado

Avocado is a great source of MUFAs (Mono-Unsaturated Fatty Acids), a huge factor in cardiovascular function. They support vitamin and mineral absorption, healthy skin, hair, and eyes, improved digestive function, and contains twenty vitamins and minerals. Avocados provide anti-inflammatory activity and are loaded with soluble fiber.

Turmeric

Highly anti-inflammatory and has potent anti-cancer properties. It has been shown to provide pain relief in arthritic conditions and supports liver health due to its high antioxidant levels. Turmeric can be hard to absorb, however taking it with black pepper improves its absorptivity.

Chia Seeds

These tiny seeds are packed full of omega 3 fatty acids and are one of the best vegan sources out there. They are also antioxidant rich and packed with protein, calcium, iron and soluble fiber. Due to this, they are recommended to reduce cardiovascular disease, diabetes, and obesity. They are healing to the digestive tract, contribute to feelings of fullness so support weight loss, help lower cholesterol and best of all, when mixed with water, they make a great egg substitute.

Legumes

A study was conducted that investigated the longest living people and cultures in the world. The only dietary thing they shared was that legumes were a huge part of their diet. In fact, the longest living people in the world eat legumes every day. Legumes are rich in protein, fiber, and complex Carbs: and contain potassium, magnesium, folate, iron, B vitamins, zinc, copper, manganese, and phosphorus. These little guys are highly nutritious and loaded with soluble fiber that benefits colon health, feed healthy bacteria and reduce the risk of colon cancer.

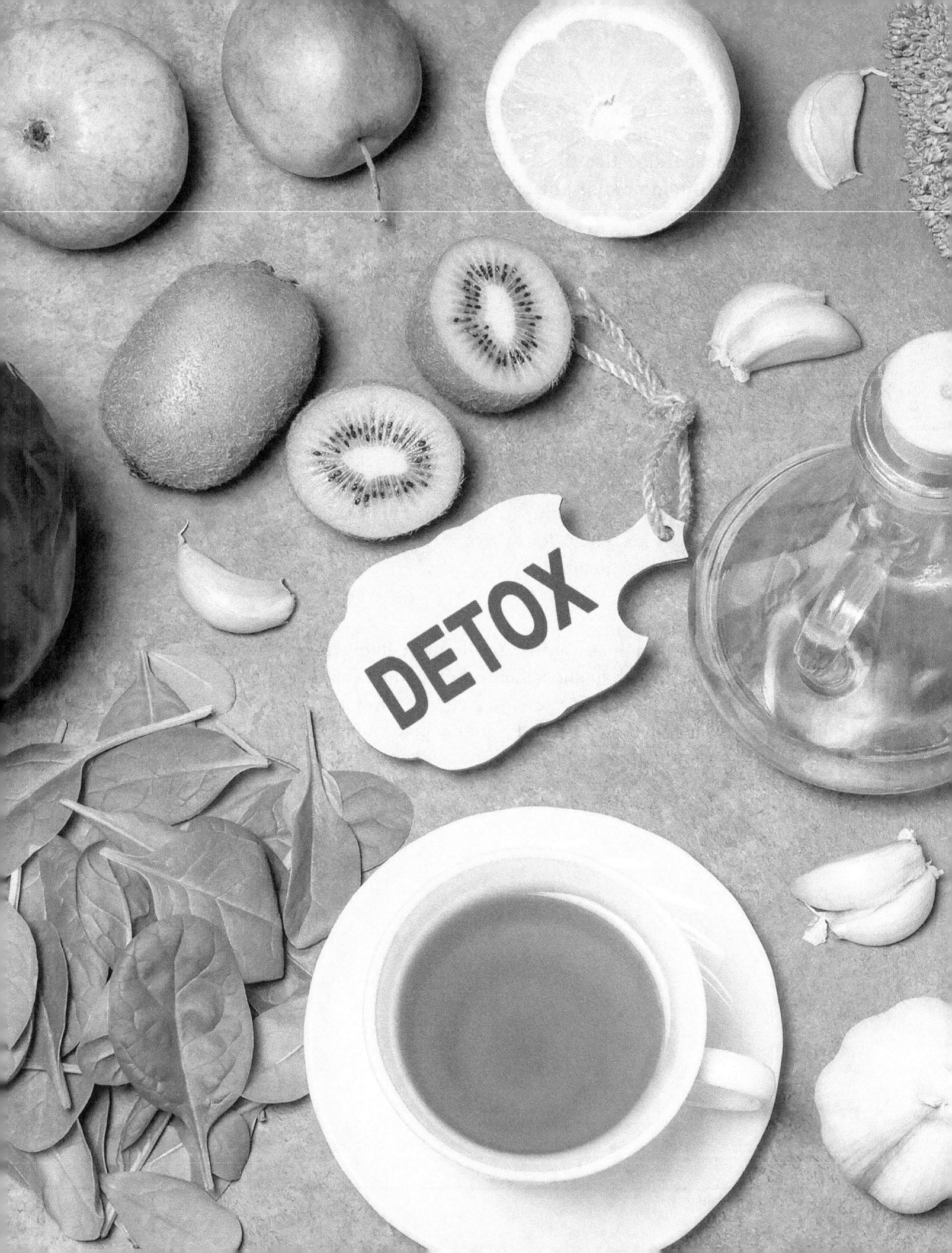

CHAPTER 5: UNDERSTANDING PLANT MICRONUTRIENTS

Plants are rich in micronutrients that come from the soil they grow in. As plants cannot move as animals do, they have a uniquely full tool chest of macro and micro-nutrients that enable them to adapt to the changing environment around them. These micronutrients are just as valuable to humans as they are to the plants but in different ways.

Below is a breakdown of the basic micronutrients found in fruits, vegetables, nuts, seeds, and legumes.

Vitamins

Vibrant vegetables and fruits are a dense source of vitamins that are essential to overall health and wellness.

- Vitamin A: Beta-carotene is a carotenoid found in yellow, orange and dark green fruits and veg, most notably carrots, spinach, and broccoli. It protects against infections and is essential for eye and skin health.

- Vitamin Bs: This group of vitamins is responsible for maintaining the nervous system and cognitive function, DNA and blood cell production.

- B1 is responsible for nervous system health and aids in the breakdown and absorption of food. Found in peas, whole grains, and most fruits and vegetables.

- B2 is responsible for energy production and healthy skin and eyes and is found in asparagus, spinach, and broccoli.

- B3 is great for healthy skin and energy production and is found in peanuts, avocados, peas, and mushrooms.

- B6 is also essential for energy production and is found in chickpeas, potatoes, banana, squash, and nuts.

- B9 is also known as folate and is essential for fetal development and growth and healthy cell division. It is found in legumes, asparagus, spinach, arugula, kale, and beets.

- B12 is predominantly sourced from animal products but you can find it in some organic soy products but most notably nutritional yeast.

- **Vitamin C:** An essential vitamin important for cell growth and energy production and tissue repair and wound healing. It is one of the most powerful antioxidants and is found in strawberries, spinach, Brussel sprouts, sweet potatoes, and tomatoes.

- **Vitamin E:** A powerful antioxidant that protects the body from free radical damage, including premature aging. It's of great support to the immune system, protecting it against external pathogens. It is found in sunflower seeds, almonds, hazelnuts, spinach, and broccoli.

- **Vitamin K:** This vitamin plays a major role in the clotting cascade and also in bone health. It is found in all green leafy veg as well as cruciferous veg and green tea.

Minerals

Macro-minerals: we need these in large quantities from our diet.

- **Calcium:** This essential mineral plays roles in bone, heart, muscle and nerve health. Foods high in calcium are spinach, collard greens, seeds, almonds, soybeans, and butter beans.

- **Chloride:** This mineral plays a part in body fluid balance, including digestive juices. It is found in sea salt, tomatoes, lettuce, celery, and rye bread.

- **Magnesium:** This mineral regulates blood sugar and assists in energy production. It also helps your muscles, kidneys, bones and heart function effectively. It is found in spinach, quinoa, dark chocolate, almonds, avocado, and black beans.

- **Phosphorous:** This mineral is found in bones and works with calcium in maintaining healthy mineral balance within the body. It is found in pumpkin, sunflower seeds, lentils, chickpeas, oatmeal, and quinoa.

- **Sodium:** The current population gets excess sodium from all pre-packaged foods and restaurant meals, so there is no need to go looking for extra sodium in the diet.

- **Potassium:** This mineral is essential in blood pressure balance, muscle health, and nerve function. It is found in avocado, bananas, apricots, grapefruit, potatoes, mushrooms, cucumbers and zucchini.

- **Trace Minerals:** We just need tiny amounts of these from our foods.

- **Copper:** Essential in the formation of red blood cells and iron absorption. It is found in whole grains, beans, potatoes, cocoa, black pepper, and dark leafy greens.

- Cobalt: This trace mineral works closely with B12 in the formation of hemoglobin. It is found in nuts, broccoli, oats, and spinach.
- Manganese: Plays many roles in enzyme activity and cellular level antioxidants. It is found in pineapple, peanuts, brown rice, spinach, sweet potato, pecans, and green tea.
- Iodine: Essential for thyroid function, you can find it in seaweed, lima beans, and prunes.
- Iron: Used to make hemoglobin and as a carrier for essential nutrients in the blood. It is found in cashews, spinach, whole grains, tofu, potatoes, and lentils in plant form.
- Selenium: A trace mineral essential in the role of reproduction, DNA production, and antioxidant function. It is found in Brazil nuts, lentils, cashew nuts, and potatoes.
- Zinc: As your body doesn't store zinc, it needs to be consumed daily because it plays important roles in nutrient metabolism, immune system maintenance, and enzyme function. It is found in legumes, nuts, seeds, potatoes, kale and green beans.

Colors

The colors in fruits and vegetables point to what kinds of nutrients they contain.

- White foods: Contain sulfur and can have anti-cancer properties. Found in cauliflower, garlic, leeks, and onions.
- Green foods: Contain lutein and vitamin K. Found in dark leafy greens, broccoli, and avocado.
- Purple foods: Contain anthocyanins, which are powerful antioxidants. Found in blueberries, eggplant, red cabbage, and blackberries.
- Red foods: Contain lycopene and has therapeutic properties for the heart. Found in strawberries, watermelon, tomatoes, and red bell peppers.

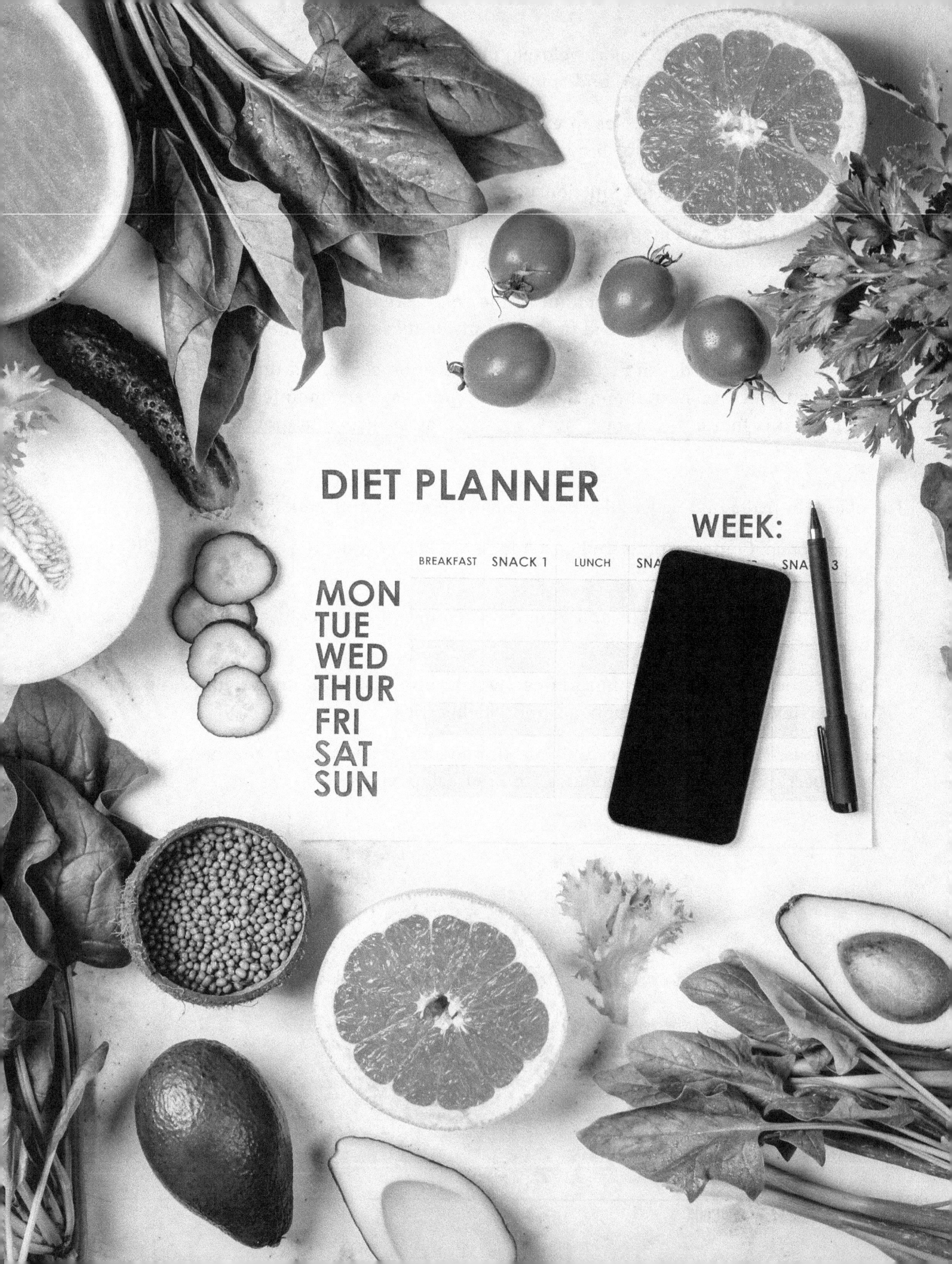

CHAPTER 6:
4-WEEK WEIGHT LOSS MEAL PLAN

Before diving into the 600 healthy recipes of this book, I want to leave you with a simple 4-week weight loss meal plan that should serve as a guideline to help with your weekly grocery shopping and meal planning.

Each daily meal combination contains no more than 2,000 calories (you can find nutritional values on the recipe's page). Feel free to add items such as small snacks and juices/smoothies as you please, and don't forget to drink any less than 3 liters of water per day. To make it easier for you to locate each recipe in the book, I added the recipe's number in between brackets. Enjoy!

WEEK 1

Days	Breakfast	Lunch	Dinner	Snack/Dessert
1	Orange French Toast (20)	Cauliflower Latke (433) Zucchini Fritters (293)	Roasted Brussels Sprouts (434) Brussels Sprouts & Cranberries (435)	Quinoa Tacos (493) Almond - Choco Cake (550)
2	Apple-Walnut Breakfast Bread (26)	Spaghetti with Chickpeas Meatballs (145) Kale and Cauliflower Salad (206)	Seitan Shawarma (331) Tofu and Pineapple in Lettuce (348)	Mint Chocolate Chip Sorbet (533)
3	Avocado and Sausage Breakfast Sandwich (13)	Ritzy Fava Bean Ratatouille (122) Creamed Green Pea Salad (187)	Amazing Chickpea and Noodle Soup (203) Coconut Cauliflower Mix (258)	Mixed Berries and Cream (548)
4	Dairy-Free Coconut Yogurt (29)	Avocado and White Bean Sandwich (338) Sweet Potato Tater Tots (328)	Green Lentil Stew with Collard Greens (172) Cucumber Edamame Salad (234)	Spicy Roasted Chickpeas (297) Apple Crumble (526)
5	Berries and Banana Smoothie Bowl (33)	Spaghetti in Spicy Tomato Sauce (152) Coconut Cauliflower Mix (258)	Mediterranean Salad (279) Mediterranean Veggie Wrap (341)	Pumpkin Flavored Popcorn (492) Banana-Coconut Ice Cream (552)
6	Sunrise Smoothie (37)	Beluga Lentil and Vegetable Mélange (167) Lebanese Potato Salad (248)	Zucchini Soup (217)	Chipotle and Lime Tortilla Chips (286) Vegan Mini Gingerbread Loaves (563)
7	Apple-Lemon Bowl (23)	Veggie Paella (105)	Tofu Salad Sandwiches (329) Basil Tomato Soup (197)	Zucchini Nuggets (495) Vegan Chocolate Turron (564)

WEEK 2

Days	Breakfast	Lunch	Dinner	Snack/Dessert
8	Sunshine Orange Smoothie (38)	Traditional Indian Rajma Dal (159) Lemongrass Rice (256)	The Garbanzo Bean Extravaganza (310)	Tomato and Pesto Toast (289) Green Buckwheat Coffee Cake (570)
9	Breakfast Muesli (43)	Hummus and Quinoa Wrap (340) Celery Dill Soup (228)	Quinoa Avocado Salad (439)	Buffalo Cashews (302)
10	Toast with Avocado and Berries (48)	5 Ingredients Pasta (158)	Old-Fashioned Lentil and Vegetable Stew (176)	Buffalo Cashews (302) Tropical Fruits Salad (573)
11	Breakfast Scramble (24)	Vegetable and Wild Rice Pilaf (106) Cauliflower Asparagus Soup (194)	Green Pesto Sandwich (336)	Hearty Brussels and Pistachio (301) Banana Nut Smoothie (57)
12	Banana Cream Pie and Chia Pudding (44)	Lentil Soup the Vegan Way (204)	Ritzy Fava Bean Ratatouille (122)	Asparagus Spanakopita (370) Avocado Pudding (315)
13	Chickpea Omelet (22)	Lentil Radish Salad (240) Vegan Chinese Noodles (150)	Broccoli Salad the Thai Way (208) Thai Vegetable and Tofu Wrap (343)	Healthy Carrot Chips (300) Fruits and Berries in Orange Juice Salad (572)
14	Gingerbread Waffles (1)	Super Summer Salad (236) Colorful Veggie Wrap (345)	Walnut-Oat Burgers (111) Potato Mash (261)	Lemony Sprouts (312) Almond - Choco Cake (550)

WEEK 3

Days	Breakfast	Lunch	Dinner	Snack
15	Easy Hummus Toast (5)	Peppers and Black Beans with Brown Rice (123)	Ratatouille Pasta shells (478) Onion Rings (314)	Veggie Crisps (507) Sweet Hummus (522)
16	Fluffy Garbanzo Bean Omelet (4)	Zucchini & Pepper Lasagna (475)	Tofu and Pineapple in Lettuce (348) Chinese-Style Soybean Salad (175)	Tamari Almonds (509) Fantastic Sticky Mango Rice (583)
17	Peach & Chia Seed Breakfast Parfait (9)	Brown Lentil Bowl (179)	Italian Stuffed Artichokes (384)	Avocado and Sprout Toast (290) Gingerbread Muffins (588)
18	Oatmeal & Peanut Butter Breakfast Bar (11)	Mediterranean-Style Chickpea Salad (165)	Veggie Kabobs (143) Creamy Cauliflower Pakora Soup (199)	Acorn Squash with Mango Chutney (299) Sweet Green Cookies (515)
19	Vegan Variety Poppy Seed Scones (15)	Shrimp Veggie Pasta Salad (281)	Chickpea and Mango Wraps (347) Tomato Gazpacho (189)	Thai Snack Mix (292) Coconut Snowballs (567)
20	Apple Oatmeal (17)	Sweet Potato & Black Bean Protein Salad (239)	Quick Lentil Wrap (342) Broccoli Fennel Soup (229)	Sweet Pistachio Bites (500)
21	Black Bean and Sweet Potato Hash (25)	Mexican-Style Bean Bowl (170)	Easy Millet Loaf (110) Lentil, Lemon & Mushroom Salad (238)	Sweet Nut Bars (497)

WEEK 4

Days	Breakfast	Lunch	Dinner	Snack
22	Sun-Butter Baked Oatmeal Cups (31)	Stir Fry Noodles (147)	Barbecued Greens & Grits (132) Cauliflower Spinach Soup (214)	Chocolate Macaroons (540)
23	Vegan Salmon Bagel (27)	Creamy Vegan Mushroom Pasta (149)	Mediterranean Chickpea Wraps (333)	Peach Crockpot Pudding (559)
24	Almond Butter Banana Overnight Oats (8)	Black Bean Buda Bowl (184)	Vegetable Broth Sans Sodium (202) Apple and Honey Toast (291)	Carrot Energy Balls (319) Mimosa Salad (599)
25	Sweet Pomegranate Porridge (16)	Sweet Potato, Corn and Jalapeno Bisque (209) Glazed Carrots (172)	Mediterranean Hummus Pizza (414) Italian Veggie Salad (252)	Blueberry and Pecan Bake (582)
26	Apple-Lemon Bowl (23)	Spicy Sweet Chili Veggie Noodles (148)	African Pineapple Peanut Stew (195) Roasted Sweet Potatoes (440)	Black Bean Orange Mousse (575)
27	No-Bake Chewy Granola Bars (6)	Loaded Creamy Vegan Pesto Pasta (155)	Greek Pizza (246) Lentil Radish Salad (240)	Quinoa Broccoli Tots (296)
28	Mint Chocolate Green Protein Smoothie (28)	Classic Italian Minestrone (171) Rosemary Beet Chips (295)	Colorful Veggie Wrap (345) Peppers Bowl (259)	Cinnamon Baked Apple Chips (298)

THE PLANT BASED DIET COOKBOOK

CHAPTER 7: BREAKFAST

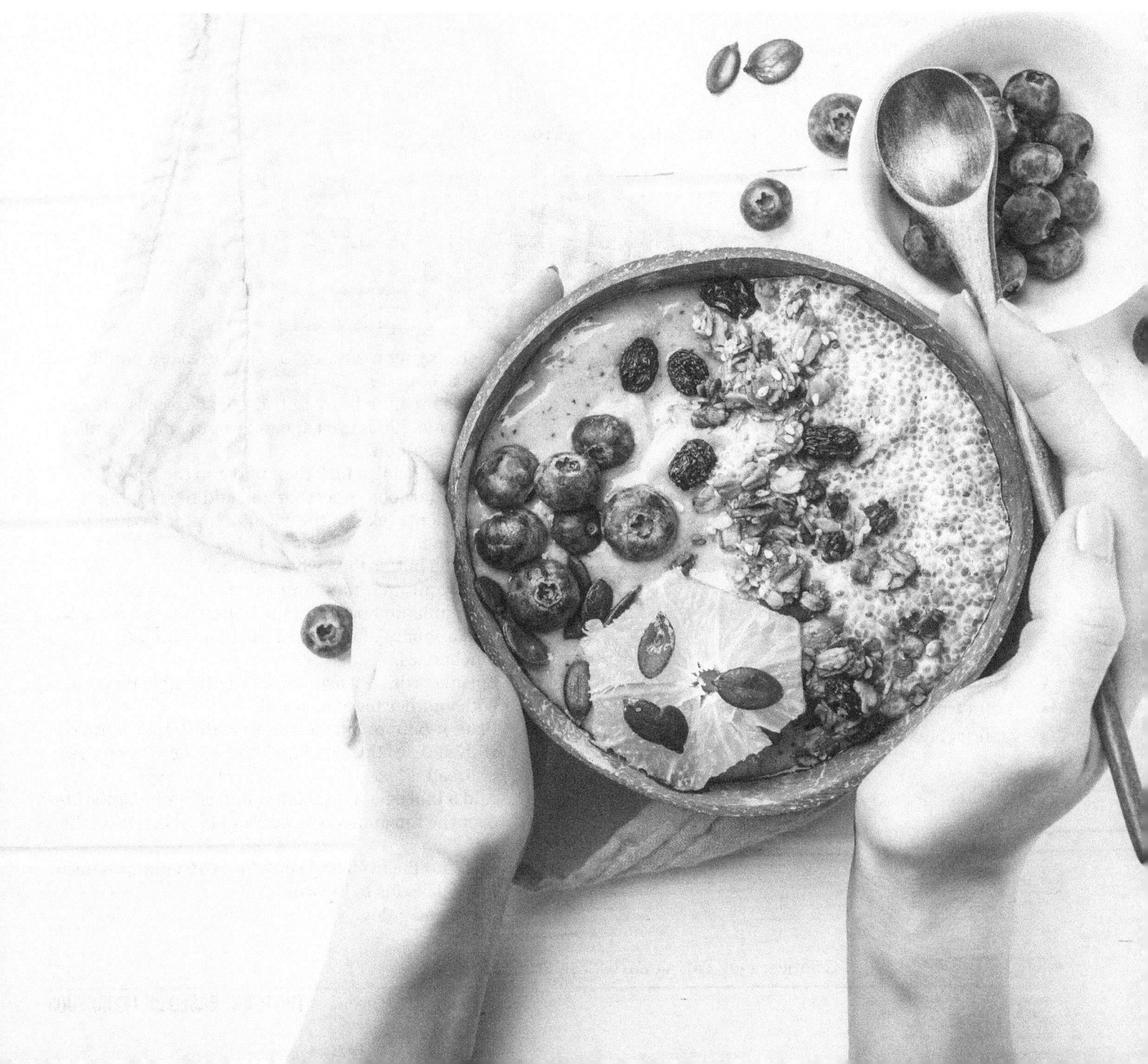

1. GINGERBREAD WAFFLES

COOKING: 20' **PREPARATION: 30'** **SERVES: 6**

INGREDIENTS

- 1 cup spelt flour
- 2 teaspoon baking powder
- ¼ teaspoon salt
- 1 tablespoon ground flax seeds
- 1 ½ teaspoon ground cinnamon
- 2 teaspoon ground ginger
- 4 tablespoon coconut sugar
- ¼ teaspoon baking soda
- 1½ tablespoon olive oil
- 1 cup non-dairy milk
- 1 tablespoon apple cider vinegar
- 2 tablespoons blackstrap molasses

DIRECTIONS

1. Take a waffle iron, oil generously, and preheat.
2. Take a large bowl and add the dry ingredients. Stir well together.
3. Put the wet ingredients into another bowl and stir until combined.
4. Stir the dry and wet together until combined.
5. Pour the mixture into the waffle iron and cook on a medium temperature for 20 minutes.
6. Open carefully and remove.
7. Serve and enjoy.

NUTRITION: Calories: 173 Fat: 5g Carbs: 29g Protein: 3g

2. BLUEBERRY FRENCH TOAST BREAKFAST MUFFINS

COOKING: 25' **PREPARATION: 20'** **SERVES: 12**

INGREDIENTS

- 1 cup unsweetened plant milk
- 1 tablespoon ground flaxseed
- 1 tablespoon almond meal
- 1 tablespoon maple syrup
- 1 teaspoon vanilla extract
- 1 teaspoon cinnamon
- 2 teaspoons nutritional yeast
- ¾th cup frozen blueberries
- 9 slices soft bread
- ¼th cup oats
- 1/3rd cup raw pecans
- ¼th cup of coconut sugar
- 3 tablespoons coconut butter, at room temperature
- 1/8th teaspoon sea salt
- 9 slices bread, each cut into 4

DIRECTIONS

1. Preheat your oven to 370°F and grease a muffin tin. Pop to one side.
2. Find a medium bowl and add the flaxseeds, almond meal, nutritional yeast, maple syrup, milk, vanilla, and cinnamon.
3. Mix well using a fork then pop into the fridge.
4. Grab your food processor and add the topping ingredients (except the coconut butter.) Whizz to combine.
5. Add the butter then whizz again.
6. Grab your muffin tin and add a teaspoon of the flax and cinnamon batter to the bottom of each space.
7. Add a square of the bread then top with 5-6 blueberries.
8. Sprinkle with 2 teaspoons of the crumble then top with another piece of bread.
9. Place 5-6 more blueberries over the bread, sprinkle with more of the topping then add the other piece of bread.
10. Add a tablespoon of the flax and cinnamon mixture over the top and add a couple of blueberries on the top.
11. Pop into the oven and cook for 20-25 minutes until the top begins to brown.
12. Serve and enjoy.

NUTRITION: Calories: 132g Fat: 5g Carbs: 14g Protein: 3g

3. GREEK GARBANZO BEANS ON TOAST

COOKING: 5'   **PREPARATION: 25'**   **SERVES: 2**

INGREDIENTS

- 2 tablespoons olive oil
- 3 small shallots, finely diced
- 2 large garlic cloves, finely diced
- ¼ teaspoon smoked paprika
- ½ teaspoon sweet paprika
- ½ teaspoon cinnamon
- ½ teaspoon salt
- ½-1 teaspoon sugar, to taste
- Black pepper, to taste
- 1 x 14oz. can peel plum tomatoes
- 2 cups cooked garbanzo beans
- 4-6 slices of crusty bread, toasted
- Fresh parsley and dill
- Pitted Kalamata olives

DIRECTIONS

1. Pop a skillet over medium heat and add the oil.
2. Add the shallots to the pan and cook for five minutes.
3. Add the garlic and cook until ready then add the other spices to the pan.
4. Stir well then add the tomatoes.
5. Lower the heat and simmer on low until the sauce thickens.
6. Add the garbanzo beans and warm through.
7. Season with the sugar, salt, and pepper, then serve and enjoy.

NUTRITION: Calories: 709g Fat: 12g Carbs: 23g Protein: 19g

4. FLUFFY GARBANZO BEAN OMELET

COOKING: 12'   **PREPARATION: 5'**   **SERVES: 1**

INGREDIENTS

- ¼ cup besan flour
- 1 tablespoon nutritional yeast
- ½ teaspoon baking power
- ¼ teaspoon turmeric
- ½ teaspoon chopped chives
- ¼ teaspoon garlic powder
- 1/8 teaspoon black pepper
- ½ teaspoon Ener-G egg replacer
- ¼ cup + 1 tablespoon water
- Leafy greens, torn with hands
- Veggies
- Salsa
- Ketchup
- Hot sauce
- Parsley

DIRECTIONS

1. Grab a medium bowl and combine all the ingredients except the greens and veggies. Leave to stand for five minutes.
2. Place a skillet over medium heat and add the oil.
3. Pour the batter into the pan, spread, and cook for 3-5 minutes until the edges pull away from the pan.
4. Add the greens and the veggies of your choice then fold the omelet over.
5. Cook for 2 more minutes than pop onto a plate.
6. Serve with the topping of your choice.
7. Serve and enjoy.

NUTRITION: Calories: 439 Fat: 8g Carbs: 35g Protein: 12g

THE PLANT BASED DIET COOKBOOK

5. EASY HUMMUS TOAST

COOKING: 10' **PREPARATION: 10'** **SERVES: 1**

INGREDIENTS

- 2 slices sprouted wheat bread
- ¼ cup hummus
- 1 tablespoon hemp seeds
- 1 tablespoon roasted unsalted sunflower seeds

DIRECTIONS

1. Start by toasting your bread.
2. Top with the hummus and seeds then eat!

NUTRITION: Calories: 316 Fat: 16g Carbs: 13g Protein: 18g

6. NO-BAKE CHEWY GRANOLA BARS

COOKING: 10' **PREPARATION: 10'** **SERVES: 8**

INGREDIENTS

- ¼ teaspoon cinnamon
- ¼ teaspoon salt
- ½ teaspoon cardamom
- ¼ cup of coconut oil
- 1 cup oats
- 1 teaspoon vanilla extract
- ½ cup raw almonds, sliced
- ¼ cup sunflower seeds
- ½ cup pumpkin seeds
- 1¼ teaspoon nutmeg
- 1 tbsp chia seeds
- ¼ cup honey
- 1 cup dried figs, chopped

DIRECTIONS

1. Line a 6" x 8" baking dish with parchment paper and pop to one side.
2. Grab a saucepan and add the salt, honey, oil, and spices.
3. Pop over medium heat and stir until it melts together.
4. Reduce the heat, add the oats, and stir.
5. Add the dried fruit, seeds, and nuts, and stir through again.
6. Cook for 10 minutes.
7. Remove from the heat and transfer the oat mixture to the pan.
8. Press down until it's packed firm.
9. Leave to cool completely then cut into 8 bars.
10. Serve and enjoy.

NUTRITION: Calories: 30 Fat: 14g Carbs: 35g Protein: 6g

7. TASTY OATMEAL AND CARROT CAKE

COOKING: 10' **PREPARATION: 5'** **SERVES: 5**

INGREDIENTS

- 1 cup of water
- ½ teaspoon of cinnamon
- 1 cup of rolled oats
- Salt
- ¼ cup of raisins
- ½ cup of shredded carrots
- 1 cup of non-dairy milk
- ¼ teaspoon of allspice
- ½ teaspoon of vanilla extract
- Toppings:
- ¼ cup of chopped walnuts
- 2 tablespoons of maple syrup
- 2 tablespoons of shredded coconut

DIRECTIONS

1. Put a small pot on low heat and bring the non-dairy milk, oats, and water to a simmer.
2. Now, add the carrots, vanilla extract, raisins, salt, cinnamon, and allspice. You need to simmer all the ingredients, but do not forget to stir them. You will know that they are ready when the liquid is fully absorbed into all the ingredients (in about 7-10 minutes).
3. Transfer the thickened dish to bowls. You can top them with coconut or walnuts.
4. This nutritious bowl will allow you to kickstart your day.

NUTRITION: Calories: 210 Fat: 11g Carbs: 42g Protein: 4g

8. ALMOND BUTTER BANANA OVERNIGHT OATS

COOKING: 10' **PREPARATION: 5'** **SERVES: 2**

INGREDIENTS

- ½ cup rolled oats
- 1 cup almond milk
- 1 tablespoon chia seeds
- ¼ teaspoon vanilla extract
- ½ teaspoon ground cinnamon
- 1 tablespoon honey or maple syrup
- 1 banana, sliced
- 2 tablespoons natural almond butter

DIRECTIONS

1. Take a large bowl and add the oats, milk, chia seeds, vanilla, cinnamon, and honey.
2. Stir to combine then divide half of the mixture between two bowls.
3. Top with the banana and peanut butter then add the remaining mixture.
4. Cover then pop into the fridge overnight.
5. Serve and enjoy.

NUTRITION: Calories: 227 Fat: 11g Carbs: 35g Protein: 7g

9. PEACH & CHIA SEED BREAKFAST PARFAIT

COOKING: 10' **PREPARATION: 5'** **SERVES: 4**

INGREDIENTS

- ¼ cup chia seeds
- 1 tablespoon pure maple syrup
- 1 cup of coconut milk
- 1 teaspoon ground cinnamon
- 3 medium peaches, diced small
- 2/3 cup granola

DIRECTIONS

1. Find a small bowl and add the chia seeds, maple syrup, and coconut milk.
2. Stir well then cover and pop into the fridge for at least one hour.
3. Find another bowl, add the peaches and sprinkle with the cinnamon. Pop to one side.
4. When it's time to serve, take two glasses, and pour the chia mixture between the two.
5. Sprinkle the granola over the top, keeping a tiny amount to one side to use to decorate later.
6. Top with the peaches and the reserved granola and serve.

NUTRITION: Calories: 260 Fat: 13g Carbs: 22g Protein: 6g

10. AVOCADO TOAST WITH WHITE BEANS

COOKING: 6' **PREPARATION: 5'** **SERVES: 4**

INGREDIENTS

- ½ cup canned white beans, drained and rinsed
- 2 teaspoons tahini paste
- 2 teaspoons lemon juice
- ½ teaspoon salt
- ½ avocado, peeled and pit removed
- 4 slices whole-grain bread, toasted
- ½ cup grape tomatoes, cut in half

DIRECTIONS

1. Grab a small bowl and add the beans, tahini, ½ the lemon juice, and ½ the salt. Mash with a fork.
2. Take another bowl and add the avocado and the remaining lemon juice and salt. Mash together.
3. Place your toast onto a flat surface and add the mashed beans, spreading well.
4. Top with the avocado and the sliced tomatoes then serve and enjoy.

NUTRITION: Calories: 140 Fat: 5g Carbs: 13g Protein: 5g

THE PLANT BASED DIET COOKBOOK

11. OATMEAL & PEANUT BUTTER BREAKFAST BAR

COOKING: 0' **PREPARATION: 10'** **SERVES: 8**

INGREDIENTS

- 1 ½ cups date, pit removed
- ½ cup peanut butter
- ½ cup old-fashioned rolled oats

DIRECTIONS

1. Grease a baking tin and pop to one side.
2. Grab your food processor, add the dates, and whizz until chopped.
3. Add the peanut butter and the oats and pulse.
4. Scoop into the baking tin then pop into the fridge or freezer until set.
5. Serve and enjoy.

NUTRITION: Calories: 232 Fat: 9g Carbs: 32g Protein: 8g

12. CHOCOLATE CHIP BANANA PANCAKE

COOKING: 3' **PREPARATION: 15'** **SERVES: 6**

INGREDIENTS

- 1 large ripe banana, mashed
- 2 tablespoons coconut sugar
- 3 tablespoons coconut oil, melted
- 1 cup of coconut milk
- 1 ½ cups whole wheat flour
- 1 teaspoon baking soda
- ½ cup vegan chocolate chips
- Olive oil, for frying

DIRECTIONS

1. Grab a large bowl and add the banana, sugar, oil, and milk. Stir well.
2. Add the flour and baking soda and stir again until combined.
3. Add the chocolate chips and fold through then pop to one side.
4. Put a skillet over medium heat and add a drop of oil.
5. Pour ¼ of the batter into the pan and move the pan to cover.
6. Cook for 3 minutes then flip and cook on the other side.
7. Repeat with the remaining pancakes then serve and enjoy.

NUTRITION: Calories: 105 Fat: 13g Carbs: 23g Protein: 5g

13. AVOCADO AND 'SAUSAGE' BREAKFAST SANDWICH

COOKING: 10' **PREPARATION: 15'** **SERVES: 1**

INGREDIENTS

- 1 vegan sausage patty
- 1 cup kale, chopped
- 2 teaspoons extra virgin olive oil
- 1 tablespoon pepitas
- Salt and pepper, to taste
- 1 tablespoon vegan mayo
- 1/8 teaspoon chipotle powder
- 1 teaspoon jalapeno chopped
- 1 English muffin, toasted
- ¼ avocado, sliced

DIRECTIONS

1. Place a sauté pan over high heat and add a drop of oil.
2. Add the vegan patty and cook for 2 minutes.
3. Flip the patty then add the kale and pepitas.
4. Season well then cook for another few minutes until the patty is cooked.
5. Find a small bowl and add the mayo, chipotle powder, and the jalapeno. Stir well to combine.
6. Place the muffin onto a flat surface, spread with the spicy mayo then top with the patty.
7. Add the sliced avocado then serve and enjoy.

NUTRITION: Calories: 573 Fat: 23g Carbs: 36g Protein: 21g

14. CINNAMON ROLLS WITH CASHEW FROSTING

COOKING: 25'   **PREPARATION: 25'**   **SERVES: 12**

INGREDIENTS

- 3 tablespoons vegan butter
- ¾ cup unsweetened almond milk
- ½ teaspoon salt
- 3 tablespoons caster sugar
- 1 teaspoon vanilla extract
- ½ cup pumpkin puree
- 3 cups all-purpose flour
- 2 ¼ teaspoons dried active yeast
- 3 tablespoons softened vegan butter
- 3 tablespoons brown sugar
- ½ teaspoon cinnamon
- ½ cup cashews
- ½ cup icing sugar
- 1 teaspoon vanilla extract
- 2/3 cup almond milk

DIRECTIONS

1. Soak the cashews for 1 hour in boiling water.
2. Grease a baking sheet and pop to one side.
3. Find a small bowl, add the butter, and pop into the microwave to melt.
4. Add the sugar and stir well then set aside to cool.
5. Grab a large bowl and add the flour, salt, and yeast. Stir well to mix.
6. Place the cooled butter into a jug, add the pumpkin puree, vanilla, and almond milk. Stir well together.
7. Pour the wet ingredients into the dry and stir well to combine.
8. Tip onto a flat surface and knead for 5 minutes, adding extra flour as needed to avoid sticking.
9. Pop back into the bowl, cover with plastic wrap, and pop into the fridge overnight.
10. Remove the dough from the fridge and punch down with your fingers.
11. Using a rolling pin, roll to form an 18" rectangle then spread with butter.
12. Find a small bowl and add the sugar and cinnamon. Mix well then sprinkle with the butter.
13. Roll the dough into a large sausage then slice into sections.
14. Place onto the greased baking sheet and leave in a dark place to rise for one hour.
15. Preheat the oven to 350°F.
16. Drain the cashews and put them to your blender. Whizz until smooth.
17. Add the sugar and the vanilla then whizz again.
18. Add the almond milk until it reaches your desired consistency.
19. Pop into the oven and bake for 20 minutes until golden.
20. Pour the glaze over the top then serve and enjoy.

NUTRITION: Calories: 243 Fat: 9g Carbs: 34g Protein: 4g

15. VEGAN VARIETY POPPY SEED SCONES

COOKING: 10'   **PREPARATION: 5'**   **SERVES: 12**

INGREDIENTS

- 1 cup white sugar
- 2 cups flour
- Juice from 1 lemon
- Zest from 1 lemon
- 4 teaspoon baking powder
- ½ teaspoon salt
- 1 cup Earth Balance or vegan butter
- 2 tablespoon poppy seeds
- ½ cup soymilk
- 1/3 cup water

DIRECTIONS

1. Begin by preheating the oven to 400°F.
2. Next, mix the sugar, the flour, the powder, and the salt in a big mixing bowl. Add the vegan butter to the mixture and cut it up until you create a sand-like mixture. Next, add the lemon juice, the lemon zest, and the poppy seeds. Add the water and the soy milk, and stir the ingredients well.
3. Portion the batter out over a baking sheet in about ¼ cup portions. Allow the scones to bake for fifteen minutes and let them cool before serving. Enjoy.

NUTRITION: Calories: 205 Fat: 3g Carbs: 12g Protein: 6g

THE PLANT BASED DIET COOKBOOK

16. SWEET POMEGRANATE PORRIDGE

COOKING: 20'   **PREPARATION: 5'**   **SERVES: 4**

INGREDIENTS

- 2 Cups Oats
- 1 ½ Cups Water
- 1 ½ Cups Pomegranate Juice
- 2 Tablespoons Pomegranate Molasses

DIRECTIONS

1. Pour all ingredients into the instant pot and mix well.
2. Seal the lid, and cook on high pressure for four minutes.
3. Use a quick release, and serve warm.

NUTRITION: Calories: 177 Fat: 6g Carbs: 23g Protein: 8g

17. APPLE OATMEAL

COOKING: 20'   **PREPARATION: 5'**   **SERVES: 4**

INGREDIENTS

- ¼ Teaspoon Sea Salt
- 1 Cup Cashew Milk
- 1 Cup Strawberries, Halved & Fresh
- 1 Tablespoon Brown Sugar
- 2 Cups Apples, Diced
- 3 Cups Water
- ¼ Teaspoon Coconut Oil
- ½ Cup Steel Cut Oats

DIRECTIONS

1. Start by greasing your instant pot with oil, and add everything to it except for the milk and berries.
2. Lock the lid and cook on high pressure for ten minutes. Allow for a natural pressure release, and then add in your milk and strawberries. Mix well, and serve warm.

NUTRITION: Calories: 435 Fat: 7g Carbs: 34g Protein: 8g

18. BREAKFAST COOKIES

COOKING: 6'   **PREPARATION: 10'**   **SERVES: 24-32**

INGREDIENTS

Dry Ingredients:
- ½ teaspoon baking powder
- 2 cups rolled oats
- ½ teaspoon baking soda
- Wet Ingredients:
- 1 teaspoon pure vanilla extract
- 2 flax eggs (2 tablespoons ground flaxseed and around 6 tablespoons of water, mix and put aside for 15 minutes)
- 2 tablespoons melted coconut oil
- 2 tablespoons pure maple syrup
- ½ cup natural creamy peanut butter
- 2 ripe bananas

Add-in Ingredients:
- ½ cup finely chopped walnuts
- ½ cup raisins

Optional Topping:
- 2 tablespoons chopped walnuts
- 2 tablespoons raisins

DIRECTIONS

1. Preheat the oven to 325°F, and then use parchment paper to line a baking sheet and put aside.
2. Add the bananas in a large bowl, and then use a fork to mash them until smooth. Add in the other wet ingredients and mix until well incorporated.
3. Add the dry ingredients and then use a rubber spatula to stir and fold them into the dry ingredients until well mixed. Stir in the walnuts and raisins.
4. Scoop the cookie dough onto the prepared baking sheet making sure that you leave adequate space between the cookies.
5. Bake in the preheated oven for around 12 minutes. Once ready, let the cookies cool on the baking sheet for around 10 minutes.
6. Lift the cookies carefully from the baking sheet onto a cooling rack to further cool.
7. Store the cookies in an airtight container in the fridge or at room temperature for up to one week.

NUTRITION: Calories: 565 Fat: 6g Carbs: 32g Protein: 8g

19. VEGAN BREAKFAST BISCUITS

COOKING: 10'   **PREPARATION: 10'**   **SERVES: 6**

INGREDIENTS

- cups Almond Flour - quantity not mentioned
- 1 tbsp Baking Powder
- ¼ teaspoon Salt
- ½ teaspoon Onion Powder
- ½ cup Coconut Milk
- ¼ cup Nutritional Yeast
- 2 tbsp Ground Flax Seeds
- ¼ cup Olive Oil

DIRECTIONS

1. Preheat oven to 450°F.
2. Whisk together all ingredients in a bowl.
3. Divide the batter into a pre-greased muffin tin.
4. Bake for 10 minutes.

NUTRITION: Calories: 432 Fat: 5g Carbs: 13g Protein: 8g

20. ORANGE FRENCH TOAST

COOKING: 30'   **PREPARATION: 5'**   **SERVES: 8**

INGREDIENTS

- 2 cups of plant milk (unflavored)
- Four tablespoon maple syrup
- 11/2 tablespoon cinnamon
- Salt (optional)
- 1 cup flour (almond)
- 1 tablespoon orange zest
- 8 bread slices

DIRECTIONS

1. Turn the oven and heat to 400°F afterwards.
2. In a cup, add ingredients and whisk until the batter is smooth.
3. Dip each piece of bread into the paste and permit to soak for a couple of seconds.
4. Put in the pan, and cook until lightly browned.
5. Put the toast on the cookie sheet and bake for ten to fifteen minutes in the oven, until it is crispy.

NUTRITION: Calories: 129 Fat: 1.1g Carbs: 21.5g Protein: 7.9g

21. CHOCOLATE CHIP COCONUT PANCAKES

COOKING: 30'   **PREPARATION: 5'**   **SERVES: 8**

INGREDIENTS

- 11/4 cup oats
- 2 teaspoons coconut flakes
- 2 cup plant milk
- 11/4 cup maple syrup
- 11/3 cup of chocolate chips
- 2 1/4 cups buckwheat flour
- 2 teaspoon baking powder
- 1 teaspoon vanilla essence
- 2 teaspoon flaxseed meal
- Salt (optional)

DIRECTIONS

1. Put the flaxseed and cook over medium heat until the paste becomes a little moist.
2. Remove seeds.
3. Stir the buckwheat, oats, coconut chips, baking powder and salt with each other in a wide dish.
4. In a large dish, stir together the retained flax water with the sugar, maple syrup, vanilla essence.
5. Transfer the wet mixture to the dry ingredients and shake to combine
6. Place over medium heat the nonstick grill pan.
7. Pour 1/4 cup flour onto the grill pan with each pancake, and scatter gently.
8. Cook for five to six minutes, before the pancakes appear somewhat crispy.

NUTRITION: Calories: 198 Fat: 9.1g Carbs: 11.5g Protein: 7.9g

THE PLANT BASED DIET COOKBOOK

22. CHICKPEA OMELET

COOKING: 30'   **PREPARATION: 10'**   **SERVES: 3**

INGREDIENTS

- 2 cup flour (chickpea)
- 1 1/2 teaspoon onion powder
- 1 1/2 teaspoon garlic powder
- 1/4 teaspoon pepper (white and black)
- 1/3 cup yeast
- 1 teaspoon baking powder
- 3 green onions (chopped)

DIRECTIONS

1. In a cup, add the chickpea flour and spices.
2. Apply 1 cup of sugar, then stir.
3. Power medium-heat and put the frying pan.
4. On each omelet, add onions and mushrooms in the batter while it heats.
5. Serve your delicious Chickpea Omelet.

NUTRITION: Calories: 399 Fat: 11.1g Carbs: 11.5g Protein: 7.9g

23. APPLE-LEMON BOWL

COOKING: 15'   **PREPARATION: 5'**   **SERVES: 1-2**

INGREDIENTS

- 6 apples
- 3 tablespoons walnuts
- 7 dates
- Lemon juice
- 1/2 teaspoon cinnamon

DIRECTIONS

1. Root the apples, then break them into wide bits.
2. In a food cup, put seeds, part of the lime juice, almonds, spices and three-quarters of the apples. Thinly slice until finely ground.
3. Apply the remaining apples and lemon juice and make slices.

NUTRITION: Calories: 249 Fat: 5.1g Carbs: 71.5g Protein: 7.9g

24. BREAKFAST SCRAMBLE

COOKING: 30'   **PREPARATION: 10'**   **SERVES: 6**

INGREDIENTS

- 1 red onion1 to
- 2 tablespoons soy sauce
- 2 cups sliced mushrooms
- Salt to taste
- 1 1/2 teaspoon black pepper
- 1 1/2 teaspoons turmeric
- 1/4 teaspoon cayenne
- 3 cloves garlic
- 1 red bell pepper
- 1 large head cauliflower
- 1 green bell pepper

DIRECTIONS

1. In a small pan, put all vegetables and cook until crispy.
2. Stir in the cauliflower and cook for four to six minutes or until it smooth.
3. Add spices to the pan and cook for another five minutes.

NUTRITION: Calories: 199 Fat: 1.1g Carbs: 14.5g Protein: 7.9g

25. BLACK BEAN AND SWEET POTATO HASH

COOKING: 30' **PREPARATION: 10'** **SERVES: 4**

INGREDIENTS

- 1 cup onion (chopped)
- 1/3 Cup vegetable broth
- 2 garlic (minced)
- 1 cup cooked black beans
- 2 teaspoons hot chili powder
- 2 cups chopped sweet potatoes

DIRECTIONS

1. Put the onions in a saucepan over medium heat and add the seasoning and mix.
2. Add potatoes and chili flakes, then mix.
3. Cook for around 12 minutes more until the vegetables are cooked thoroughly.
4. Add the green onion, beans, and salt
5. Cook for more 2 minutes and serve.

NUTRITION: Calories: 239 Fat: 1.1g Carbs: 71.5g Protein: 7.9g

26. APPLE-WALNUT BREAKFAST BREAD

COOKING: 60' **PREPARATION: 15'** **SERVES: 8**

INGREDIENTS

- 1 1/2 cups apple sauce
- 1/3 cup plant milk
- 2 cups all-purpose flour
- Salt to taste
- 1 teaspoon ground cinnamon
- 1 tablespoon flax seeds mixed with 2 tablespoons warm water
- 3/4 cup brown sugar
- 1 teaspoon baking powder
- 1/2 cup chopped walnuts

DIRECTIONS

1. Preheat to 375°F.
2. Combine the apple sauce, sugar, milk, and flax mixture in a jar and mix.
3. Combine the flour, baking powder, salt, and cinnamon in a separate bowl.
4. Simply add dry ingredients into the wet ingredients and combine to make slices.
5. Bake for 25 minutes until it becomes light brown.

NUTRITION: Calories: 309 Fat: 9.1g Carbs: 16.5g Protein: 6.9g

27. VEGAN SALMON BAGEL

COOKING: 30' **PREPARATION: 10'** **SERVES: 2**

INGREDIENTS

- 4 cups of water
- 1 1/2 red onion
- Vegan cream cheese
- Salt, pepper
- 4 bagels
- 1 1/2 cup of apple cider vinegar
- 7 carrots

DIRECTIONS

1. Preheat oven to 390°F.
2. Slice the carrots.
3. In a mixer to mix, combine sugar, vinegar, and ground pepper.
4. Put the carrot strips in a stir fry bowl, apply the marinade and stir.
5. Cover the carrots with foil and bake for twenty minutes, then switch heat down to 210°F and cook for 40 minutes more.

NUTRITION: Calories: 232 Fat: 9.1g Carbs: 71.5g Protein: 7.9g

THE PLANT BASED DIET COOKBOOK

28. MINT CHOCOLATE GREEN PROTEIN SMOOTHIE

COOKING: 10'   **PREPARATION: 5'**   **SERVES: 1**

INGREDIENTS

- 1 scoop chocolate powder
- 1 tablespoon flaxseed
- 1 banana
- 1 mint leaf
- 3/4 cup almond milk
- 3 tablespoons dark chocolate (chopped)

DIRECTIONS

1. Blend all the ingredients except the dark chocolate.
2. Garnish dark chocolate when ready.

NUTRITION: Calories: 300 Fat: 19.1g Carbs: 21.5g Protein: 27.9g

29. DAIRY-FREE COCONUT YOGURT

COOKING: 10'   **PREPARATION: 5'**   **SERVES: 2**

INGREDIENTS

- 1 can coconut milk
- 4 vegan probiotic capsules

DIRECTIONS

1. Shake coconut milk with a whole tube.
2. Remove the plastic of capsules and mix in.
3. Cut a 12-inch cheesecloth until stirred.
4. Freeze or eat immediately.

NUTRITION: Calories: 219 Fat: 10.1g Carbs: 1.5g Protein: 7.9g

30. VEGAN GREEN AVOCADO SMOOTHIE

COOKING: 10'   **PREPARATION: 5'**   **SERVES: 2**

INGREDIENTS

- 1 banana
- 1 cup water
- 1/2 avocado
- 1/2 lemon juice
- 1/2 cup coconut yoghurt

DIRECTIONS

1. Blend all ingredients until smooth.

NUTRITION: Calories: 299 Fat: 1.1g Carbs: 1.5g Protein: 7.9g

31. SUN-BUTTER BAKED OATMEAL CUPS

COOKING: 35'   **PREPARATION: 10'**   **SERVES: 12**

INGREDIENTS

- 1/4 cup coconut sugar
- 11/2 rolled oats
- 2 tablespoon chia seeds
- 1/4 teaspoon salt
- 1 teaspoon cinnamon
- 1/2 cup non-dairy milk
- 1/2 cup Sun-Butter
- 1/2 cup apple sauce

DIRECTIONS

1. Preheat oven to 350°F.
2. Mix all ingredients and blend well.
3. Add in muffins and insert extra toppings.
4. Bake 25 minutes, or until golden brown.

NUTRITION: Calories: 129 Fat: 1.1g Carbs: 1.5g Protein: 4.9g

32. CHOCOLATE PEANUT BUTTER SHAKE

COOKING: 5' **PREPARATION: 5'** **SERVES: 2**

INGREDIENTS

- 2 bananas
- 3 Tablespoons peanut butter
- 1 cup almond milk
- 3 Tablespoons cacao powder

DIRECTIONS

1. Combine ingredients in a blender until smooth.

NUTRITION: Calories: 149 Fat: 1.1g Carbs: 1.5g Protein: 7.9g

33. BERRIES AND BANANA SMOOTHIE BOWL

COOKING: 0' **PREPARATION: 5'** **SERVES: 4**

INGREDIENTS

- For the Smoothie:
- 4 cups frozen mixed berries
- 4 small frozen bananas, sliced
- 4 scoops of vanilla Protein: powder
- 12 tablespoons almond milk, unsweetened
- For the Toppings:
- 4 tablespoons chia seeds
- 4 tablespoons shredded coconut, unsweetened
- 4 tablespoons hemp seeds
- ½ cup Granola
- Fresh strawberries, sliced, as needed

DIRECTIONS

1. Add mixed berries into a food processor and banana and then pulse at low speed for 1 to 2 minutes until broken.
2. Add remaining ingredients for the smoothie and then pulse again for 1 minute at low speed until creamy, scraping the container's sides frequently.
3. Distribute the smoothie among four bowls, then top with chia seeds, coconut, hemp seeds, granola, and strawberries and serve.

NUTRITION: Calories: 214 Fat: 2.5g Carbs: 47.5g Protein: 2.8g

34. KALE AND PEANUT BUTTER SMOOTHIE

COOKING: 0' **PREPARATION: 5'** **SERVES: 4**

INGREDIENTS

- 4 frozen bananas, sliced
- 2 cups kale
- ½ cup peanut butter
- 2 2/3 cups coconut milk, unsweetened

DIRECTIONS

1. Add all the ingredients in the order into a food processor or blender and then pulse for 1 to 2 minutes until blended, scraping the container's sides frequently.
2. Distribute the smoothie among glasses and then serve.

NUTRITION: Calories: 390 Fat: 19g Carbs: 42g Sugars 22g Protein: 15g

THE PLANT BASED DIET COOKBOOK

35. MINT CHOCOLATE PROTEIN SMOOTHIE

COOKING: 0'   **PREPARATION: 5'**   **SERVES: 4**

INGREDIENTS

- 4 tablespoons ground flaxseed
- 4 cups fresh spinach
- 4 frozen bananas, sliced
- 4 scoops of chocolate Protein: powder
- 4 tablespoons chopped dark chocolate, vegan
- ½ cup melted dark chocolate
- 1 teaspoon peppermint extract, unsweetened
- 4 tablespoons honey
- 3 cups almond milk, unsweetened
- 1 cup ice cubed

DIRECTIONS

1. Add all the ingredients in the order into a food processor or blender and then pulse for 1 to 2 minutes until blended, scraping the container's sides frequently.
2. Distribute the smoothie among glasses and then serve.

NUTRITION: Calories: 480.5 Fat: 20.3g Carbs: 45.6g Sugars: 22.5 Protein: 31.2g

---

36. BERRY BREAKFAST SMOOTHIE

COOKING: 0'   **PREPARATION: 0'**   **SERVES: 4**

INGREDIENTS

- 1 cup of frozen mixed berries
- 1 cup quick oats
- 1 frozen banana
- 2 cups vanilla almond milk, unsweetened

DIRECTIONS

1. Add all the ingredients in the order into a food processor or blender and then pulse for 1 to 2 minutes until blended, scraping the container's sides frequently.
2. Distribute the smoothie among glasses and then serve.

NUTRITION: Calories: 138.5g Fat: 2.5g Carbs: 25.6g Sugars: 6.6g Protein: 3.5g

---

37. SUNRISE SMOOTHIE

COOKING: 0'   **PREPARATION: 5'**   **SERVES: 4**

INGREDIENTS

- 4 tablespoons chia seed
- 2 frozen banana
- 2 lemons, peeled
- 2 cups diced carrots
- 4 clementine, peeled
- 4 cups frozen strawberries, unsweetened
- 12 tablespoons pomegranate tendrils
- 2 cup almond milk, unsweetened

DIRECTIONS

1. Add all the ingredients in the order into a food processor or blender and then pulse for 1 to 2 minutes until blended, scraping the container's sides frequently.
2. Distribute the smoothie among glasses and then serve.

NUTRITION: Calories: 274 Fat: 5.4g Carbs: 57.3g Sugars: 33.8g Protein: 0.5g

38. SUNSHINE ORANGE SMOOTHIE

COOKING: 0'   **PREPARATION: 5'**   **SERVES: 4**

INGREDIENTS

- 2 medium oranges, zested, juiced
- 4 frozen bananas
- 4 tablespoons goji berries
- ½ cup hemp seeds
- 1 teaspoon grated ginger
- 1 cup almond milk, unsweetened
- ½ cup of ice cubes

DIRECTIONS

1. Add all the ingredients in the order into a food processor or blender and then pulse for 1 to 2 minutes until blended, scraping the container's sides frequently.
2. Distribute the smoothie among glasses and then serve.

NUTRITION: Calories: 131 Fat: 2.3g Carbs: 26.7g Sugars: 11g Protein: 2.6g

39. CHOCOLATE AND HAZELNUT SMOOTHIE

COOKING: 0'   **PREPARATION: 5'**   **SERVES: 4**

INGREDIENTS

- 1 frozen banana
- 1 cup hazelnuts, unsalted, roasted
- 8 teaspoons maple syrup
- 4 tablespoons cocoa powder, unsweetened
- 1/2 teaspoon hazelnut extract, unsweetened
- 2 cups almond milk, unsweetened
- 1 cup of ice cubes

DIRECTIONS

1. Add all the ingredients in the order into a food processor or blender and then pulse for 1 to 2 minutes until blended, scraping the container's sides frequently.
2. Distribute the smoothie among glasses and then serve.

NUTRITION: Calories: 198 Fat: 12g Carbs: 21g Sugars: 12g Protein: 5g

40. BLUEBERRY OATMEAL SMOOTHIE

COOKING: 0'   **PREPARATION: 5'**   **SERVES: 4**

INGREDIENTS

- 2 cups frozen blueberries
- 1 cup old-fashioned oats
- 2 teaspoons cinnamon
- 2 tablespoons maple syrup
- 1 cup spinach
- 2 cup almond milk, unsweetened
- 8 ice cubes

DIRECTIONS

1. Add all the ingredients in the order into a food processor or blender and then pulse for 1 to 2 minutes until blended, scraping the container's sides frequently.
2. Distribute the smoothie among glasses and then serve.

NUTRITION: Calories: 194 Fat: 5g Carbs: 34g Sugars: 15g Protein: 5g

41. COOKIE DOUGH SMOOTHIE

COOKING: 0'   **PREPARATION: 5'**   **SERVES: 4**

INGREDIENTS

- 4 frozen banana
- 8 tablespoons hemp seeds
- 8 tablespoons chocolate chips, vegan
- 4 scoops of salted caramel Protein:
- 2 teaspoons cinnamon
- 8 teaspoons honey
- 8 tablespoons peanut butter powder
- 4 cups almond milk, unsweetened
- 4 cups of ice cubes

DIRECTIONS

1. Add all the ingredients in the order into a food processor or blender and then pulse for 1 to 2 minutes until blended, scraping the container's sides frequently.
2. Distribute the smoothie among glasses and then serve.

NUTRITION: Calories: 442 Fat: 19.5g Carbs: 41.3g Sugars: 22.2g Protein: 31.2g

42. COFFEE SMOOTHIE

COOKING: 0'   **PREPARATION: 5'**   **SERVES: 4**

INGREDIENTS

- 4 cups baby spinach
- 4 tablespoons hemp hearts
- 12 Medjool dates, pitted
- 4 tablespoons cashew butter
- 2 cup brewed coffee, chilled
- 6 cups of ice cubes

DIRECTIONS

1. Place pitted dates in a medium bowl, cover with hot water and let them soak for 15 minutes.
2. Drain the dates, add them into a food processor and the remaining ingredients, and then pulse for 1 to 2 minutes until blended, scraping the sides of the container frequently.
3. Distribute the smoothie among glasses and then serve.

NUTRITION: Calories: 138.5g Fat: 2.5g Carbs: 25.6g Sugars: 6.6g Protein: 3.5g

43. BREAKFAST MUESLI

COOKING: 0'   **PREPARATION: 5'**   **SERVES: 4**

INGREDIENTS

- 2 bananas, peeled, sliced
- 1 cup raspberries
- 2 cups sliced strawberries
- 1 cup blueberries
- 4 tablespoons crushed pistachios
- 4 tablespoons hemp seeds
- 4 tablespoons chia seeds
- 4 teaspoons honey
- 2 cups of coconut yogurt
- 2 cups muesli, unsweetened
- Mint leaves as needed for garnish

DIRECTIONS

1. Take a large bowl, place yogurt in it, and then add muesli.
2. Top with raspberries, strawberries, blueberries, and banana slices, drizzle with honey and then sprinkle with pistachios.
3. Garnish with mint, hemp seeds, and chia seeds and then serve.

NUTRITION: Calories: 411 Fat: 18g Carbs: 53g Sugars: 17 Protein: 8g

44. BANANA CREAM PIE AND CHIA PUDDING

COOKING: 0'   **PREPARATION: 1H 10'**   **SERVES: 4**

INGREDIENTS

- 2 bananas, peeled, mashed
- 2 bananas, peeled, chopped
- 1/2 cup chia seeds
- 2 teaspoons cinnamon
- 4 tablespoons coconut flakes
- 1 cup coconut milk, unsweetened
- 2 tablespoons maple syrup
- 1 cup almond milk, unsweetened

DIRECTIONS

1. Take a large bowl, add chia seeds and mashed bananas, add maple syrup and cinnamon, pour in almond and coconut milk, and whisk until well combined.
2. Cover the bowl with lid, and then place it in the refrigerator for a minimum of 1 hour until firm.
3. When ready to eat, distribute pudding evenly among 4 bowls, top with chopped banana, and sprinkle with coconut flakes and then serve.

NUTRITION: Calories: 350 Fat: 17g Carbs: 37 g Sugars: 19g Protein: 5g

45. BROWN RICE BREAKFAST PUDDING

COOKING: 15'   **PREPARATION: 5'**   **SERVES: 4**

INGREDIENTS

- 4 cups baby spinach
- 4 tablespoons hemp hearts
- 12 Medjool dates, pitted
- 4 tablespoons cashew butter
- 2 cup brewed coffee, chilled
- 6 cups of ice cubes

DIRECTIONS

1. Place pitted dates in a medium bowl, cover with hot water and let them soak for 15 minutes.
2. Drain the dates, add them into a food processor and the remaining ingredients, and then pulse for 1 to 2 minutes until blended, scraping the sides of the container frequently.
3. Distribute the smoothie among glasses and then serve.

NUTRITION: Calories: 391 Fat: 4.8g Carbs: 81.1g Sugars: 24.8g Protein: 6g

46. OATS WITH CHIA

COOKING: 0'   **PREPARATION: 6H 10'**   **SERVES: 4**

INGREDIENTS

- 3 cups rolled oats
- 4 tablespoons chia seeds and more for topping
- 4 tablespoons maple syrup
- 1 teaspoon cinnamon
- 1 teaspoon vanilla extract, unsweetened
- 1 cup almond milk, unsweetened
- 2 cups of water
- 1 cup sliced strawberries

DIRECTIONS

1. Take a large container, add oats and chia seeds in it, add cinnamon, vanilla extract, and maple syrup, then pour in water and almond milk and stir until mixed.
2. Cover the bowl with lid, and then place it in the refrigerator for a minimum of 6 hours.
3. When ready to eat, distribute oats and chia mixture evenly among 4 bowls, top with some chia seeds and sliced strawberries, and then serve.

NUTRITION: Calories: 351.8 Fat: 7.4g Carbs: 62.4g Sugars: 14.6g Protein: 8.8g

THE PLANT BASED DIET COOKBOOK

47. CARROT CAKE OATS

COOKING: 0'   **PREPARATION: 6H 10'**   **SERVES: 4**

INGREDIENTS

- ¼ cup shredded carrot
- 1/3 cup rolled oats
- 2 tablespoons chopped pineapple
- 1 tablespoon shredded coconut, unsweetened and more for topping
- 1 tablespoon ground flaxseed
- 1 tablespoon raisins and more for topping
- 2 tablespoons maple syrup and more for topping
- 1/8 teaspoon ground nutmeg
- ¼ teaspoon ground cinnamon and more for topping
- ¼ teaspoon vanilla extract, unsweetened
- 1 tablespoon chopped walnuts and more for topping
- ½ cup almond milk, unsweetened

DIRECTIONS

1. Take a large bowl, place all the ingredients in it, and stir until well mixed.
2. Cover the bowl with lid, and then place it in the refrigerator for a minimum of 6 hours.
3. When ready to eat, distribute oats mixture evenly among 4 bowls, top with some shredded coconut, raisins, and walnuts, sprinkle with cinnamon, drizzle with maple syrup and then serve.

NUTRITION: Calories: 242 Fat: 9g Carbs: 35g Sugars: 12g Protein: 7g

48. TOAST WITH AVOCADO AND BERRIES

COOKING: 10'   **PREPARATION: 10'**   **SERVES: 4**

INGREDIENTS

- 1 cup sliced strawberries
- 2 large avocados, peeled, pitted, sliced
- 4 tablespoons honey
- 4 slices of whole-grain bread
- 4oz. block of vegan cheddar cheese, thinly sliced

DIRECTIONS

1. Take a skillet pan, place it over medium heat, and heat bread slices for 2 to 3 minutes until toasted.
2. Peel the avocados, remove the pit, cut the flesh in slices, place into a bowl, and then mash with a fork.
3. Spread mashed avocado on one side of the toasted slices, then top with berries and cover with cheese slices.
4. Drizzle with honey and then serve.

NUTRITION: Calories: 379 Fat: 21g Carbs: 35g Sugars: 9g Protein: 18g

49. CHOCOLATE CHIP AND COCONUT PANCAKES

COOKING: 40' **PREPARATION: 10'** **SERVES: 8**

INGREDIENTS

- 1¼ cups buckwheat flour
- 1 tablespoon flaxseeds
- 2 tablespoons coconut flakes, unsweetened
- ¼ cup rolled oats
- 1/8 teaspoon sea salt
- 1 tablespoon baking powder
- 1/3 cup mini chocolate chips, vegan
- ¼ cup maple syrup
- 1 teaspoon vanilla extract, unsweetened
- ½ cup applesauce, unsweetened
- 1 cup almond milk, unsweetened
- ½ cup of water
- 2 bananas, peeled, sliced

DIRECTIONS

1. Take a small saucepan, place it over medium heat, add flaxseeds, pour in water, and then cook for 4 to 5 minutes until sticky mixture comes together.
2. Strain the flaxseeds mixture immediately into a cup, discard the seeds, and set aside the collected flax water until required.
3. Take a large bowl, add buckwheat flour and oats in it, and then stir in salt, baking powder, and coconut until mixed.
4. Take a medium bowl, add 2 tablespoons of reserved flax water along with maple syrup and vanilla, pour in applesauce and milk, and whisk until combined.
5. Pour the milk mixture into the flour mixture, whisk well until thick batter comes together, and fold in chocolate chips.
6. Take a griddle pan, place it over medium-low heat, spray it with oil and when hot, pour in 1/3 cup of the prepared batter, spread it gently and cook for 5 to 7 minutes until the bottom turns golden brown; pour in more batter if there is a space on the pan.
7. Flip the pancake, continue cooking for 5 minutes, and when done, transfer pancake to a plate and then repeat with the remaining batter.
8. Serve pancakes with sliced bananas.

NUTRITION: Calories: 190 Fat: 14g Carbs: 8 g Sugars: 18.2g Protein: 8g

THE PLANT BASED DIET COOKBOOK

CHAPTER 8: SMOOTHIES AND FRESH JUICES

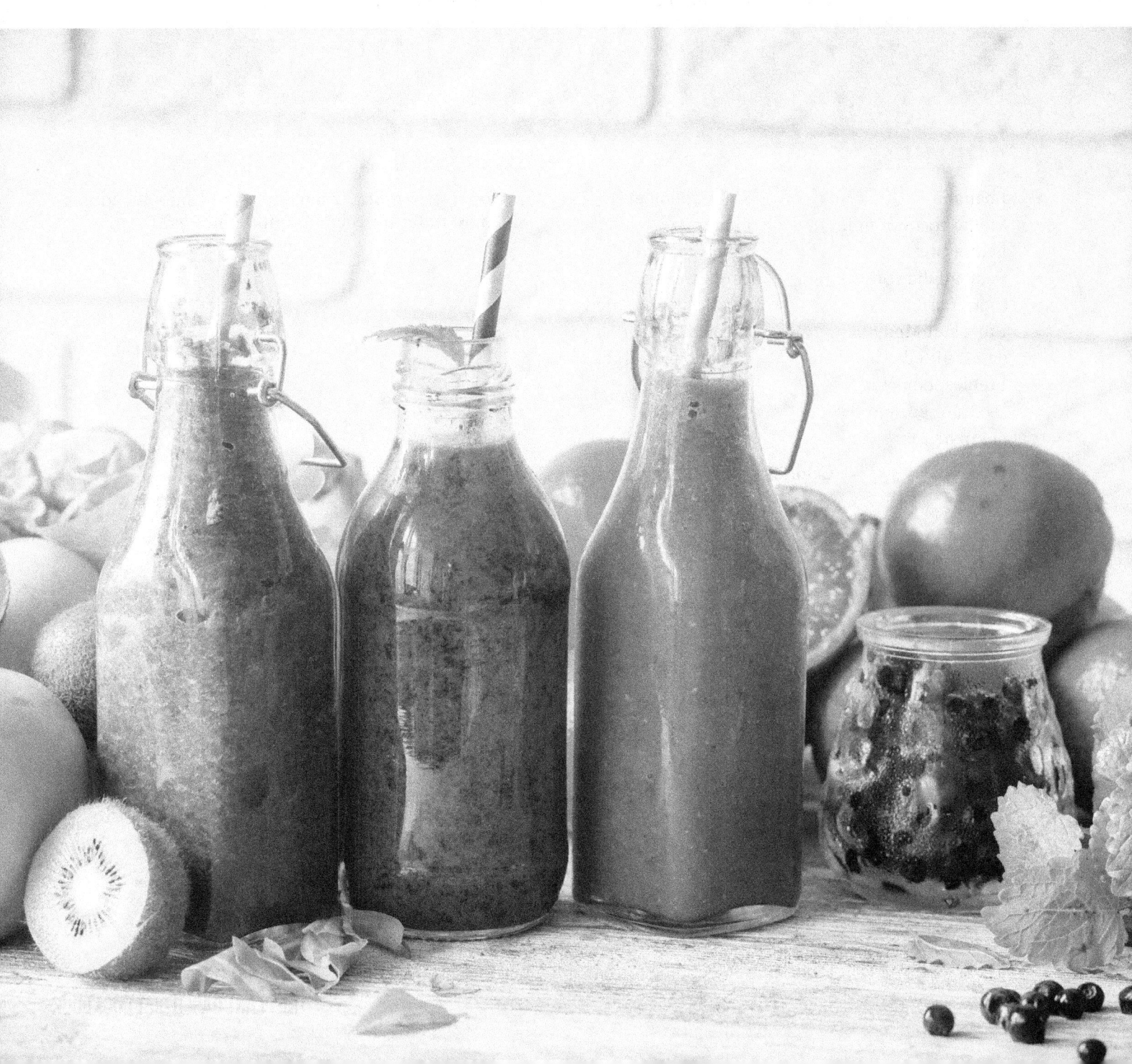

50. MAX POWER SMOOTHIE

COOKING: 0'   **PREPARATION: 5'**   **SERVES: 3-4 CUPS**

INGREDIENTS

- 1 banana
- ¼ cup rolled oats, or 1 scoop plant Protein: powder
- 1 tablespoon flaxseed, or chia seeds
- 1 cup raspberries, or other berries
- 1 cup chopped mango (frozen or fresh)
- ½ cup non-dairy milk (optional)
- 1 cup water

DIRECTIONS

1. Purée everything in a blender until smooth, adding more water (or non-dairy milk) if needed.
2. Add none, some, or all of the bonus boosters, as desired. Purée until blended.

NUTRITION: Calories: 550 Fat: 9 Carbs: 116g Fiber: 29g Protein: 13g

51. CHAI CHIA SMOOTHIE

COOKING: 0'   **PREPARATION: 5'**   **SERVES: 3 CUPS**

INGREDIENTS

- 1 banana
- ½ cup coconut milk
- 1 cup water
- 1 cup alfalfa sprouts (optional)
- 1 to 2 soft Medjool dates, pitted
- 1 tablespoon chia seeds, or ground flax or hemp hearts
- ¼ teaspoon ground cinnamon
- Pinch ground cardamom
- 1 tablespoon grated fresh ginger, or ¼ teaspoon ground ginger

DIRECTIONS

1. Purée everything in a blender until smooth, adding more water (or coconut milk) if needed.

NUTRITION: Calories: 477 Fat: 29g Carbs: 57g Fiber: 14g Protein: 8g

52. TROPE-KALE BREEZE

COOKING: 0'   **PREPARATION: 5'**   **SERVES: 3-4 CUPS**

INGREDIENTS

- 1 cup chopped pineapple (frozen or fresh)
- 1 cup chopped mango (frozen or fresh)
- ½ to 1 cup chopped kale
- ½ avocado
- ½ cup coconut milk
- 1 cup water, or coconut water
- 1 teaspoon matcha green tea powder (optional)

DIRECTIONS

1. Purée everything in a blender until smooth, adding more water (or coconut milk) if needed.

NUTRITION: Calories: 566 Fat: 36g Carbs: 66g Fiber: 12g Protein: 8g

53. HYDRATION STATION

COOKING: 0'   **PREPARATION: 5'**   **SERVES: 3-4 CUPS**

INGREDIENTS

- 1 banana
- 1 orange, peeled and sectioned, or 1 cup pure orange juice
- 1 cup strawberries (frozen or fresh)
- 1 cup chopped cucumber
- ½ cup coconut water
- 1 cup water
- ½ cup ice

DIRECTIONS

1. Purée everything in a blender until smooth, adding more water if needed.

Add bonus boosters, as desired. Purée until blended.

NUTRITION: Calories: 320 Fat: 3g Carbs: 76g Fiber: 13g Protein: 6g

54. MANGO MADNESS

COOKING: 0'   **PREPARATION: 5'**   **SERVES: 3-4 CUPS**

INGREDIENTS

- 1 banana
- 1 cup chopped mango (frozen or fresh)
- 1 cup chopped peach (frozen or fresh)
- 1 cup strawberries
- 1 carrot, peeled and chopped (optional)
- 1 cup water

DIRECTIONS

1. Purée everything in a blender until smooth, adding more water if needed.

NUTRITION: Calories: 376 Fat: 2g Carbs: 95g Fiber: 14g Protein: 5g

55. CHOCOLATE PB SMOOTHIE

COOKING: 0'   **PREPARATION: 5'**   **SERVES: 3-4 CUPS**

INGREDIENTS

- 1 banana
- ¼ cup rolled oats, or 1 scoop plant Protein: powder
- 1 tablespoon flaxseed, or chia seeds
- 1 tablespoon unsweetened cocoa powder
- 1 tablespoon peanut butter, or almond or sunflower seed butter
- 1 tablespoon maple syrup (optional)
- 1 cup alfalfa sprouts, or spinach, chopped (optional)
- ½ cup non-dairy milk (optional)
- 1 cup water

DIRECTIONS

1. Take a large bowl, place yogurt in it, and then add muesli.
2. Top with raspberries, strawberries, blueberries, and banana slices, drizzle with honey and then sprinkle with pistachios.
3. Garnish with mint, hemp seeds, and chia seeds and then serve.

NUTRITION: Calories: 474 Fat: 16g Carbs: 79g Fiber: 18g Protein: 13g

THE PLANT BASED DIET COOKBOOK

56. TPINK PANTHER SMOOTHIE

COOKING: 0'   **PREPARATION: 5'**   **SERVES: 3 CUPS**

INGREDIENTS

- 1 cup strawberries
- 1 cup chopped melon (any kind)
- 1 cup cranberries, or raspberries
- 1 tablespoon chia seeds
- ½ cup coconut milk, or other non-dairy milk
- 1 cup water

DIRECTIONS

1. Purée everything in a blender until smooth, adding more water (or coconut milk) if needed.
2. Add bonus boosters, as desired. Purée until blended.

NUTRITION: Calories: 459 Fat: 30g Carbs: 52g Fiber: 19g Protein: 8g

57. BANANA NUT SMOOTHIE

COOKING: 0'   **PREPARATION: 5'**   **SERVES: 3 CUPS**

INGREDIENTS

- 1 banana
- 1 tablespoon almond butter, or sunflower seed butter
- ¼ teaspoon ground cinnamon
- Pinch ground nutmeg
- 1 to 2 tablespoons dates, or maple syrup
- 1 tablespoon ground flaxseed, or chia, or hemp hearts
- ½ cup non-dairy milk (optional)
- 1 cup water

DIRECTIONS

1. Purée everything in a blender until smooth, adding more water (or non-dairy milk) if needed.

NUTRITION: Calories: 343 Fat: 14g Carbs: 55g Fiber: 8g Protein: 6g

58. OVERNIGHT OATS ON THE GO

COOKING: 5' OR OVERNIGHT   **PREPARATION: 5'**   **SERVES: 1**

INGREDIENTS

BASIC OVERNIGHT OATS
- ½ cup rolled oats, or quinoa flakes for gluten-free
- 1 tablespoon ground flaxseed, or chia seeds, or hemp hearts
- 1 tablespoon maple syrup, or coconut sugar (optional)
- ¼ teaspoon ground cinnamon (optional)

TOPPING OPTIONS
- 1 apple, chopped, and 1 tablespoon walnuts
- 2 tablespoons dried cranberries and 1 tablespoon pumpkin seeds
- 1 pear, chopped, and 1 tablespoon cashews
- 1 cup sliced grapes and 1 tablespoon sunflower seeds
- 1 banana, sliced, and 1 tablespoon peanut butter
- 2 tablespoons raisins and 1 tablespoon hazelnuts
- 1 cup berries and 1 tablespoon unsweetened coconut flakes

DIRECTIONS

1. Mix the oats, flax, maple syrup, and cinnamon (if using) in a bowl or to-go container (a travel mug or short thermos works beautifully).
2. Pour enough cool water over the oats to submerge them, and stir to combine. Leave to soak for a minimum of half an hour, or overnight.
3. Add your choice of toppings.

NUTRITION: Calories: 244 Fat: 6g Carbs: 30g Fiber: 6g Protein: 7g

59. OATMEAL BREAKFAST COOKIES

COOKING: 12' **PREPARATION: 15'** **SERVES: 5 BIG COOKIES**

INGREDIENTS

- 1 tablespoon ground flaxseed
- 2 tablespoons almond butter, or sunflower seed butter
- 2 tablespoons maple syrup
- 1 banana, mashed
- 1 teaspoon ground cinnamon
- ¼ teaspoon ground nutmeg (optional)
- Pinch sea salt
- ½ cup rolled oats
- ¼ cup raisins, or dark chocolate chips

DIRECTIONS

1. Preheat the oven to 350°F. Line a large baking sheet with parchment paper.
2. Mix the ground flax with just enough water to cover it in a small dish, and leave it to sit.
3. In a large bowl, mix the almond butter and maple syrup until creamy, then add the banana. Add the flax-water mixture.
4. Sift the cinnamon, nutmeg, and salt into a separate medium bowl, then stir into the wet mixture.
5. Add the oats and raisins, and fold in.
6. From 3 to 4 tablespoons batter into a ball and press lightly to flatten onto the baking sheet. Repeat, spacing the cookies 2 to 3 inches apart.
7. Bake for 12 minutes, or until golden brown.
8. Store the cookies in an airtight container in the fridge, or freeze them for later.

NUTRITION: Calories: 192 Fat: 6 Carbs: 34g Fiber: 4g Protein: 4g

60. SUNSHINE MUFFINS

COOKING: 30' **PREPARATION: 15'** **SERVES: 6 MUFFINS**

INGREDIENTS

- 1 teaspoon coconut oil, for greasing muffin tins (optional)
- 2 tablespoons almond butter, or sunflower seed butter
- ¼ cup non-dairy milk
- 1 orange, peeled
- 1 carrot, coarsely chopped
- 2 tablespoons chopped dried apricots, or other dried fruit
- 3 tablespoons molasses
- 2 tablespoons ground flaxseed
- 1 teaspoon apple cider vinegar
- 1 teaspoon pure vanilla extract
- ½ teaspoon ground cinnamon
- ½ teaspoon ground ginger (optional)
- ¼ teaspoon ground nutmeg (optional)
- ¼ teaspoon allspice (optional)
- ¾ cup rolled oats, or whole-grain flour
- 1 teaspoon baking powder
- ½ teaspoon baking soda

DIRECTIONS

1. Preheat the oven to 350°F. Prepare a 6-cup muffin tin by rubbing the cups' insides with coconut oil or using silicone or paper muffin cups.
2. Purée the nut butter, milk, orange, carrot, apricots, molasses, flaxseed, vinegar, vanilla, cinnamon, ginger, nutmeg, and allspice in a food processor or blender until somewhat smooth.
3. Grind the oats in a clean coffee grinder until they're consistent with flour (or use whole-grain flour). In a large bowl, mix the oats with the baking powder and baking soda.
4. Mix the wet ingredients into the dry ingredients until just combined. Fold in the mix-ins (if using).
5. Spoon about ¼ cup batter into each muffin cup and bake for 30 minutes, or until a toothpick inserted into the center comes out clean. The orange creates a very moist base, so the muffins may take longer than 30 minutes, depending on how heavy your muffin tin is.

NUTRITION: Calories: 287 Fat: 12 Carbs: 41 gFiber: 6g Protein: 8g

61. APPLESAUCE CRUMBLE MUFFINS

COOKING: 15-20' **PREPARATION:** 15' **SERVES:** 12 MUFFINS

INGREDIENTS

- 1 teaspoon coconut oil, for greasing muffin tins (optional)
- 2 tablespoons nut butter, or seed butter
- 1½ cups unsweetened applesauce
- 1/3 cup coconut sugar
- ½ cup non-dairy milk
- 2 tablespoons ground flaxseed
- 1 teaspoon apple cider vinegar
- 1 teaspoon pure vanilla extract
- 2 cups whole-grain flour
- 1 teaspoon baking soda
- ½ teaspoon baking powder
- 1 teaspoon ground cinnamon
- Pinch sea salt
- ½ cup walnuts, chopped

DIRECTIONS

1. Preheat the oven to 350°F. Prepare two 6-cup muffin tins by rubbing the cups' insides with coconut oil, or using silicone or paper muffin cups.
2. In a large bowl, mix the nut butter, applesauce, coconut sugar, milk, flaxseed, vinegar, and vanilla until thoroughly combined, or purée in a food processor or blender.
3. In another large bowl, sift together the flour, baking soda, baking powder, cinnamon, salt, and chopped walnuts.
4. Mix the dry ingredients into the wet ingredients until just combined.
5. Spoon about ¼ cup batter into each muffin cup and sprinkle with the topping of your choice (if using). Bake for 15 to 20 minutes, or until a toothpick inserted into the center comes out clean. The applesauce creates a very moist base, so the muffins may take longer, depending on how heavy your muffin tins are.

NUTRITION: Calories: 287 Fat: 12 Carbs: 41g Fiber: 6g Protein: 8g

62. BAKED BANANA FRENCH TOAST WITH RASPBERRY SYRUP

COOKING: 30' **PREPARATION:** 10' **SERVES:** 8

INGREDIENTS

FOR THE FRENCH TOAST
- 1 banana
- 1 cup coconut milk
- 1 teaspoon pure vanilla extract
- ¼ teaspoon ground nutmeg
- ½ teaspoon ground cinnamon
- 1½ teaspoons arrowroot powder, or flour
- Pinch sea salt
- 8 slices whole-grain bread

FOR THE RASPBERRY SYRUP
- 1 cup fresh or frozen raspberries, or other berries
- 2 tablespoons water, or pure fruit juice
- 1 to 2 tablespoons maple syrup, or coconut sugar (optional)

DIRECTIONS

TO MAKE THE FRENCH TOAST
1. Preheat the oven to 350°F.
2. In a shallow bowl, purée or mash the banana well. Mix in the coconut milk, vanilla, nutmeg, cinnamon, arrowroot, and salt.
3. Dip the slices of bread in the banana mixture, and then lay them out in a 13-by-9-inch baking dish. They should cover the bottom of the dish and overlap slightly but shouldn't be stacked on top of each other. Pour any leftover banana mixture over the bread, and put the dish in the oven. Bake about 30 minutes, or until the tops are lightly browned.
4. Serve topped with raspberry syrup.

TO MAKE THE RASPBERRY SYRUP
5. Heat the raspberries in a small pot with the water and the maple syrup (if using) on medium heat.
6. Leave to simmer, stirring occasionally and breaking up the berries, until the liquid has reduced for 15 to 20 minutes.

NUTRITION: Calories: 166 Fat: 7g Carbs: 23g Fiber: 4g Protein: 5g

63. KALE SMOOTHIE

COOKING: 0'   **PREPARATION: 5'**   **SERVES: 2**

INGREDIENTS

- 2 cups chopped kale leaves
- 1 banana, peeled
- 1 cup frozen strawberries
- 1 cup unsweetened almond milk
- 4 Medjool dates, pitted and chopped

DIRECTIONS

1. Put all the ingredients in a food processor, then blitz until glossy and smooth.
2. Serve immediately or chill in the refrigerator for an hour before serving.

NUTRITION: Calories: 663 Fat: 10.0g Carbs: 142.5g Fiber: 19.0g Protein: 17.4g

---

64. HOT TROPICAL SMOOTHIE

COOKING: 0'   **PREPARATION: 5'**   **SERVES: 4**

INGREDIENTS

- 1 cup frozen mango chunks
- 1 cup frozen pineapple chunks
- 1 small tangerine, peeled and pitted
- 2 cups spinach leaves
- 1 cup coconut water
- ¼ teaspoon cayenne pepper, optional

DIRECTIONS

1. Add all the ingredients in a food processor, then blitz until the mixture is smooth and combine well.
2. Serve immediately or chill in the refrigerator for an hour before serving.

NUTRITION: Calories: 283 Fat: 1.9g Carbs: 67.9g Fiber: 10.4g Protein: 6.4g

---

65. BERRY SMOOTHIE

COOKING: 0'   **PREPARATION: 5'**   **SERVES: 4**

INGREDIENTS

- 1 cup berry mix (strawberries, blueberries, and cranberries)
- 4 Medjool dates, pitted and chopped
- 1½ cups unsweetened almond milk, plus more as needed

DIRECTIONS

1. Add all the ingredients in a blender, then process until the mixture is smooth and well mixed.
2. Serve immediately or chill in the refrigerator for an hour before serving.

NUTRITION: Calories: 473 Fat: 4.0g Carbs: 103.7g Fiber: 9.7g Protein: 14.8g

---

66. CRANBERRY AND BANANA SMOOTHIE

COOKING: 0'   **PREPARATION: 5'**   **SERVES: 4**

INGREDIENTS

- 1 cup frozen cranberries
- 1 large banana, peeled
- 4 Medjool dates, pitted and chopped
- 1½ cups unsweetened almond milk

DIRECTIONS

1. Add all the ingredients in a food processor, then process until the mixture is glossy and well mixed.
2. Serve immediately or chill in the refrigerator for an hour before serving.

NUTRITION: Calories: 616 Fat: 8.0g Carbs: 132.8g Fiber: 14.6g Protein: 15.7g

67. PUMPKIN SMOOTHIE

COOKING: 0'   **PREPARATION: 5'**   **SERVES: 5**

INGREDIENTS

- ½ cup pumpkin purée
- 4 Medjool dates, pitted and chopped
- 1 cup unsweetened almond milk
- ¼ teaspoon vanilla extract
- ¼ teaspoon ground cinnamon
- ½ cup ice
- Pinch ground nutmeg

DIRECTIONS

1. Add all the ingredients in a blender, then process until the mixture is glossy and well mixed.
2. Serve immediately.

NUTRITION: Calories: 417 Fat: 3.0g Carbs: 94.9g Fiber: 10.4g Protein: 11.4g

68. SUPER SMOOTHIE

COOKING: 0'   **PREPARATION: 5'**   **SERVES: 4**

INGREDIENTS

- 1 banana, peeled
- 1 cup chopped mango
- 1 cup raspberries
- ¼ cup rolled oats
- 1 carrot, peeled
- 1 cup chopped fresh kale
- 2 tablespoons chopped fresh parsley
- 1 tablespoon flaxseeds
- 1 tablespoon grated fresh ginger
- ½ cup unsweetened soy milk
- 1 cup water

DIRECTIONS

1. Put all the ingredients in a food processor, then blitz until glossy and smooth.
2. Serve immediately or chill in the refrigerator for an hour before serving.

NUTRITION: Calories: 550 Fat: 39.0 Carbs: 31.0g Fiber: 15.0g Protein: 13.0g

69. KIWI AND STRAWBERRY SMOOTHIE

COOKING: 0'   **PREPARATION: 5'**   **SERVES: 3**

INGREDIENTS

- 1 kiwi, peeled
- 5 medium strawberries
- ½ frozen banana
- 1 cup unsweetened almond milk
- 2 tablespoons hemp seeds
- 2 tablespoons peanut butter
- 1 to 2 teaspoons maple syrup
- ½ cup spinach leaves
- Handful broccoli sprouts

DIRECTIONS

1. Put all the ingredients in a food processor, then blitz until creamy and smooth.
2. Serve immediately or chill in the refrigerator for an hour before serving.

NUTRITION: Calories: 562 Fat: 28.6g Carbs: 63.6g Fiber: 15.1g Protein: 23.3g

70. BANANA AND CHAI CHIA SMOOTHIE

COOKING: 0'   **PREPARATION: 5'**   **SERVES: 3**

INGREDIENTS

- 1 banana
- 1 cup alfalfa sprouts
- 1 tablespoon chia seeds
- ½ cup unsweetened coconut milk
- 1 to 2 soft Medjool dates, pitted
- ¼ teaspoon ground cinnamon
- 1 tablespoon grated fresh ginger
- 1 cup water
- Pinch ground cardamom

DIRECTIONS

1. Add all the ingredients in a blender, then process until the mixture is smooth and creamy. Add water or coconut milk if necessary.
2. Serve immediately.

NUTRITION: Calories: 477 Fat: 41.0g Carbs: 31.0 gFiber: 14.0g Protein: 8.0g

71. CHOCOLATE AND PEANUT BUTTER SMOOTHIE

COOKING: 0'   **PREPARATION: 5'**   **SERVES: 4**

INGREDIENTS

- 1 tablespoon unsweetened cocoa powder
- 1 tablespoon peanut butter
- 1 banana
- 1 teaspoon maca powder
- ½ cup unsweetened soy milk
- ¼ cup rolled oats
- 1 tablespoon flaxseeds
- 1 tablespoon maple syrup
- 1 cup water

DIRECTIONS

1. Add all the ingredients in a blender, then process until the mixture is smooth and creamy. Add water or soy milk if necessary.
2. Serve immediately.

NUTRITION: Calories: 474 Fat: 16.0 Carbs: 27.0g Fiber: 18.0g Protein: 13.0g

72. GOLDEN MILK

COOKING: 0'   **PREPARATION: 5'**   **SERVES: 4**

INGREDIENTS

- ¼ teaspoon ground cinnamon
- ½ teaspoon ground turmeric
- ½ teaspoon grated fresh ginger
- 1 teaspoon maple syrup
- 1 cup unsweetened coconut milk
- Ground black pepper, to taste
- 2 tablespoon water

DIRECTIONS

1. Combine all the ingredients in a saucepan. Stir to mix well.
2. Heat over medium heat for 5 minutes. Keep stirring during the heating.
3. Allow to cool for 5 minutes, then pour the mixture in a blender. Pulse until creamy and smooth. Serve immediately.

NUTRITION: Calories: 577 Fat: 57.3g Carbs: 19.7g Fiber: 6.1g Protein: 5.7g

THE PLANT BASED DIET COOKBOOK

73. MANGO AGUA FRESCA

COOKING: 0'   **PREPARATION: 5'**   **SERVES: 5**

INGREDIENTS

- 2 fresh mangoes, diced
- 1½ cups water
- 1 teaspoon fresh lime juice
- Maple syrup, to taste
- 2 cups ice
- 2 slices fresh lime, for garnish
- 2 fresh mint sprigs, for garnish

DIRECTIONS

1. Put the mangoes, lime juice, maple syrup, and water in a blender. Process until creamy and smooth.
2. Divide the beverage into two glasses, then garnish each glass with ice, lime slice, and mint sprig before serving.

NUTRITION: Calories: 230 Fat: 1.3g Carbs: 57.7g Fiber: 5.4g Protein: 2.8g

74. LIGHT GINGER TEA

COOKING: 10-15'   **PREPARATION: 5'**   **SERVES: 2**

INGREDIENTS

- 1 small ginger knob, sliced into four 1-inch chunks
- 4 cups water
- Juice of 1 large lemon
- Maple syrup, to taste

DIRECTIONS

1. Add the ginger knob and water in a saucepan, then simmer over medium heat for 10 to 15 minutes.
2. Turn off the heat, then mix in the lemon juice. Strain the liquid to remove the ginger, then fold in the maple syrup and serve.

NUTRITION: Calories: 32 Fat: 0.1g Carbs: 8.6g Fiber: 0.1g Protein: 0.1g

75. CLASSIC SWITCHEL

COOKING: 0'   **PREPARATION: 5'**   **SERVES: 4**

INGREDIENTS

- 1-inch piece ginger, minced
- 2 tablespoons apple cider vinegar
- 2 tablespoons maple syrup
- 4 cups water
- ¼ teaspoon sea salt, optional

DIRECTIONS

1. Put all the ingredients in a food processor, then blitz until creamy and smooth.
2. Serve immediately or chill in the refrigerator for an hour before serving.

NUTRITION: Calories: 110 Fat: 0g Carbs: 28.0g Fiber: 0g Protein: 0g

76. LIME AND CUCUMBER ELECTROLYTE DRINK

COOKING: 0'   **PREPARATION: 5'**   **SERVES: 4**

INGREDIENTS

- ¼ cup chopped cucumber
- 1 tablespoon fresh lime juice
- 1 tablespoon apple cider vinegar
- 2 tablespoons maple syrup
- ¼ teaspoon sea salt, optional
- 4 cups water

DIRECTIONS

1. Combine all the ingredients in a glass. Stir to mix well.
2. Refrigerate overnight before serving.

NUTRITION: Calories: 114 Fat: 0.1g Carbs: 28.9g Fiber: 0.3g Protein: 0.3g

77. EASY AND FRESH MANGO MADNESS

COOKING: 0' **PREPARATION: 5'** **SERVES: 4**

INGREDIENTS

- 1 cup chopped mango
- 1 cup chopped peach
- 1 banana
- 1 cup strawberries
- 1 carrot, peeled and chopped
- 1 cup water

DIRECTIONS

1. Put all the ingredients in a food processor, then blitz until glossy and smooth.
2. Serve immediately or chill in the refrigerator for an hour before serving.

NUTRITION: Calories: 376 Fat: 22.0g Carbs: 19.0g Fiber: 14.0g Protein: 5.0g

78. SIMPLE DATE SHAKE

COOKING: 0' **PREPARATION: 10'** **SERVES: 2**

INGREDIENTS

- 5 Medjool dates, pitted, soaked in boiling water for 5 minutes
- ¾ cup unsweetened coconut milk
- 1 teaspoon vanilla extract
- ½ teaspoon fresh lemon juice
- ¼ teaspoon sea salt, optional
- 1½ cups ice

DIRECTIONS

1. Put all the ingredients in a food processor, then blitz until it has a milkshake and smooth texture.
2. Serve immediately.
3.

NUTRITION: Calories: 380 Fat: 21.6 Carbs: 50.3g Fiber: 6.0g Protein: 3.2g

79. BEET AND CLEMENTINE PROTEIN SMOOTHIE

COOKING: 0' **PREPARATION: 10'** **SERVES: 3**

INGREDIENTS

- 1 small beet, peeled and chopped
- 1 clementine, peeled and broken into segments
- ½ ripe banana
- ½ cup raspberries
- 1 tablespoon chia seeds
- 2 tablespoons almond butter
- ¼ teaspoon vanilla extract
- 1 cup unsweetened almond milk
- 1/8 teaspoon fine sea salt, optional

DIRECTIONS

1. Combine all the ingredients in a food processor, then pulse on high for 2 minutes or until glossy and creamy.
2. Refrigerate for an hour and serve chilled.

NUTRITION: Calories: 526 Fat: 25.4g Carbs: 61.9g Fiber: 17.3g Protein: 20.6g

THE PLANT BASED DIET COOKBOOK

80. MATCHA LIMEADE

COOKING: 0' **PREPARATION: 10'** **SERVES: 4**

INGREDIENTS

- 2 tablespoons matcha powder
- ¼ cup raw agave syrup
- 3 cups water, divided
- 1 cup fresh lime juice
- 3 tablespoons chia seeds

DIRECTIONS

1. Lightly simmer the matcha, agave syrup, and 1 cup of water in a saucepan over medium heat. Keep stirring until no matcha lumps.
2. Pour the matcha mixture in a large glass, add the remaining ingredients, and mix well.
3. Refrigerate for at least an hour before serving.

NUTRITION: Calories: 152 Fat: 4.5g Carbs: 26.8g Fiber: 5.3g Protein: 3.7g

81. FRUIT INFUSED WATER

COOKING: 0' **PREPARATION: 5'** **SERVES: 2**

INGREDIENTS

- 3 strawberries, sliced
- 5 mint leaves
- ½ of orange, sliced
- 2 cups of water

DIRECTIONS

1. Divide fruits and mint between two glasses, pour in water, stir until just mixed, and refrigerate for 2 hours.
2. Serve straight away.

NUTRITION: Calories: 5.4 Fat: 0.1g Carbs: 1.3g Protein: 0.1g Fiber: 0.4g

82. HAZELNUT AND CHOCOLATE MILK

COOKING: 0' **PREPARATION: 5'** **SERVES: 2**

INGREDIENTS

- 2 tablespoons cocoa powder
- 4 dates, pitted
- 1 cup hazelnuts
- 3 cups of water

DIRECTIONS

1. Place all the ingredients in the order in a food processor or blender and then pulse for 2 to 3 minutes at high speed until smooth.
2. Pour the smoothie into two glasses and then serve.

NUTRITION: Calories: 120 Fat: 5g Carbs: 19g Protein: 2g Fiber: 1g

83. BANANA MILK

COOKING: 0' **PREPARATION: 5'** **SERVES: 2**

INGREDIENTS

- 2 dates
- 2 medium bananas, peeled
- 1 teaspoon vanilla extract, unsweetened
- 1/2 cup ice
- 2 cups of water

DIRECTIONS

1. Place all the ingredients in the order in a food processor or blender and then pulse for 2 to 3 minutes at high speed until smooth.
2. Pour the smoothie into two glasses and then serve.

NUTRITION: Calories: 79 Fat: 0g Carbs: 19.8g Protein: 0.8g Fiber: 6g

84. APPLE, CARROT, CELERY AND KALE JUICE

COOKING: 0' | **PREPARATION: 5'** | **SERVES: 2**

INGREDIENTS
- 5 curly kale
- 2 green apples, cored, peeled, chopped
- 2 large stalks celery
- 4 large carrots, cored, peeled, chopped

DIRECTIONS
1. Process all the ingredients in the order in a juicer or blender and then strain it into two glasses.
2. Serve straight away.

NUTRITION: Calories: 183 Fat: 2.5g Carbs: 46g Protein: 13g Fiber: 3g

85. SWEET AND SOUR JUICE

COOKING: 0' | **PREPARATION: 5'** | **SERVES: 2**

INGREDIENTS
- 2 medium apples, cored, peeled, chopped
- 2 large cucumbers, peeled
- 4 cups chopped grapefruit
- 1 cup mint

DIRECTIONS
1. Process all the ingredients in the order in a juicer or blender and then strain it into two glasses.
2. Serve straight away.

NUTRITION: Calories: 90 Fat: 0g Carbs: 23g Protein: 0g Fiber: 9g

86. GREEN LEMONADE

COOKING: 0' | **PREPARATION: 5'** | **SERVES: 2**

INGREDIENTS
- 10 large stalks of celery, chopped
- 2 medium green apples, cored, peeled, chopped
- 2 medium cucumbers, peeled, chopped
- 2 inches' piece of ginger
- 10 stalks of kale, chopped
- 2 cups parsley

DIRECTIONS
1. Process all the ingredients in the order in a juicer or blender and then strain it into two glasses.
2. Serve straight away.

NUTRITION: Calories: 102.3 Fat: 1.1g Carbs: 26.2g Protein: 4.7g Fiber: 8.5g

87. PINEAPPLE AND SPINACH JUICE

COOKING: 0' | **PREPARATION: 5'** | **SERVES: 2**

INGREDIENTS
- 2 medium red apples, cored, peeled, chopped
- 3 cups spinach
- ½ of a medium pineapple, peeled
- 2 lemons, peeled

DIRECTIONS
1. Process all the ingredients in the order in a juicer or blender and then strain it into two glasses.
2. Serve straight away.

NUTRITION: Calories: 131 Fat: 0.5g Carbs: 34.5g Protein: 1.7g Fiber: 5g

88. STRAWBERRY, BLUEBERRY AND BANANA SMOOTHIE

COOKING: 0'   **PREPARATION: 5'**   **SERVES: 2**

INGREDIENTS
- 1 tablespoon hulled hemp seeds
- ½ cup of frozen strawberries
- 1 small frozen banana
- ½ cup frozen blueberries
- 2 tablespoons cashew butùter
- ¾ cup cashew milk, unsweetened

DIRECTIONS
1. Place all the ingredients in the order in a food processor or blender and then pulse for 2 to 3 minutes at high speed until smooth.
2. Pour the smoothie into two glasses and then serve.

NUTRITION: Calories: 334 Fat: 17g Carbs: 46g Protein: 7g Fiber: 7g

89. MANGO, PINEAPPLE AND BANANA SMOOTHIE

COOKING: 0'   **PREPARATION: 5'**   **SERVES: 2**

INGREDIENTS
- 2 cups pineapple chunks
- 2 frozen bananas
- 2 medium mangoes, destoned, cut into chunks
- 1 cup almond milk, unsweetened
- Chia seeds as needed for garnishing

DIRECTIONS
1. Place all the ingredients in the order in a food processor or blender and then pulse for 2 to 3 minutes at high speed until smooth.
2. Pour the smoothie into two glasses and then serve.

NUTRITION: Calories: 287 Fat: 1.2g Carbs: 73.3g Protein: 3.5g Fiber: 8g

90. BLUEBERRY AND BANANA SMOOTHIE

COOKING: 0'   **PREPARATION: 5'**   **SERVES: 2**

INGREDIENTS
- 2 frozen bananas
- 2 cups frozen blueberries
- 2 cups almond milk, unsweetened
- 1/2 teaspoon or so cinnamon
- dash of vanilla extract

DIRECTIONS
1. Place all the ingredients in the order in a food processor or blender and then pulse for 2 to 3 minutes at high speed until smooth.
2. Pour the smoothie into two glasses and then serve.

NUTRITION: Calories: 244 Fat: 3.8g Carbs: 51.5g Protein: 4g Fiber: 7.3g

91. CHARD, LETTUCE AND GINGER SMOOTHIE

COOKING: 0'   **PREPARATION: 5'**   **SERVES: 2**

INGREDIENTS
- 10 Chard leaves, chopped
- 1-inch piece of ginger, chopped
- 10 lettuce leaves, chopped
- ½ teaspoon black salt
- 2 pears, chopped
- 2 teaspoons coconut sugar
- ¼ teaspoon ground black pepper
- ¼ teaspoon salt
- 2 tablespoons lemon juice
- 2 cups of water

DIRECTIONS
1. Place all the ingredients in the order in a food processor or blender and then pulse for 2 to 3 minutes at high speed until smooth.
2. Pour the smoothie into two glasses and then serve.

NUTRITION: Calories: 514 Fat: 0g Carbs: 15g Protein: 4g Fiber: 4g

92. RED BEET, PEAR AND APPLE SMOOTHIE

COOKING: 0' **PREPARATION: 5'** **SERVES: 2**

INGREDIENTS
- 1/2 of medium beet, peeled, chopped
- 1 tablespoon chopped cilantro
- 1 orange, juiced
- 1 medium pear, chopped
- 1 medium apple, cored, chopped
- 1/4 teaspoon ground black pepper
- 1/8 teaspoon rock salt
- 1 teaspoon coconut sugar
- 1/4 teaspoons salt
- 1 cup of water

DIRECTIONS
1. Place all the ingredients in the order in a food processor or blender and then pulse for 2 to 3 minutes at high speed until smooth.
2. Pour the smoothie into two glasses and then serve.

NUTRITION: Calories: 132 Fat: 0g Carbs: 34g Protein: 1g Fiber: 5g

93. BERRY AND YOGURT SMOOTHIE

COOKING: 0' **PREPARATION: 5'** **SERVES: 2**

INGREDIENTS
- 2 small bananas
- 3 cups frozen mixed berries
- 1 ½ cup cashew yogurt
- 1/2 teaspoon vanilla extract, unsweetened
- 1/2 cup almond milk, unsweetened

DIRECTIONS
1. Place all the ingredients in the order in a food processor or blender and then pulse for 2 to 3 minutes at high speed until smooth.
2. Pour the smoothie into two glasses and then serve.

NUTRITION: Calories: 326 Fat: 6.5g Carbs: 65.6g Protein: 8g Fiber: 8.4g

94. CHOCOLATE AND CHERRY SMOOTHIE

COOKING: 0' **PREPARATION: 5'** **SERVES: 2**

INGREDIENTS
- 4 cups frozen cherries
- 2 tablespoons cocoa powder
- 1 scoop of Protein: powder
- 1 teaspoon maple syrup
- 2 cups almond milk, unsweetened

DIRECTIONS
1. Place all the ingredients in the order in a food processor or blender and then pulse for 2 to 3 minutes at high speed until smooth.
2. Pour the smoothie into two glasses and then serve.

NUTRITION: Calories: 324 Fat: 5g Carbs: 75.1g Protein: 7.2g Fiber: 11.3g

95. STRAWBERRY AND CHOCOLATE MILKSHAKE

COOKING: 0' **PREPARATION: 5'** **SERVES: 2**

INGREDIENTS
- 2 cups frozen strawberries
- 3 tablespoons cocoa powder
- 1 scoop Protein: powder
- 2 tablespoons maple syrup
- 1 teaspoon vanilla extract, unsweetened
- 2 cups almond milk, unsweetened

DIRECTIONS
1. Place all the ingredients in the order in a food processor or blender and then pulse for 2 to 3 minutes at high speed until smooth.
2. Pour the smoothie into two glasses and then serve.

NUTRITION: Calories: 199 Fat: 4.1g Carbs: 40.5g Protein: 3.7g Fiber: 5.5g

96. ZOBO DRINK

COOKING: 10'   **PREPARATION: 5'**   **SERVES: 8**

INGREDIENTS

- 2 cups dried hibiscus petals (zobo leaves), rinsed
- Pineapple rind from 1 pineapple
- 1 cup of granulated sugar
- 1 tsp. fresh ginger, grated
- 10 cups of water

DIRECTIONS

1. Add water, ginger, and sugar into the pot and mix well.
2. Then add zobo leaves and pineapple rind.
3. Cover and cook on High for 10 minutes. Open and discard solids.
4. Chill and serve.

NUTRITION: Calories: 65, Carbs: 7g, Fat: 2.6g, Protein: 1.14g

97. BASIL LIME GREEN TEA

COOKING: 4'   **PREPARATION: 5'**   **SERVES: 8**

INGREDIENTS

- 8 cups of filtered water
- 10 bags of green tea
- ¼ cup of honey
- A pinch of baking soda
- Lime slices to taste
- Lemon slices to taste
- Basil leaves to taste

DIRECTIONS

1. Add water, honey, and baking soda in the pot and mix. Add the tea bags and cover. Cook on High for 4 minutes. Open and serve with lime slices, lemon slices, and basil leaves.

NUTRITION: Calories: 32, Carbs: 8g, Fat: 0g, Protein: 0g

98. TURMERIC COCONUT MILK

COOKING: 15'   **PREPARATION: 5'**   **SERVES: 8**

INGREDIENTS

- 13.5oz. coconut milk
- 3 cups of filtered water
- 2 tsps. turmeric powder
- 3 whole cloves
- 2 cinnamon sticks
- ½ tsp. ginger powder
- A pinch of pepper
- 2 tbsp. honey

DIRECTIONS

1. Place everything except the honey in the pot. Cover and cook on High for 15 minutes. Remove cloves and cinnamon sticks. Add honey, mix and serve.

NUTRITION: Calories: 42, Carbs: 9g, Fat: 0g, Protein: 0g

99. BERRY LEMONADE TEA

COOKING: 12'   **PREPARATION: 5'**   **SERVES: 4**

INGREDIENTS

- 3 tea bags
- 2 cups of natural lemonade
- 1 cup of frozen mixed berries
- 2 cups of water
- 1 lemon, sliced

DIRECTIONS

1. Put everything in the Instant Pot and cover. Cook on High for 12 minutes. Open, strain, and serve.

NUTRITION: Calories: 21 Carbs: 8g Fat: 0.2g Protein: 0.4g

100. SWEDISH GLÖGG

COOKING: 15'   **PREPARATION: 5'**   **SERVES: 1**

INGREDIENTS

- ½ cup of orange juice
- ½ cup of water
- 1 piece of ginger cut into ½ pieces
- 1 whole clove
- 1 opened cardamom pods
- 2 tbsps. orange zest
- 1 cinnamon stick
- 1 whole allspice
- 1 vanilla bean

DIRECTIONS

1. Add everything in the pot. Cover and cook on High for 15 minutes. Open and serve.

NUTRITION: Calories: 194 Carbs: 41g Fat: 3g Protein: 1.7g

CHAPTER 9: GRAINS

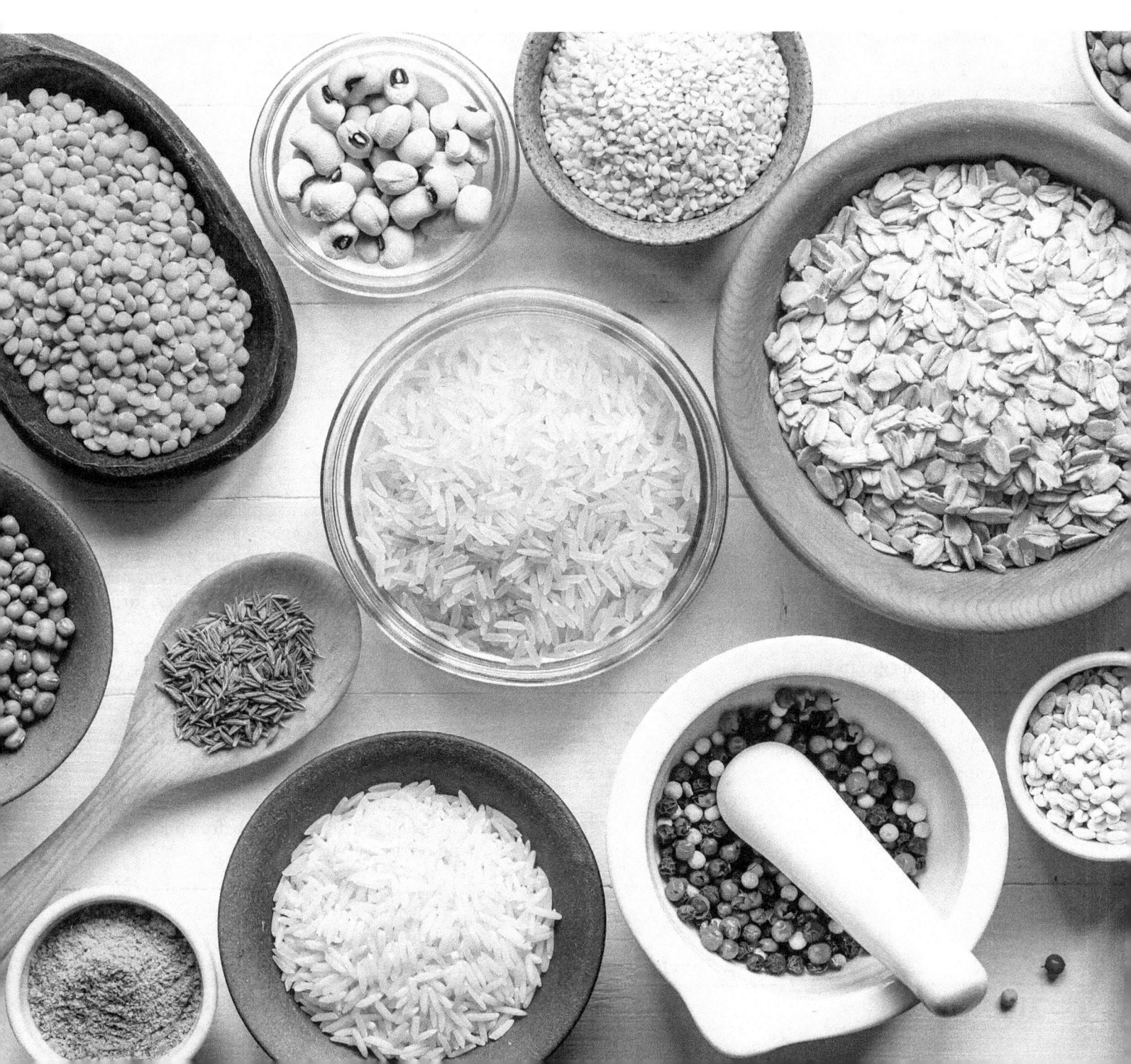

101. VEGGIE BARLEY BOWL

COOKING: 1H 11'   **PREPARATION: 10'**   **SERVES: 8**

INGREDIENTS

- 1 cup barley
- 3 cups low-sodium vegetable broth
- 2 cups sliced mushrooms
- 2 cups broccoli florets
- 1 cup snow peas, trimmed
- ½ cup sliced scallion
- ¼ cup chopped green bell pepper
- ¼ cup chopped red bell pepper
- 1 cup bean sprouts
- ¼ cup soy sauce
- ¼ cup water
- ¼ teaspoon ground ginger
- 1 tablespoon cornstarch, mixed with 2 tablespoons cold water

DIRECTIONS

1. In a saucepan over medium heat, place the barley and vegetable stock. Cover and cook for 1 hour.
2. Combine all the vegetables, except for the bean sprouts, in a large pot with the soy sauce, water and ginger. Cook for 5 minutes, stirring constantly.
3. Add the bean sprouts and cook, stirring, for another 5 minutes. Add the cornstarch mixture and cook for about 1 minute, stirring, or until thickened.
4. Remove from the heat. Toss the vegetables with the cooked barley.
5. Serve hot.

NUTRITION: Calories: 190 Fat: 2.6g Carbs: 35.7g Protein: 5.9g Fiber: 6.9g

102. INDIAN LENTIL DAHL

COOKING: 25'   **PREPARATION: 10'**   **SERVES: 6**

INGREDIENTS

- 3 cup cooked basmati rice
- 2 tablespoons olive oil (optional)
- 6 garlic cloves, minced
- 2 yellow onions, finely diced
- 1-inch piece fresh ginger, minced
- 2 tomatoes, diced
- 2 tablespoons ground cumin
- 1 tablespoon ground coriander
- 1 tablespoon ground turmeric
- 1 tablespoon paprika
- 4 cups water
- 2 cups uncooked green lentils, rinsed
- 1 teaspoon salt (optional)

DIRECTIONS

1. In a large pot, heat the olive oil (if desired) over medium heat. Add the garlic, onions, and ginger. Cook for 3 minutes, or until onions are golden. Add the tomatoes and cook for 2 minutes more, stirring occasionally. Stir in the cumin, coriander, turmeric and paprika.
2. Add the water and lentils. Cover and bring to a boil over high heat. Once boiling, stir and reduce the heat to a simmer. Cook, covered, for 20 minutes, stirring every 5 minutes, or until the lentils are fully cooked and beginning to break down. Season with salt (if desired) and stir.
3. Divide the rice evenly among 6 meal prep containers. Add an equal portion of the dahl to each container. Let cool completely before putting on lids and refrigerating.

NUTRITION: Calories: 432 Fat: 17.2g Carbs: 58.8g Protein: 10.9g Fiber: 8.9g

103. KALE AND SWEET POTATO QUINOA

COOKING: 19' — **PREPARATION: 10'** — **SERVES: 4**

INGREDIENTS

- ¼ cup olive oil (optional)
- 1 yellow onion, diced
- 2 tablespoons ground coriander
- 2 tablespoons ground cumin
- 2 tablespoons mustard powder
- 2 tablespoons ground turmeric
- 2 teaspoons ground cinnamon
- 1 large sweet potato, diced
- 1¼ cup uncooked quinoa
- 4 cups water
- 1 bunch kale, rinsed and chopped
- Salt, to taste (optional)
- Freshly ground black pepper, to taste

DIRECTIONS

1. In a large pot, heat the oil (if desired) over medium-high heat. Add the onion and sauté for 3 minutes. Stir in the coriander, cumin, mustard powder, turmeric and cinnamon. Cook for about 1 minute, or until fragrant. Add the sweet potatoes and stir until well coated with the spices.
2. Stir in the quinoa and water. Cover with a lid and bring to a boil over high heat, stirring occasionally. Once the liquid is boiling, remove the lid and reduce the heat to medium-low. Simmer for 15 minutes.
3. Once the water is mostly absorbed and the sweet potato is cooked through, stir in the kale. Remove from the heat and cover with a lid. Let sit for 10 to 15 minutes. The residual heat will cook the kale and the quinoa will absorb the remaining water.
4. Taste and season with salt (if desired) and pepper. Divide evenly among 4 meal prep containers and let cool completely before putting on lids and refrigerating.

NUTRITION: Calories: 457 Fat: 16.2g Carbs: 67.9g Protein: 10.1g Fiber: 12.2g

104. BROWN RICE WITH MUSHROOMS

COOKING: 20' — **PREPARATION: 5'** — **SERVES: 6-8**

INGREDIENTS

- ½ pound (227 g) mushrooms, sliced
- 1 green bell pepper, chopped
- 1 onion, chopped
- 1 bunch scallions, chopped
- 2 cloves garlic, minced
- ½ cup water
- 5 cups cooked brown rice
- 1 (16-oz. / 454-g) can chopped tomatoes
- 1 (4-oz. / 113-g) can chopped green chilies
- 2 teaspoons chili powder
- 1 teaspoon ground cumin

DIRECTIONS

1. In a large pot, sauté the mushrooms, green pepper, onion, scallions, and garlic in the water for 10 minutes.
2. Stir in the remaining ingredients. Cook over low heat for about 10 minutes, or until heated through, stirring frequently.
3. Serve immediately.

NUTRITION: Calories: 185 Fat: 2.6g Carbs: 34.5g Protein: 6.1g Fiber: 4.3g

105. VEGGIE PAELLA

COOKING: 52-58' **PREPARATION:** 15' **SERVES:** 4

INGREDIENTS

- 1 onion, coarsely chopped
- 8 medium mushrooms, sliced
- 2 small zucchinis, cut in half, then sliced ½ inch thick
- 1 leek, rinsed and sliced
- 2 large cloves garlic, crushed
- 1 medium tomato, coarsely chopped
- 3 cups low-sodium vegetable broth
- 1¼ cups long-grain brown rice
- ½ teaspoon crushed saffron threads
- Freshly ground black pepper, to taste
- ½ cup frozen green peas
- ½ cup water
- Chopped fresh parsley, for garnish

DIRECTIONS

1. Pour the water in a large wok. Add the onion and sauté for 5 minutes, or until most of the liquid is absorbed.
2. Stir in the mushrooms, zucchini, leek, and garlic, cook for 2 to 3 minutes, or soften slightly.
3. Add the tomato, broth, rice, saffron, and pepper. Bring to a boil. Reduce the heat and simmer, covered, for 30 minutes.
4. Add the peas and continue to cook for another 5 to 10 minutes. Remove from the heat and let rest for 10 minutes to allow any excess moisture to be absorbed.
5. Sprinkle with the parsley before serving.

NUTRITION: Calories: 418 Fat: 3.9g Carbs: 83.2g Protein: 12.7g Fiber: 9.2g

106. VEGETABLE AND WILD RICE PILAF

COOKING: 48-49' **PREPARATION:** 10' **SERVES:** 6

INGREDIENTS

- 1 banana
- ½ cup coconut milk
- 1 cup water
- 1 cup alfalfa sprouts (optional)
- 1 to 2 soft Medjool dates, pitted
- 1 tablespoon chia seeds, or ground flax or hemp hearts
- ¼ teaspoon ground cinnamon
- Pinch ground cardamom
- 1 tablespoon grated fresh ginger, or ¼ teaspoon ground ginger

DIRECTIONS

1. Purée everything in a blender until smooth, adding more water (or coconut milk) if needed.

NUTRITION: Calories: 477 Fat: 29g Carbs: 57g Fiber: 14g Protein: 8g

52. TROPE-KALE BREEZE

COOKING: 0' **PREPARATION:** 5' **SERVES:** 4

INGREDIENTS

- 1 potato, scrubbed and chopped
- 1 cup chopped cauliflower
- 1 cup chopped scallion
- 1 cup chopped broccoli
- 1 to 2 cloves garlic, minced
- 2 tablespoons soy sauce
- 3 cups low-sodium vegetable broth
- 1 cup long-grain brown rice
- 1/3 cup wild rice
- 2 small zucchinis, chopped
- ½ cup grated carrot
- 1/8 teaspoon sesame oil (optional)
- ¼ cup chopped fresh cilantro
- ½ cup water

DIRECTIONS

1. Bring the water to a boil in a large saucepan. Add the potato, cauliflower, scallion, broccoli and garlic and sauté for 2 to 3 minutes.
2. Add the soy sauce and cook for 1 minute. Add the vegetable broth, brown rice and wild rice. Bring to a boil. Reduce the heat, cover, and cook for 15 minutes.
3. Stir in the zucchinis. After another 15 minutes, stir in the carrot. Continue to cook for 15 minutes. Stir in the sesame oil (if desired) and cilantro.
4. Serve immediately.

NUTRITION: Calories: 376 Fat: 3.6g Carbs: 74.5g Protein: 11.8g Fiber: 8.1g

107. BROWN RICE WITH SPICED VEGETABLES

COOKING: 16-8' **PREPARATION:** 10' **SERVES:** 6

INGREDIENTS

- 2 teaspoons grated fresh ginger
- 2 cloves garlic, crushed
- ½ cup water
- ¼ pound (113 g) green beans, trimmed and cut into 1-inch pieces
- 1 carrot, scrubbed and sliced
- ½ pound mushrooms, sliced
- 2 zucchinis, cut in half lengthwise and sliced
- 1 bunch scallions, cut into 1-inch pieces
- 4 cups cooked brown rice
- 3 tablespoons soy sauce

DIRECTIONS

1. Place the ginger and garlic in a large pot with the water. Add the green beans and carrot and sauté for 3 minutes.
2. Add the mushrooms and sauté for another 2 minutes. Stir in the zucchini and scallions. Reduce the heat. Cover and cook for 6 to 8 minutes, or until the vegetables are tender-crisp, stirring frequently.
3. Stir in the rice and soy sauce. Cook over low heat for 5 minutes, or until heated through.
4. Serve warm.

NUTRITION: Calories: 205 Fat: 3.0g Carbs: 38.0g Protein: 6.4g Fiber: 4.4g

108. SPICED TOMATO BROWN RICE

COOKING: 15'   **PREPARATION: 10'**   **SERVES: 4-6**

INGREDIENTS

- 1 onion, diced
- 1 green bell pepper, diced
- 3 cloves garlic, minced
- ¼ cup water
- 15 to 16oz. (425 to 454g) tomatoes, chopped
- 1 tablespoon chili powder
- 2 teaspoons ground cumin
- 1 teaspoon dried basil
- ½ teaspoon Parsley Patch seasoning, general blend
- ¼ teaspoon cayenne
- 2 cups cooked brown rice

DIRECTIONS

1. Combine the onion, green pepper, garlic and water in a saucepan over medium heat. Cook for about 5 minutes, stirring constantly, or until softened.
2. Add the tomatoes and seasonings. Cook for another 5 minutes. Stir in the cooked rice. Cook for another 5 minutes to allow the flavors to blend.
3. Serve immediately.

NUTRITION: Calories: 107 Fat: 1.1g Carbs: 21.1g Protein: 3.2g Fiber: 2.9g

---

109. NOODLE AND RICE PILAF

COOKING: 33-44'   **PREPARATION: 5'**   **SERVES: 6-8**

INGREDIENTS

- 1 cup whole-wheat noodles, broken into 1/8 inch pieces
- 2 cups long-grain brown rice
- 6½ cups low-sodium vegetable broth
- 1 teaspoon ground cumin
- ½ teaspoon dried oregano

DIRECTIONS

1. Combine the noodles and rice in a saucepan over medium heat and cook for 3 to 4 minutes, or until they begin to smell toasted.
2. Stir in the vegetable broth, cumin and oregano. Bring to a boil. Reduce the heat to medium-low. Cover and cook for 30 to 40 minutes, or until all water is absorbed.

NUTRITION: Calories: 287 Fat: 2.5g Carbs: 58.1g Protein: 7.9g Fiber: 5.0g

---

110. EASY MILLET LOAF

COOKING: 33-44'   **PREPARATION: 5'**   **SERVES: 6-8**

INGREDIENTS

- 1¼ cups millet
- 4 cups unsweetened tomato juice
- 1 medium onion, chopped
- 1 to 2 cloves garlic
- ½ teaspoon dried sage
- ½ teaspoon dried basil
- ½ teaspoon poultry seasoning

DIRECTIONS

1. Preheat the oven to 350°F.
2. Place the millet in a large bowl.
3. Place the remaining ingredients in a blender and pulse until smooth. Add to the bowl with the millet and mix well.
4. Pour the mixture into a shallow casserole dish. Cover and bake in the oven for 1¼ hours, or until set.
5. Serve warm.

NUTRITION: Calories: 315 Fat: 3.4g Carbs: 61.6g Protein: 10.2g Fiber: 9.6g

111. WALNUT-OAT BURGERS

COOKING: 20-30' **PREPARATION: 5'** **SERVES: 6-8**

INGREDIENTS

- 1 medium onion, finely chopped
- 2 cups rolled oats
- 2 cups unsweetened low-Fat: soy milk
- 1 cup finely chopped walnuts
- 1 tablespoon soy sauce
- ½ teaspoon dried sage
- ½ teaspoon garlic powder
- ½ teaspoon onion powder
- ½ teaspoon dried thyme
- ¼ teaspoon dried marjoram

DIRECTIONS

1. Stir together all the ingredients in a large bowl. Let rest for 20 minutes.
2. Form the mixture into six or eight patties. Cook the patties on a nonstick griddle over medium heat for 20 to 30 minutes, or until browned on each side.
3. Serve warm.

NUTRITION: Calories: 341 Fat: 13.9g Carbs: 42.4g Protein: 13.9g Fiber: 6.8g

112. SPICY BEANS AND RICE

COOKING: 45' **PREPARATION: 5'** **SERVES: 4-6**

INGREDIENTS

- 1½ cups long-grain brown rice
- 1 (19-oz.) can kidney beans, rinsed and drained
- 2 cups chopped onion
- 1 cup mild salsa
- 1 teaspoon ground cumin
- 16 oz. tomatoes, chopped
- 3 cups water

DIRECTIONS

1. In a pot, bring the water to a boil. Stir in the rice. Bring to a boil again and stir in the remaining ingredients, except for the tomatoes. Return to a boil. Reduce the heat to low. Cover and simmer for 45 minutes.
2. Remove from the heat and stir in the tomatoes. Let sit for 5 minutes, covered.

NUTRITION: Calories: 386 Fat: 7.1g Carbs: 71.1g Protein: 11.1g Fiber: 5.8g

113. BLACK-EYED PEAS AND CORN SALAD

COOKING: 50' **PREPARATION: 30'** **SERVES: 4**

INGREDIENTS

- 2½ cups cooked black-eyed peas
- 3 ears corn, kernels removed
- 1 medium ripe tomato, diced
- ½ medium red onion, peeled and diced small
- ½ red bell pepper, deseeded and diced small
- 1 jalapeño pepper, deseeded and minced
- ½ cup finely chopped cilantro
- ¼ cup plus 2 tablespoons balsamic vinegar
- 3 cloves garlic, peeled and minced
- 1 teaspoon toasted and ground cumin seeds

DIRECTIONS

1. Stir together all the ingredients in a large bowl and refrigerate for about 1 hour, or until well chilled.
2. Serve chilled.

NUTRITION: Calories: 247 Fat: 1.8g Carbs: 47.6g Protein: 12.9g Fiber: 11.7g

114. INDIAN TOMATO AND GARBANZO STEW

COOKING: 50' **PREPARATION: 15'** **SERVES: 4-6**

INGREDIENTS

- 1 large onion, quartered and thinly sliced
- 1-inch fresh ginger, peeled and minced
- 2 cloves garlic, peeled and minced
- 1 teaspoon curry powder
- 1 teaspoon cumin seeds
- 1 teaspoon black mustard seeds
- 1 teaspoon coriander seeds,
- 1½ lb. (680 g) tomatoes, deseeded and puréed
- 1 red bell pepper, cut into ½-inch dice
- 1 green bell pepper, cut into ½-inch dice
- 3 cups cooked garbanzo beans
- 1 tablespoon garam masala
- 1/3 cup water

DIRECTIONS

1. Heat the water in a medium saucepan over medium-low heat. Add the onion, ginger, garlic, curry powder, and seeds to the pan. Sauté for about 10 minutes, or until the onion is tender, stirring frequently.
2. Add the tomatoes and simmer, uncovered, for 10 minutes. Add the peppers and garbanzo beans. Reduce heat. Cover and simmer for 30 minutes, stirring occasionally. Stir in the garam masala and serve.

NUTRITION: Calories: 100 Fat: 1.2g Carbs: 20.9g Protein: 5.1g Fiber: 7.0g

115. SIMPLE BAKED NAVY BEANS

COOKING: 2 1/2 - 3H **PREPARATION: 10'**

INGREDIENTS

- 1½ cups navy beans
- 8 cups water
- 1 bay leaf
- ½ cup finely chopped green bell pepper
- ½ cup finely chopped onion
- 1 teaspoon minced garlic
- ½ cup unsweetened tomato purée
- 3 tablespoons molasses
- 1 tablespoon fresh lemon juice

DIRECTIONS

1. Preheat the oven to 300°F (150°C).
2. Place the beans and water in a large pot, along with the bay leaf, green pepper, onion and garlic. Cover and cook for 1½ to 2 hours, or until the beans are softened. Remove from the heat and drain, reserving the cooking liquid. Discard the bay leaf.
3. Transfer the mixture to a casserole dish with a cover. Stir in the remaining ingredients and 1 cup of the reserved cooking liquid. Bake in the oven for 1 hour, covered. Stir occasionally during baking and add a little more cooking liquid if needed to keep the beans moist.
4. Serve warm.

NUTRITION: Calories: 162 Fat: 0.6g Carbs: 31.3g Protein: 9.1g Fiber: 6.4g

116. VINEGARY BLACK BEANS

COOKING: 2H | **PREPARATION: 10'** | **SERVES: 8**

INGREDIENTS

- 1 pound (454 g) black beans, soaked overnight and drained
- 10½ cups water, divided
- 1 green bell pepper, cut in half
- 1 onion, finely chopped
- 1 green bell pepper, finely chopped
- 4 cloves garlic, pressed
- 1 tablespoon maple syrup (optional)
- 1 tablespoon Mrs. Dash seasoning
- 1 bay leaf
- ¼ teaspoon dried oregano
- 2 tablespoons cider vinegar

DIRECTIONS

1. Place the beans, 10 cups of the water, and green bell pepper in a large pot. Cook over medium heat for about 45 minutes, or until the green pepper is tendered. Remove the green pepper and discard.
2. Meanwhile, in a different pot, combine the onion, chopped green pepper, garlic and the remaining ½ cup of the water. Sauté for 15 to 20 minutes, or until soft.
3. Add 1 cup of the cooked beans to the pot with vegetables. Mash the beans and vegetables with a potato masher. Add to the pot with the beans, maple syrup (if desired), Mrs. Dash, bay leaf and oregano. Cover and cook over low heat for 1 hour.
4. Drizzle in the vinegar and continue to cook for another hour.
5. Serve warm.

NUTRITION: Calories: 226 Fat: 0.9g Carbs: 42.7g Protein: 12.9g Fiber: 9.9g

117. SPICED LENTIL BURGERS

COOKING: 43' | **PREPARATION: 10'** | **SERVES: 4**

INGREDIENTS

- ¼ cup minced onion
- 1 clove garlic, minced
- 2 tablespoons water
- 1 cup chopped boiled potatoes
- 1 cup cooked lentils
- 2 tablespoons minced fresh parsley
- 1 teaspoon onion powder
- 1 teaspoon minced fresh basil
- 1 teaspoon dried dill
- 1 teaspoon paprika

DIRECTIONS

1. Preheat the oven to 350°F.
2. In a pot, sauté the onion and garlic in the water for about 3 minutes, or until soft.
3. Combine the lentils and potatoes in a large bowl and mash together well. Add the cooked onion and garlic and the remaining ingredients to the lentil-potato mixture and stir until well combined.
4. Form the mixture into four patties and place on a nonstick baking sheet. Bake in the oven for 20 minutes. Turnover and bake for an additional 20 minutes.
5. Serve hot.

NUTRITION: Calories: 101 Fat: 0.4g Carbs: 19.9g Protein: 5.5g Fiber: 5.3g

THE PLANT BASED DIET COOKBOOK

118. PECAN-MAPLE GRANOLA

COOKING: 50'   **PREPARATION: 5'**   **SERVES: 4**

INGREDIENTS

- 1½ cups rolled oats
- ¼ cup maple syrup (optional)
- ¼ cup pecan pieces
- 1 teaspoon vanilla extract
- ½ teaspoon ground cinnamon

DIRECTIONS

1. Preheat the oven to 300°F. Line a baking sheet with parchment paper.
2. In a large bowl, stir together all the ingredients until the oats and pecan pieces are completely coated.
3. Spread the mixture on the baking sheet in an even layer. Bake in the oven for 20 minutes, stirring once halfway through cooking.
4. Remove from the oven and allow to cool on the countertop for 30 minutes before serving.

NUTRITION: Calories: 221 Fat: 17.2g Carbs: 5.1g Protein: 4.9g Fiber: 3.8g

119. BEAN AND SUMMER SQUASH SAUTÉ

COOKING: 15-16'   **PREPARATION: 10'**   **SERVES: 4**

INGREDIENTS

- 1 medium red onion, peeled and thinly sliced
- 4 yellow squash, cut into ½-inch rounds
- 4 medium zucchinis, cut into ½-inch rounds
- 1 (15-oz. / 425-g) can navy beans, drained and rinsed
- 2 cups corn kernels
- Zest of 2 lemons
- 1 cup finely chopped basil
- Salt, to taste (optional)
- Freshly ground black pepper, to taste

DIRECTIONS

1. Place the onion in a large saucepan and sauté over medium heat for 7 to 8 minutes. Add water 1 to 2 tablespoons at a time to keep the onion from sticking to the pan.
2. Add the squash, zucchini, beans, and corn and cook for about 8 minutes, or until the squash is softened.
3. Remove from the heat. Stir in the lemon zest and basil. Season with salt (if desired) and pepper.
4. Serve hot.

NUTRITION: Calories: 298 Fat: 2.2g Carbs: 60.4g Protein: 17.2g Fiber: 13.6g

120. PEPPERY BLACK BEANS

COOKING: 33-34'   **PREPARATION: 5'**   **SERVES: 4**

INGREDIENTS

- 1 red bell pepper, deseeded and chopped
- 1 medium yellow onion, peeled and chopped
- 2 jalapeño peppers, deseeded and minced
- 4 cloves garlic, peeled and minced
- 1 tablespoon thyme
- 1 tablespoon curry powder
- 1½ teaspoons ground allspice
- 1 teaspoon freshly ground black pepper
- 1 (15-oz. / 425-g) can diced tomatoes
- 4 cups cooked black beans

DIRECTIONS

1. Add the red bell pepper and onion to a saucepan and sauté over medium heat for 10 minutes, or until the onion is softened. Add water 1 to 2 tablespoons at a time to keep the vegetables from sticking to the pan.
2. Stir in the jalapeño peppers, garlic, thyme, curry powder, allspice and black pepper. Cook for 3 to 4 minutes, then add the tomatoes and black beans. Cook over medium heat for 20 minutes, covered.
3. Serve immediately.

NUTRITION: Calories: 283 Fat: 1.7g Carbs: 52.8g Protein: 17.4g Fiber: 19.8g

121. WALNUT, COCONUT, AND OAT GRANOLA

COOKING: 1H 40' | **PREPARATION: 15'** | **SERVES: 4**

INGREDIENTS

- 1 cup chopped walnuts
- 1 cup unsweetened, shredded coconut
- 2 cups rolled oats
- 1 teaspoon ground cinnamon
- 2 tablespoons hemp seeds
- 2 tablespoons ground flaxseeds
- 2 tablespoons chia seeds
- ¾ teaspoon salt (optional)
- ¼ cup maple syrup
- ¼ cup water
- 1 teaspoon vanilla extract
- ½ cup dried cranberries

DIRECTIONS

1. Preheat the oven to 250ºF. Line a baking sheet with parchment paper.
2. Mix the walnuts, coconut, rolled oats, cinnamon, hemp seeds, flaxseeds, chia seeds, and salt (if desired) in a bowl.
3. Combine the maple syrup and water in a saucepan. Bring to a boil over medium heat, then pour in the bowl of walnut mixture.
4. Add the vanilla extract to the bowl of mixture. Stir to mix well. Pour the mixture in the baking sheet, then level with a spatula so the mixture coats the bottom evenly.
5. Place the baking sheet in the preheated oven and bake for 90 minutes or until browned and crispy. Stir the mixture every 15 minutes.
6. Remove the baking sheet from the oven. Allow to cool for 10 minutes, then serve with dried cranberries on top.

NUTRITION: Calories: 1870 Fat: 115.8g Carbs: 238.0g Protein: 59.8g Fiber: 68.9g

122. RITZY FAVA BEAN RATATOUILLE

COOKING: 40' | **PREPARATION: 15'** | **SERVES: 4**

INGREDIENTS

- 1 medium red onion, peeled and thinly sliced
- 2 tablespoons low-sodium vegetable broth
- 1 large eggplant, stemmed and cut into ½-inch dice
- 1 red bell pepper, seeded and diced
- 2 cups cooked fava beans
- 2 Roma tomatoes, chopped
- 1 medium zucchini, diced
- 2 cloves garlic, peeled and finely chopped
- ¼ cup finely chopped basil
- Salt, to taste (optional)
- Ground black pepper, to taste

DIRECTIONS

1. Add the onion to a saucepan and sauté for 7 minutes or until caramelized.
2. Add the vegetable broth, eggplant and red bell pepper to the pan and sauté for 10 more minutes.
3. Add the fava beans, tomatoes, zucchini, and garlic to the pan and sauté for an additional 5 minutes.
4. Reduce the heat to medium-low. Put the pan lid on and cook for 15 minutes or until the vegetables are soft. Stir the vegetables halfway through.
5. Transfer them onto a large serving plate. Sprinkle with basil, salt (if desired), and black pepper before serving.

NUTRITION: Calories: 114 Fat: 1.0g Carbs: 24.2g Protein: 7.4g Fiber: 10.3g

THE PLANT BASED DIET COOKBOOK

123. PEPPERS AND BLACK BEANS WITH BROWN RICE

COOKING: 20'   **PREPARATION: 15'**   **SERVES: 4**

INGREDIENTS

- 2 jalapeño peppers, diced
- 1 red bell pepper, seeded and diced
- 1 medium yellow onion, peeled and diced
- 2 tablespoons low-sodium vegetable broth
- 1 teaspoon toasted and ground cumin seeds
- 1½ teaspoons toasted oregano
- 5 cloves garlic, peeled and minced
- 4 cups cooked black beans
- Salt, to taste (optional)
- Ground black pepper, to taste
- 3 cups cooked brown rice
- 1 lime, quartered
- 1 cup chopped cilantro

DIRECTIONS

1. Add the jalapeño peppers, bell pepper, and onion to a saucepan and sauté for 7 minutes or until the onion is well browned and caramelized.
2. Add vegetable broth, cumin, oregano, and garlic to the pan and sauté for 3 minutes or until fragrant.
3. Add the black beans and sauté for 10 minutes or until the vegetables are tender. Sprinkle with salt (if desired) and black pepper halfway through.
4. Arrange the brown rice on a platter, then top with the cooked vegetables. Garnish with lime wedges and cilantro before serving.

NUTRITION: Calories: 426 Fat: 2.6g Carbs: 82.4g Protein: 20.2g Fiber: 19.5g

124. BLACK-EYED PEA, BEET, AND CARROT STEW

COOKING: 40'   **PREPARATION: 15'**   **SERVES: 2**

INGREDIENTS

- ½ cup black-eyed peas, soaked in water overnight
- 3 cups water
- 1 large beet, peeled and cut into ½-inch pieces (about ¾ cup)
- 1 large carrot, peeled and cut into ½-inch pieces (about ¾ cup)
- ¼ teaspoon turmeric
- ¼ teaspoon toasted and ground cumin seeds
- 1/8 teaspoon asafetida
- ¼ cup finely chopped parsley
- ¼ teaspoon cayenne pepper
- ¼ teaspoon salt (optional)
- ½ teaspoon fresh lime juice

DIRECTIONS

1. Pour the black-eyed peas and water in a pot, then cook over medium heat for 25 minutes.
2. Add the beet and carrot to the pot and cook for 10 more minutes. Add more water if necessary.
3. Add the turmeric, cumin, asafetida, parsley, and cayenne pepper to the pot and cook for an additional 6 minutes or until the vegetables are soft. Stir the mixture periodically. Sprinkle with salt, if desired.
4. Drizzle the lime juice on top before serving in a large bowl.

NUTRITION: Calories: 84, Fat: 0.7g, Carbs: 16.6g, Protein: 4.1g, Fiber: 4.5g

125. KOSHARI

COOKING: 2H 10' **PREPARATION: 15'** **SERVES: 6**

INGREDIENTS

- 1 cup green lentils, rinsed
- 3 cups water
- Salt, to taste (optional)
- 1 large onion, peeled and minced
- 2 tablespoons low-sodium vegetable broth
- 4 cloves garlic, peeled and minced
- ½ teaspoon ground allspice
- 1 teaspoon ground coriander
- 1 teaspoon ground cumin
- 2 tablespoons tomato paste
- ½ teaspoon crushed red pepper flakes
- 3 large tomatoes, diced
- 1 cup cooked medium-grain brown rice
- 1 cup whole-grain elbow macaroni, cooked, drained, and kept warm
- 1 tablespoon brown rice vinegar

DIRECTIONS

1. Put the lentils and water in a saucepan, and sprinkle with salt, if desired. Bring to a boil over high heat. Reduce the heat to medium, then put the pan lid on and cook for 45 minutes or until the water is mostly absorbed. Pour the cooked lentils in the bowl and set aside.
2. Add the onion to a nonstick skillet, then sauté over medium heat for 15 minutes or caramelized.
3. Add vegetable broth and garlic to the skillet and sauté for 3 minutes or until fragrant.
4. Add the allspice, coriander, cumin, tomato paste, and red pepper flakes to the skillet and sauté for an additional 3 minutes until aromatic.
5. Add the tomatoes to the skillet and sauté for 15 minutes or until the tomatoes are wilted. Sprinkle with salt, if desired.
6. Arrange the cooked brown rice on the bottom of a large platter, then top the rice with macaroni, and then spread the lentils over. Pour the tomato mixture and brown rice vinegar over before serving.

NUTRITION: Calories: 201 Fat: 1.6g Carbs: 41.8g Protein: 6.5g Fiber: 3.6g

126. BLACK BEAN & SWEET POTATO HASH

COOKING: 20' **PREPARATION: 20'** **SERVES: 4 BOWLS**

INGREDIENTS

- 1 cup onion, chopped
- 2 garlic cloves, minced
- 2 cups sweet potatoes, chopped and peeled
- 2 tsp hot chili powder
- 1/3 cup vegetable broth
- 1 cup cooked black beans
- ¼ cup chopped scallions
- Chopped cilantro, for garnish
- Hot sauce (optional)

DIRECTIONS

1. In a nonstick skillet, place the onion and sauté over medium heat. Stir occasionally for 2 to 3 minutes. Add the garlic and stir.
2. Add the chili pepper and sweet potatoes. Stir to coat the vegetables with chili powder.
3. Add the broth and stir. Cook the contents for 12 minutes and stir occasionally until the potatoes are well-cooked.
4. Add some liquid. This will keep the vegetables from sticking to the pan. Add the scallions, black beans, and salt. Cook for 1 or 2 minutes until the beans are well-heated.
5. Add the hot sauce, if you are using it. Stir. Check the taste and adjust accordingly with the seasoning.
6. Top it with cilantro.

NUTRITION: Calories: 270 Fat: 7g Protein: 13g Carbs: 35g Fiber: 7g

THE PLANT BASED DIET COOKBOOK

127. SWEET AND SALTY PINEAPPLE FRIED RICE

COOKING: 15'   **PREPARATION: 5'**   **SERVES: 4**

INGREDIENTS

- 2 tbsp coconut oil
- 2/3 cup frozen green peas, thawed
- ½ cup sunflower seeds (raw)
- Red pepper (one large), diced
- 3 cups canned or fresh pineapple chunks
- 2 garlic cloves, minced
- 1 tbsp ginger, minced
- 2 cups long-grain brown rice, cooked
- Green onions (one bunch)
- Sauce:
- 1 cup pineapple juice
- 4 tbsp tamari
- 1 tsp sesame oil
- Lime juice (half a lime)
- Chili sauce to taste (sriracha is a good option)

DIRECTIONS

1. On medium heat in a large pan, toast the sunflower seeds for about 2 minutes. Set aside when the content is lightly browned.
2. On medium heat using the same pan, heat the coconut oil. Add the red pepper, pineapple chunks, and 2/3 of the green onion. Stir for about 5 minutes.
3. Now add the garlic and ginger. Stir so the tastes can meld.
4. Keep the heat on high. Add the cold rice and cook for 5 minutes until it is toasty.
5. Fold in the green peas as well as the toasted seeds
6. With the pan still on medium heat, pour in the tamari, sesame oil, and pineapple juice. Stir.
7. Season as required with the chili sauce.
8. For a better taste, add more lime juice and salt as required.

NUTRITION: Calories: 180 Fat: 11g Protein: 18g Carbs: 38g Fiber: 12g

128. RICE & VEGGIE BOWL RICE

COOKING: 15'   **PREPARATION: 5'**   **SERVES: 6**

INGREDIENTS

- 2 tbsp coconut oil
- 1 tsp ground cumin
- 1 tsp ground turmeric
- 1 tsp chili powder
- 1 red bell pepper, chopped
- 1 tsp tomato paste
- 1 bunch of broccoli, cut into bite-sized florets with short stems
- 1 tsp salt, to taste
- 1 large red onion, sliced
- 2 garlic cloves, minced
- 1 head of cauliflower, cut into bite-sized florets
- 2 cups cooked rice (or other cooked grain)
- Freshly ground black pepper to taste

DIRECTIONS

1. In a large pan or skillet, heat the coconut oil over medium-high heat.
2. When the oil is hot, stir in the turmeric, cumin, chili powder, salt, and tomato paste.
3. Cook the content for 1 minute. Stir repeatedly until the spices are fragrant.
4. Add the garlic and onion. Sauté for 2 to 3 minutes until the onions are softened.
5. Add the broccoli, cauliflower, and bell pepper. Cover. Cook for 3 to 4 minutes and stir occasionally.
6. Add the cooked rice. Stir so it will combine well with the vegetables. Cook for 2 to 3 minutes. Stir until the rice is warmed through.
7. Check the seasoning and adjust to taste if desired.
8. Lower the heat and cook on low for 2 to 3 more minutes so the flavors will meld.
9. Serve with freshly ground black pepper.

NUTRITION: Calories: 260 Fat: 9g Protein: 9g Carbs: 36g Fiber: 5g

THE PLANT BASED DIET COOKBOOK

129. RED BEANS AND RICE RICE

COOKING: 25' — **PREPARATION: 5'** — **SERVES: 4**

INGREDIENTS

- 3½ cups water, divided
- 1 tsp red pepper flakes
- 3 stalks celery, diced
- 1 green pepper, chopped
- ½ yellow onion, diced
- 2 small cans kidney beans, drained and rinsed
- 1 cup brown rice
- 3 garlic cloves, minced
- 1 bay leaf
- 1 tsp sage
- ½ tsp oregano
- ½ tsp cayenne
- Optional for heat: 1-2 jalapenos, diced

DIRECTIONS

1. Add 1 cup of rice and 2 cups of water to a pot. Bring the contents to a boil, turn down the heat, and cover to simmer until the water is absorbed.
2. Once the rice is cooked, put all the remaining ingredients in a large saucepan and cover for 20 to 30 minutes on low-medium heat. Stir occasionally until the onions are cooked and the 1 cup of water has boiled off.

NUTRITION: Calories: 221 Fat: 1g Protein: 11g Carbs: 25g Fiber: 4g

130. RAW NOODLES WITH AVOCADO 'N NUTS

COOKING: 10' — **PREPARATION: 5'** — **SERVES: 2**

INGREDIENTS

- 1 zucchini
- 1½ cup basil
- 1/3 cup water
- 5 tbsps. pine nuts
- 2 tbsps. lemon juice
- 1 avocado, peeled, pitted, sliced
- Optional: 2 tbsps. olive oil
- 6 yellow cherry tomatoes, halved
- Optional: 6 red cherry tomatoes, halved
- Sea salt and black pepper

DIRECTIONS

1. Add the basil, water, nuts, lemon juice, avocado slices, optional olive oil (if desired), salt, and pepper to a blender.
2. Blend the ingredients into a smooth mixture. Season with more pepper and salt and blend again.
3. Divide the sauce and the zucchini noodles between two medium-sized bowls for serving, and combine in each.
4. Top the mixtures with the halved yellow cherry tomatoes, and the optional red cherry tomatoes (if desired);

NUTRITION: Calories: 317, Carbs: 7.4 g, Fat: 28.1 g, Protein: 7.2g

THE PLANT BASED DIET COOKBOOK

131. RICE & BEAN BURRITOS

COOKING: 15'   **PREPARATION: 10'**   **SERVES: 8**

INGREDIENTS

- 32 oz. fat-free refried beans
- 6 tortillas
- 2 cups cooked rice
- ½ cup salsa
- 1 tbsp. olive oil
- 1 bunch green onions, chopped
- 2 bell peppers, chopped
- Guacamole

DIRECTIONS

1. Preheat the oven to 375°F.
2. Dump the refried beans into a saucepan and place over medium heat to warm.
3. Heat the tortillas and lay them out on a flat surface.
4. Spoon the beans in a long mound that runs across the tortilla, just a little off from center.
5. Spoon some rice and salsa over the beans; add the green pepper and onions to taste, along with any other finely chopped vegetables you like.
6. Fold over the shortest edge of the plain tortilla and roll it up, folding in the sides as you go.
7. Place each burrito, seam side down, on a nonstick-sprayed baking sheet.
8. Brush with olive oil and bake for 15 minutes.

NUTRITION: Calories: 290, Carbs: 49 g, Fat: 6 g, Protein: 9g

---

132. BARBECUED GREENS & GRITS

COOKING: 4H   **PREPARATION: 20'**   **SERVES: 4**

INGREDIENTS

- 14 oz. tempeh, sliced
- 3 cups vegetable broth
- 3 cups collard greens, chopped
- ½ cup BBQ sauce
- 1 cup gluten-free grits
- ¼ cup white onion, diced
- 2 tbsps. olive oil
- 2 garlic cloves, minced
- 1 tsp. salt

DIRECTIONS

1. Preheat the oven to 400°F.
2. Mix tempeh slices with the BBQ sauce in a shallow baking dish. Set aside and let marinate for up to 3 hours.
3. Heat 1 tablespoon of olive oil in a frying pan over medium heat and then add the garlic and sauté until it is fragrant.
4. Add the collard greens and ½ teaspoon of salt and cook until the collards are wilted and dark. Set the pan from heat and set aside.
5. Cover the tempeh and BBQ sauce mixture with aluminum foil. In your oven, set the baking dish in place and bake the ingredients for 15 minutes. Uncover and continue to bake for another 10 minutes until the tempeh is browned and crispy.
6. While the tempeh cooks heat the remaining tablespoon of olive oil in the previously used frying pan over medium heat.
7. Cook the onions until brown and fragrant, around 10 minutes.
8. Pour in the vegetable broth, bring it to a boil; then turn the heat down to low.
9. Slowly whisk the grits into the simmering broth. Add the remaining ½ teaspoon of salt before covering the pan with a lid.
10. Let the ingredients simmer for about 8 minutes until the grits are soft and creamy.
11. Serve the tempeh and collard greens on top of a bowl of grits and enjoy, or store for later!

NUTRITION: Calories: 374, Fat: 19.1g, Carbs: 31.1g, Protein: 23.7g

133. CHICKPEA AND SPINACH CUTLETS

COOKING: 30' | **PREPARATION: 10'** | **SERVES: 2**

INGREDIENTS

- 1 Red Bell Pepper
- 19 oz. Chickpeas, Rinsed & Drained
- 1 cup ground Almonds
- 2 tsps. Dijon Mustard
- 1 tsp. Oregano
- ½ tsp. Sage
- 1 cup Spinach, Fresh
- 1½ cup Rolled Oats
- 1 Clove Garlic, Pressed
- ½ Lemon, Juiced
- 2 tsps. Maple Syrup, Pure

DIRECTIONS

1. Get out a baking sheet. Line it with parchment paper.
2. Cut your red pepper in half and then take the seeds out. Place it on your baking sheet, and roast in the oven while you prepare your other ingredients.
3. Process your chickpeas, almonds, mustard, and maple syrup together in a food processor.
4. Add in your lemon juice, oregano, sage, garlic, and spinach, processing again. Make sure it's combined, but don't puree it.
5. Once your red bell pepper is softened, which should roughly take ten minutes, add this to the processor as well. Add in your oats, mixing well.
6. Form twelve patties, cooking in the oven for a half hour. They should be browned.

NUTRITION: Calories: 200 Protein: 8g Fat: 11g Carbs: 21g

134. FLAVORFUL REFRIED BEANS

COOKING: 6H | **PREPARATION: 10'** | **SERVES: 8**

INGREDIENTS

- 3 cups rinsed pinto beans
- 1 seeded jalapeno pepper, chopped
- 1 sliced white onion, peeled
- 2 tbsps. minced garlic
- 5 tsps. salt
- 2 tsps. ground black pepper
- ¼ tsps. ground cumin
- 9 cups water

DIRECTIONS

1. Using a 6-quarts slow cooker, place all the ingredients and stir until it mixes properly.
2. Cover the top, plug in the slow cooker, adjust the cooking time to 6 hours, let it cook on high heat setting, and add more water if the beans get too dry.
3. When beans are done, drain and reserve the liquid.
4. Use a potato masher to mash the beans and pour in the reserved cooking liquid until it reaches your desired mixture.

NUTRITION: Calories: 105 Carbs: 36g Protein: 13g Fat: 1g

135. SMOKY RED BEANS AND RICE

COOKING: 4H **PREPARATION:** 10' **SERVES:** 6

INGREDIENTS

- 30 oz. cooked red beans
- 1 cup brown rice, uncooked
- 1 cup green pepper, chopped
- 1 cup chopped celery
- 1 cup white onion, chopped
- 1 ½ tsps. minced garlic
- ½ tsp. salt
- ¼ tsp. cayenne pepper
- 1 tsp. smoked paprika
- 2 tsps. dried thyme
- 1 bay leaf
- 2 1/3 cups vegetable broth

DIRECTIONS

1. Using a 6-quarts slow cooker, place all the ingredients except for the rice, salt, and cayenne pepper.
2. Stir until it mixes properly and then cover the top.
3. Plug in the slow cooker; adjust the cooking time to 4 hours, and steam on a low heat setting.
4. Then pour in and stir the rice, salt, cayenne pepper and continue cooking for an additional 2 hours at a high heat setting.

NUTRITION: Calories: 425 Carbs: 62g Protein: 27g Fat: 22g

136. SAVORY SPANISH RICE

COOKING: 5H **PREPARATION:** 5' **SERVES:** 10

INGREDIENTS

- 1 cup long grain rice, uncooked
- ½ cup green bell pepper, chopped
- 14 oz. diced tomatoes
- ½ cup chopped white onion
- 1 tsp. minced garlic
- ½ tsp. salt
- 1 tsp. red chili powder
- 1 tsp. ground cumin
- 4 oz. tomato puree
- 8 fl. oz. water

DIRECTIONS

1. Grease a 6-quarts slow cooker with a non-stick cooking spray and add all the ingredients into it.
2. Stir properly and cover the top.
3. Plug in the slow cooker; adjust the cooking time to 5 hours, and cook on high or until the rice absorbs all the liquid.

NUTRITION: Calories: 210 Cal, Carbs: 11g, Protein: 12g, Fat: 10g

137. DELIGHTFUL COCONUT VEGETARIAN CURRY

COOKING: 5H **PREPARATION: 10'** **SERVES: 6**

INGREDIENTS

- 5 potatoes, peeled and cubed
- ¼ cup curry powder
- 2 tbsps. flour
- 1 tbsp. chili powder
- ½ tsp. red pepper flakes
- ½ tsp. cayenne pepper
- 1 green bell pepper, chopped
- 1 red bell pepper, chopped
- 2 tbsps. onion soup mix
- 14 oz. coconut cream, unsweetened
- 3 cups vegetable broth
- 2 carrots, peeled and sliced
- 1 cup green peas
- ¼ cup chopped cilantro

DIRECTIONS

1. Take a 6-quarts slow cooker, grease it with a non-stick cooking spray and place the potatoes pieces in the bottom.
2. Set in the rest of the ingredients except for peas, cilantro, and carrots.
3. Stir properly and cover the top.
4. Plug in the slow cooker; adjust the cooking time to 4 hours and let it cook on the low heat setting or until it cooks thoroughly.
5. When the cooking time is over, add the carrots to the curry and continue cooking for 30 minutes.
6. Stir in the peas to cook for 30 more minutes or until the peas get tender.
7. Garnish it with cilantro and serve.

NUTRITION: Calories: 369 Carbs: 39g, Protein: 7g, Fat: 23g

138. COMFORTING CHICKPEA TAGINE

COOKING: 4H **PREPARATION: 5'** **SERVES: 6**

INGREDIENTS

- 14 oz. cooked chickpeas
- 12 dried apricots
- 1 red bell pepper, cored and sliced
- 1 cored butternut squash, peeled and chopped
- 2 stemmed zucchinis, chopped
- 1 white onion, peeled and chopped
- 1 tsp. minced garlic
- 1 tsp. ground ginger
- 1 ½ tsps. salt
- 1 tsp. ground black pepper
- 1 tsp. ground cumin
- 2 tsps. paprika
- 1 tsp. harissa paste
- 2 tsps. honey
- 2 tbsps. olive oil
- 1 lb. passata
- ¼ cup chopped coriander

DIRECTIONS

1. Take a 6-quarts slow cooker, grease it with a non-stick cooking spray and place the chickpeas, apricots, bell pepper, butternut squash, zucchini, and onion into it.
2. Sprinkle it with salt, black pepper, and set it aside until it is called for.
3. Place a large non-stick skillet pan over an average temperature of heat; add the oil, garlic, cumin, and paprika.
4. Stir properly and cook for 1 minutes or until it starts producing fragrance.
5. Then pour in the harissa paste, honey, passata, and boil the mixture.
6. When the mixture is done boiling, pour this mixture over the vegetables in the slow cooker and cover it with the lid.
7. Plug in the slow cooker; adjust the cooking time to 4 hours and let it cook on the high heat setting or until the vegetables gets tender.
8. When done, add the seasoning, garnish it with the coriander, and serve right away.

NUTRITION: Calories: 237 Carbs: 45g Protein: 9g Fat: 2g

139. BLACK BEAN STUFFED SWEET POTATOES

COOKING: 1H   **PREPARATION: 5'**   **SERVES: 4**

INGREDIENTS

- 4 sweet potatoes
- 15 oz. cooked black beans
- ½ tsp. ground black pepper
- ½ red onion, peeled, diced
- ½ tsp. sea salt
- ¼ tsp. onion powder
- ¼ tsp. garlic powder
- ¼ tsp. red chili powder
- ¼ tsp. cumin
- 1 tsp. lime juice
- 1 ½ tbsps. olive oil
- ½ cup cashew cream sauce

DIRECTIONS

1. Spread sweet potatoes on a baking tray greased with foil and bake for 65 minutes at 350°F until tender.
2. Meanwhile, prepare the sauce, and for this, whisk together the cream sauce, black pepper, and lime juice until combined, set aside until required.
3. When 10 minutes of the baking time of potatoes are left, heat a skillet pan with oil. Add in onion to cook until golden for 5 minutes.
4. Then stir in spice, cook for another 3 minutes, stir in bean until combined and cook for 5 minutes until hot.
5. Let roasted sweet potatoes cool for 10 minutes, then cut them open, mash the flesh and top with bean mixture, cilantro and avocado, and then drizzle with cream sauce.
6. Serve straight away.

NUTRITION: Calories: 387, Fat: 16.1 g, Carbs: 53 g, Protein: 10.4g

140. BLACK BEAN AND QUINOA SALAD

COOKING: 0   **PREPARATION: 10'**   **SERVES: 10**

INGREDIENTS

- 15 oz. cooked black beans
- 1 chopped red bell pepper, cored
- 1 cup quinoa, cooked
- 1 cored green bell pepper, chopped
- ½ cup vegan feta cheese, crumbled

DIRECTIONS

1. In a bowl, set in all ingredients, except for cheese, and stir until incorporated.
2. Top the salad with cheese and serve straight away.

NUTRITION: Calories: 64, Fat: 1g, Carbs: 8g, Protein: 3g

141. COCONUT CHICKPEA CURRY

COOKING: 15'   **PREPARATION: 5'**   **SERVES: 4**

INGREDIENTS

- 2 tsps. coconut flour
- 16 oz. cooked chickpeas
- 14 oz. tomatoes, diced
- 1 red onion, sliced
- 1 ½ tsps. minced garlic
- ½ tsp. sea salt
- 1 tsp. curry powder
- 1/3 tsp. ground black pepper
- 1 ½ tbsps. garam masala
- ¼ tsp. cumin
- 1 lime, juiced
- 13.5 oz. coconut milk, unsweetened
- 2 tbsps. coconut oil

DIRECTIONS

1. Take a large pot, place it over medium-high heat, add oil and when it melts, add onions and tomatoes, season with salt and black pepper and cook for 5 minutes.
2. Switch heat to medium-low level, cook for 10 minutes until tomatoes have released their liquid, then add chickpeas and stir in garlic, curry powder, garam masala, and cumin until combined.
3. Stir in milk and flour, bring the mixture to boil, switch heat to medium heat and simmer the curry for 12 minutes until cooked.
4. Taste to adjust seasoning, drizzle with lime juice, and serve.

NUTRITION: Calories: 225 Fat: 9.4 g Carbs: 28.5g Protein: 7.3g

142. SWEET POTATO AND WHITE BEAN SKILLET

COOKING: 20'   **PREPARATION: 5'**   **SERVES: 4**

INGREDIENTS

- 1 bunch kale, chopped
- 2 sweet potatoes, peeled, cubed
- 12 oz. cannellini beans
- 1 peeled onion, diced
- 1/8 tsp. red pepper flakes
- 1 tsp. salt
- 1 tsp. cumin
- ½ tsp. ground black pepper
- 1 tsp. curry powder
- 1 ½ tbsps. coconut oil
- 6 oz. coconut milk, unsweetened

DIRECTIONS

1. Take a large skillet pan, place it over medium heat, add ½ tablespoon oil and when it melts, add onion and cook for 5 minutes.
2. Then stir in sweet potatoes, stir well, cook for 5 minutes, then season with all the spices, cook for 1 minute and remove the pan from heat.
3. Take another pan, add remaining oil in it, place it over medium heat and when oil melts, add kale, season with some salt and black pepper, stir well, pour in the milk and cook for 15 minutes until tender.
4. Then add beans, beans, and red pepper, stir until mixed and cook for 5 minutes until hot.
5. Serve straight away.

NUTRITION: Calories: 263 Fat: 4 g Carbs: 44 g Protein: 13g

143. VEGGIE KABOBS

COOKING: 10'   **PREPARATION: 10'**   **SERVES: 10**

INGREDIENTS

- 8 oz. button mushrooms, halved
- 2 lbs. summer squash, peeled, 1-inch cubed
- 12 oz. small broccoli florets
- 2 cups grape tomatoes
- 1 tsp. salt
- ½ tsp. smoked paprika
- 1 tsp. ground cumin
- 6 tbsps. olive oil
- 1/2 tsp. ground coriander
- 1 lime, juiced

DIRECTIONS

1. Toss broccoli florets with 1 tablespoon oil, toss tomatoes and squash pieces with 2 tablespoons oil, toss mushrooms with 1 tablespoon oil and thread these vegetables onto skewers.
2. Grill mushrooms and broccoli for 7 to 10 minutes, squash and tomatoes and 8 minutes, and when done, transfer the skewers to a plate and drizzle with lime juice and remaining oil.
3. Prepared the spice mix and for this, stir together salt, paprika, cumin, and coriander, sprinkle half of the mixture over grilled veggies, cover them with foil for 5 minutes, and then sprinkle with the remaining spice mix.
4. Serve straight away.

NUTRITION: Calories: 110, Fat: 9g, Carbs: 8g, Protein: 3g

144. PILAF WITH GARBANZOS AND DRIED APRICOTS

COOKING: 20'   **PREPARATION: 5'**   **SERVES: 4**

INGREDIENTS

- 1 cup bulgur
- 6 oz. cooked chickpeas
- ½ cup dried apricot
- 1 white onion, peeled, diced
- ½ tsps. minced garlic
- 2 tsps. curry powder
- ½ tsp. salt
- 1 tbsp. olive oil
- ¼ cup fresh parsley leaves
- 2 cups vegetable broth
- ¾ cup water

DIRECTIONS

1. Take a saucepan, place it over high heat, pour in water and 1 ½ cup broth, and bring it to a boil.
2. Then stir in bulgur, switch heat to medium-low level and simmer for 15 minutes until most of the liquid has absorbed.
3. Meanwhile, take a skillet pan, place it over medium heat, add oil and when hot, add onion, cook for 10 minutes, then stir in garlic and curry powder and cook for another minute.
4. Then add apricots, beans, and salt, pour in remaining broth and bring the mixture to boiling.
5. Remove pan from heat, fluff the bulgur with a fork, add to the onion-apricot mixture and stir until mixed.
6. Garnish with parsley and serve.

NUTRITION: Calories: 222 Fat: 4.5g Carbs: 35g Protein: 9.5g

145. SPAGHETTI WITH CHICKPEAS MEATBALLS

COOKING: 40' **PREPARATION: 10'** **SERVES: 8**

INGREDIENTS

- ½ cup Breadcrumbs
- 1 tsp. Italian Seasoning
- 3 cups Chickpeas, drained & rinsed
- ½ tsp. Salt
- 3 tbsps. Flax Seed, grounded
- 2 tsps. Onion Powder
- 8 tbsps. Water
- ½ tbsp. Garlic Powder
- ¼ cup Nutritional Yeast
- For the pasta:
- 1 lb. Spaghetti
- 25 oz. Pasta Sauce

DIRECTIONS

1. First, preheat the oven to 325°F.
2. After that, combine the flax seeds with water in a small bowl and set it aside for 5 minutes.
3. Next, place the chickpeas and salt in the food processor and process them for one minute or until you get a smooth mixture.
4. Now, transfer the chickpea mixture and the flaxseed mixture to a large mixing bowl. Stir well.
5. Once combined, add all the remaining ingredients needed to the bowl.
6. Give everything a good stir and mix well.
7. Then, make balls out of this mixture and arrange them on a parchment paper-lined baking sheet while leaving ample space in between.
8. Bake them for 33 to 35 minutes. Turn them once halfway through.
9. In the meantime, make the spaghetti by following the instructions given on the packet. Cook until al dente.
10. Finally, place the spaghetti on the serving plate and top it with the meatballs and pasta sauce.
11. Serve and enjoy.

NUTRITION: Calories: 323, Proteins: 15g, Carbs: 63g, Fat: 4g

146. BLACK BEAN WRAP WITH HUMMUS

COOKING: 30' **PREPARATION: 5'** **SERVES: 2 WRAPS**

INGREDIENTS

- 1 Poblano Pepper, roasted
- ½ packet Spinach
- 1 Onion, chopped
- 2 Whole Grain Wraps
- ½ can Black Beans
- 1 Bell Pepper, seeded & chopped
- 4 oz. Mushrooms, sliced
- ½ cup Corn
- 8 oz. Red Bell Pepper Hummus, roasted

DIRECTIONS

1. First, preheat the oven to 450°F.
2. Next, spoon in oil to a heated skillet and stir in the onion.
3. Cook them for 2 to 3 minutes or until softened.
4. After that, stir in the bell pepper and sauté for another 3 minutes.
5. Then, add mushrooms and corn to the skillet. Sauté for 2 minutes.
6. In the meantime, spread the hummus over the wraps.
7. Now, place the sautéed vegetables, spinach, Poblano strips, and beans.
8. Roll them into a burrito and place on a baking sheet with the seam side down.
9. Finally, bake them for 9 to 10 minutes.
10. Serve them warm.

NUTRITION: Calories: 293, Proteins: 13.7g, Carbs: 42.8g, Fat: 8.8g

THE PLANT BASED DIET COOKBOOK

CHAPTER 10: PASTA & NOODLES

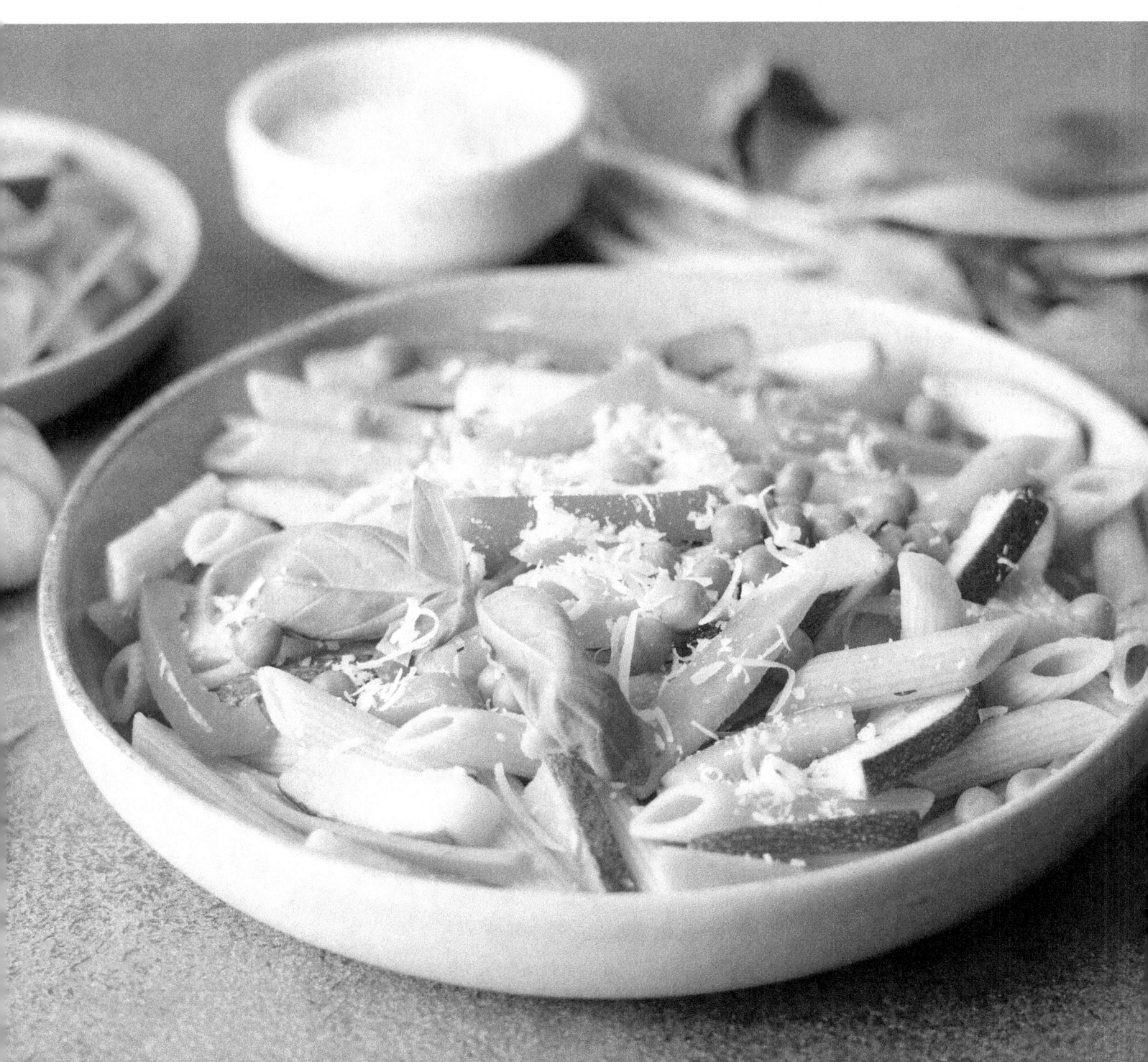

147. STIR FRY NOODLES

COOKING: 8'   **PREPARATION: 10'**   **SERVES: 4**

INGREDIENTS

- 1 cup broccoli, chopped
- 1 cup red bell pepper, chopped
- 1 cup mushrooms, chopped
- 1 large onion, chopped
- 1 batch Stir Fry Sauce, prepared
- Salt and black pepper, to taste
- 2 cups spaghetti, cooked
- 4 garlic cloves, minced
- 2 tablespoons sesame oil

DIRECTIONS

1. Heat sesame oil in a pan over medium heat and add garlic, onions, bell pepper, broccoli, mushrooms.
2. Sauté for about 5 minutes and add spaghetti noodles and stir fry sauce.
3. Mix well and cook for 3 more minutes.
4. Dish out in plates and serve to enjoy.

NUTRITION: Calories: 567 Fat: 48g Carbs: 6g Fiber: 4g Protein: 33g

148. SPICY SWEET CHILI VEGGIE NOODLES

COOKING: 7'   **PREPARATION: 10'**   **SERVES: 2**

INGREDIENTS

- 1 head of broccoli, cut into bite sized florets
- 1 onion, finely sliced
- 1 tablespoon olive oil
- 1 courgette, halved
- 2 nests of whole-wheat noodles
- 5 oz. mushrooms, sliced

For Sauce:

- 3 tablespoons soy sauce
- ¼ cup sweet chili sauce
- 1 teaspoon Sriracha
- 1 tablespoon peanut butter
- 2 tablespoons boiled water

For Topping

- 2 teaspoons sesame seeds
- 2 teaspoons dried chili flakes

DIRECTIONS

1. Heat olive oil on medium heat in a saucepan and add onions.
2. Sauté for about 2 minutes and add broccoli, courgette and mushrooms.
3. Cook for about 5 minutes, stirring occasionally.
4. Whisk sweet chili sauce, soy sauce, Sriracha, water and peanut butter in a bowl.
5. Cook the noodles according to packet instructions and add to the vegetables.
6. Stir in the sauce and top with dried chili flakes and sesame seeds to serve.

NUTRITION: Calories: 351 Fat: 27g Protein: 25g Carbs: 2g Fiber: 1g

149. CREAMY VEGAN MUSHROOM PASTA

COOKING: 30'   **PREPARATION: 10'**   **SERVES: 6**

INGREDIENTS

- 2 cups frozen peas, thawed
- 3 tablespoons flour, unbleached
- 3 cups almond breeze, unsweetened
- 1 tablespoon nutritional yeast
- 1/3 cup fresh parsley, chopped, plus extra for garnish
- ¼ cup olive oil
- 1-pound pasta of choice
- 4 cloves garlic, minced
- 2/3 cup shallots, chopped
- 8 cups mixed mushrooms, sliced
- Salt and black pepper, to taste

DIRECTIONS

1. Take a bowl and boil pasta in salted water.
2. Heat olive oil in a pan over medium heat.
3. Add mushrooms, garlic, shallots and ½ tsp salt and cook for 15 minutes.
4. Sprinkle flour on the vegetables and stir for a minute while cooking.
5. Add almond beverage, stir constantly.
6. Let it simmer for 5 minutes and add pepper to it.
7. Cook for 3 more minutes and remove from heat.
8. Stir in nutritional yeast.
9. Add peas, salt, and pepper.
10. Cook for another minute and add
11. Add pasta to this sauce.
12. Garnish and serve!

NUTRITION: Calories: 364 Fat: 28g Protein: 24g Carbs: 24g Fiber: 2g

150. VEGAN CHINESE NOODLES

COOKING: 8'   **PREPARATION: 15'**   **SERVES: 4**

INGREDIENTS

- 10 oz. mixed oriental mushrooms, such as oyster, shiitake and enoki, cleaned and sliced
- 7 oz. thin rice noodles, cooked according to packet instructions and drained
- 2 garlic cloves, minced
- 1 fresh red chili
- 7 oz. courgettes, sliced
- 6 spring onions, reserving the green part
- 1 teaspoon corn flour
- 1 tablespoon agave syrup
- 1 teaspoon sesame oil
- 100g baby spinach, chopped
- Hot chili sauce, to serve
- 2(1-inch) pieces of ginger
- ½ bunch fresh coriander, chopped
- 4 tablespoons vegetable oil
- 2 tablespoons low-salt soy sauce
- ½ tablespoon rice wine
- 2 limes, to serve

DIRECTIONS

1. Heat sesame oil over high heat in a large wok and add the mushrooms.
2. Sauté for about 4 minutes and add garlic, chili, ginger, courgette, coriander stalks and the white part of the spring onions.
3. Sauté for about 3 minutes until softened and lightly golden.
4. Meanwhile, combine the corn flour and 2 tablespoons of water in a bowl.
5. Add soy sauce, agave syrup, sesame oil and rice wine to the corn flour mixture.
6. Put this mixture in the pan to the veggie mixture and cook for about 3 minutes until thickened.
7. Add the spinach and noodles and mix well.
8. Stir in the coriander leaves and top with lime wedges, hot chili sauce and reserved spring onions to serve.

NUTRITION: Calories: 314 Fat: 22g Protein: 26g Carbs: 8g Fiber: 0.3g

THE PLANT BASED DIET COOKBOOK

151. VEGETABLE PENNE PASTA

COOKING: 20' **PREPARATION: 15'** **SERVES: 6**

INGREDIENTS

- ½ large onion, chopped
- 2 celery sticks, chopped
- ½ tablespoon ginger paste
- ½ cup green bell pepper
- 1½ tablespoons soy sauce
- ½ teaspoon parsley
- Salt and black pepper, to taste
- ½ pound penne pasta, cooked
- 2 large carrots, diced
- ½ small leek, chopped
- 1 tablespoon olive oil
- ½ teaspoon garlic paste
- ½ tablespoon Worcester sauce
- ½ teaspoon coriander
- 1 cup water

DIRECTIONS

1. Heat olive oil in a wok on medium heat and add onions, garlic and ginger paste.
2. Sauté for about 3 minutes and stir in all bell pepper, celery sticks, carrots and leek.
3. Sauté for about 5 minutes and add remaining ingredients except for pasta.
4. Cover the lid and cook for about 12 minutes.
5. Stir in the cooked pasta and dish out to serve warm.

NUTRITION: Calories: 385 Fat: 29g Protein: 26g Carbs: 12g Fiber: 1g

152. SPAGHETTI IN SPICY TOMATO SAUCE

COOKING: 40' **PREPARATION: 15'** **SERVES: 4**

INGREDIENTS

- 1 pound dried spaghetti
- 1 red bell pepper, diced
- 4 garlic cloves, minced
- 1 teaspoon red pepper flakes, crushed
- 2 (14-oz.) cans diced tomatoes
- 1 (6-oz.) can tomato paste
- 2 teaspoons vegan sugar, granulated
- 2 tablespoons olive oil
- 1 medium onion, diced
- 1 cup dry red wine
- 1 teaspoon dried thyme
- ½ teaspoon fennel seed, crushed
- 1½ cups coconut milk, full-fat
- Salt and black pepper, to taste

DIRECTIONS

1. Boil water in a large pot and add pasta.
2. Cook according to the package directions and drain the pasta into a colander.
3. Dish out the pasta in a large serving bowl and add a dash of olive oil to prevent sticking.
4. Heat 2 tablespoons of olive oil over medium heat in a large pot and add garlic, onion and bell pepper.
5. Sauté for about 5 minutes and stir in the wine, thyme, fennel and red pepper flakes.
6. Allow to simmer on high heat for about 5 minutes until the liquid is reduced by about half.
7. Add diced tomatoes and tomato paste and allow to simmer for about 20 minutes, stirring occasionally.
8. Stir in the coconut milk and sugar and simmer for about 10 more minutes.
9. Season with salt and black pepper and pour the sauce over the pasta.
10. Toss to coat well and dish out in plates to serve.

NUTRITION: Calories: 313 Fat: 7 Protein: 21g Carbs: 21g

153. 20 MINUTES VEGETARIAN PASTA

COOKING: 16' **PREPARATION: 5'** **SERVES: 4**

INGREDIENTS

- 3 shallots, chopped
- ¼ teaspoon red pepper flakes
- ¼ cup vegan parmesan cheese
- 2 tablespoons olive oil
- 2 garlic cloves, minced
- 8-oz. spinach leaves
- 8-oz. linguine pasta
- 1 pinch salt
- 1 pinch black pepper

DIRECTIONS

1. Boil salted water in a large pot and add pasta.
2. Cook for about 6 minutes and drain the pasta in a colander.
3. Heat olive oil over medium heat in a large skillet and add the shallots.
4. Cook for about 5 minutes until soft and caramelized and stir in the spinach, garlic, red pepper flakes, salt and black pepper.
5. Cook for about 5 minutes and add pasta and 2 spoons of pasta water.
6. Stir in the parmesan cheese and dish out in a bowl to serve.

NUTRITION: Calories: 284 Fat: 18g Protein: 19g Carbs: 15g Fiber: 4g

154. CREAMY VEGAN PUMPKIN PASTA

COOKING: 5' **PREPARATION: 15'** **SERVES: 6**

INGREDIENTS

- 1 tablespoon olive oil
- 1 cup raw cashews, soaked in water 4-8 hours, drained and rinsed
- 12 oz. dried penne pasta
- 1 cup pumpkin puree, canned
- 1 cup almond milk, plus more as needed
- 3 garlic cloves
- ¼ teaspoon ground nutmeg
- Fresh parsley, for garnish
- 1 tablespoon lemon juice
- ¾ teaspoon salt
- 1 tablespoon fresh sage, chopped

DIRECTIONS

1. Boil salted water in a large pot and add pasta.
2. Cook according to the package directions and drain the pasta into a colander.
3. Dish out the pasta in a large serving bowl and add a dash of olive oil to prevent sticking.
4. Put the pumpkin, cashews, milk, lemon juice, garlic, salt and nutmeg into the food processor and blend until smooth.
5. Stir in the sauce and sage over the pasta and toss to coat well.
6. Garnish with fresh parsley and dish out to serve hot.

NUTRITION: Calories: 431 Fat: 21g Protein: 25g Carbs: 15g Fiber: 5g

THE PLANT BASED DIET COOKBOOK

155. LOADED CREAMY VEGAN PESTO PASTA

COOKING: 10'   **PREPARATION: 15'**   **SERVES: 6**

INGREDIENTS

- ¼ onion, finely chopped
- 8 romaine lettuce leaves
- 1 celery stalk, thinly sliced
- ½ cup blue cheese, crumbled
- 1 tablespoon olive oil, plus a dash
- 1 cup almond milk, unflavored and unsweetened
- ½ cup vegan pesto
- 1 cup chickpeas, cooked
- 1 cup fresh arugula, packed
- 2 tablespoons lemon juice
- Salt and black pepper, to taste
- 6-oz. orecchiette pasta, dried
- 1 cup full-fat coconut milk
- 2 tablespoons whole wheat flour
- 1½ cups cherry tomatoes, halved
- ½ cup Kalamata olives, halved
- Red pepper flakes, to taste

DIRECTIONS

1. Boil salted water in a large pot and add pasta.
2. Cook according to the package directions and drain the pasta into a colander.
3. Dish out the pasta in a large serving bowl and add a dash of olive oil to prevent sticking.
4. Put olive oil over medium heat in a large pot and whisk in the flour.
5. Cook for about 4 minutes, until the mixture begins to smell nutty and stir in the coconut milk and almond milk.
6. Let the sauce simmer for about 1 minute and add the chickpeas, olives and arugula.
7. Stir well and season with lemon juice, red pepper flakes, and salt and black pepper.
8. Dish out into plates and serve hot.

NUTRITION: Calories: 420 Fat: 10g Protein: 31g Carbs: 19g Fiber: 9g

156. CREAMY VEGAN SPINACH PASTA

COOKING: 5'   **PREPARATION: 20'**   **SERVES: 4**

INGREDIENTS

- 1 cup raw cashews, soaked in water for 8 hours
- 2 tablespoons lemon juice
- 1 tablespoon olive oil
- 1½ cups vegetable broth
- 2 tablespoons fresh dill, chopped
- Red pepper flakes, to taste
- 10 oz. dried fusilli
- ½ cup almond milk, unflavored and unsweetened
- 2 tablespoons white miso paste
- 4 garlic cloves, divided
- 8-oz. fresh spinach, finely chopped
- ¼ cup scallions, chopped
- Salt and black pepper, to taste

DIRECTIONS

1. Boil salted water in a large pot and add pasta.
2. Cook according to the package directions and drain the pasta into a colander.
3. Dish out the pasta in a large serving bowl and add a dash of olive oil to prevent sticking.
4. Put the cashews, milk, miso, lemon juice, and 1 garlic clove into the food processor and blend until smooth.
5. Put olive oil over medium heat in a large pot and add the remaining 3 cloves of garlic.
6. Sauté for about 1 minute and stir in the spinach and broth.
7. Raise the heat and simmer for about 4 minutes until the spinach is bright green and wilted.
8. Stir in the pasta and cashew mixture and season with salt and black pepper.
9. Top with scallions and dill and dish out into plates to serve.

NUTRITION: Calories: 94 Fat: 10g Protein: 8g Carbs: 17g Fiber: 6g

157. VEGAN BAKE PASTA WITH BOLOGNESE SAUCE AND CASHEW CREAM

COOKING: 20'   **PREPARATION: 1H 10'**   **SERVES: 7**

INGREDIENTS

For the Pasta:
- 1 packet penne pasta
- For the Bolognese Sauce:
- 1 tablespoon soy sauce
- 1 small can lentils
- 1 tablespoon brown sugar
- ½ cup tomato paste
- 1 teaspoon garlic, crushed
- 1 tablespoon olive oil
- 2 tomatoes, chopped
- 1 onion, chopped
- 2 cups mushrooms, sliced
- Salt, to taste
- Pepper, to taste

For the Cashew Cream:
- 1 cup raw cashews
- ½ lemon, squeezed
- ½ teaspoon salt
- ½ cup water

For the White Sauce:
- 1 teaspoon black pepper
- 1 teaspoon Dijon mustard
- ¼ cup nutritional yeast
- Sea salt, as required
- 2 cups coconut milk
- 3 tablespoons vegan butter
- 2 tablespoons all-purpose flour
- 1/3 cup vegetable broth

DIRECTIONS

1. Take a pot and boil water, add pasta to it, boil for 3 minutes and set aside.
2. Fry onion and garlic, mushroom in olive oil and add soy sauce to it.
3. Add sugar tomato paste, lentils, and canned tomato to it and let it simmer, Bolognese sauce is prepared.
4. Season it with salt and black pepper.
5. Add the lemon juice, cashews, water and salt to the blender, blend for 2 minutes.
6. Add this to the sauce you have prepared and stir pasta in it.
7. Melt the vegan butter in a saucepan, add in the flour and stir.
8. Add vegetable stock and coconut milk to it and whisk well.
9. Stir continuously and let it boil for about 5 minutes, then remove from heat.
10. Add Dijon mustard, nutritional yeast, black pepper, and sea salt.
11. Preheat the oven to 430°F.
12. Prepare rectangular oven-safe dish by placing pasta and Bolognese sauce to it.
13. Pour the white sauce on it and bake for a time of 20-25 minutes.

NUTRITION: Calories: 314 Fat: 20g Protein: 21g Carbs: 15g Fiber: 6g

158. 5 INGREDIENTS PASTA

COOKING: 25'   **PREPARATION: 15'**   **SERVES: 5**

INGREDIENTS

- 1 (25 oz.) jar marinara sauce
- Olive oil, as needed
- 1-pound dry vegan pasta
- 1 pound assorted vegetables, like red onion, zucchini and tomatoes
- ¼ cup prepared hummus
- Salt, to taste

DIRECTIONS

1. Preheat the oven to 400°F and grease a large baking sheet.
2. Arrange the vegetables in a single layer on the baking sheet and sprinkle with olive oil and salt.
3. Transfer into the oven and roast the vegetables for about 15 minutes.
4. Boil salted water in a large pot and cook the pasta according to the package directions.
5. Drain the water when the pasta is tender and put the pasta in a colander.
6. Mix the marinara sauce and hummus in a large pot to make a creamy sauce.
7. Stir in the cooked vegetables and pasta to the sauce and toss to coat well.
8. Dish out in a bowl and serve warm.

NUTRITION: Calories: 415 Fat: 29g Protein: 33g Carbs: 5.5g Fiber: 2g

THE PLANT BASED DIET COOKBOOK

CHAPTER 11: LEGUMES

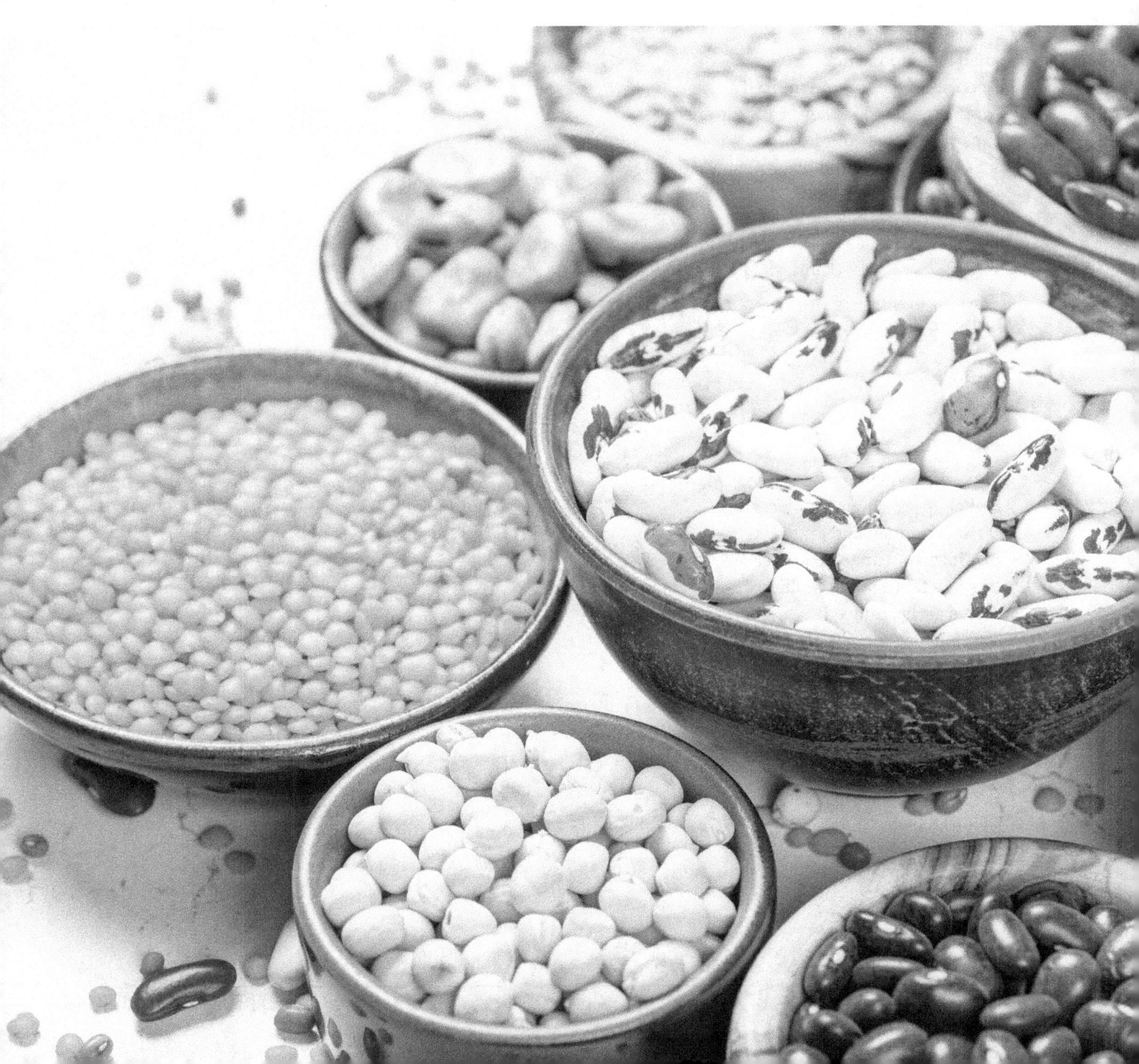

159. TRADITIONAL INDIAN RAJMA DAL

COOKING: 10' **PREPARATION: 10'** **SERVES: 4**

INGREDIENTS

- 3 tablespoons sesame oil
- 1 teaspoon ginger, minced
- 1 teaspoon cumin seeds
- 1 teaspoon coriander seeds
- 1 large onion, chopped
- 1 celery stalk, chopped
- 1 teaspoon garlic, minced
- 1 cup tomato sauce
- 1 teaspoon garam masala
- 1/2 teaspoon curry powder
- 1 small cinnamon stick
- 1 green chili, seeded and minced
- 2 cups canned red kidney beans, drained
- 2 cups vegetable broth
- Kosher salt and ground black pepper, to taste

DIRECTIONS

1. In a saucepan, heat the sesame oil over medium-high heat; now, sauté the ginger, cumin seeds and coriander seeds until fragrant or about 30 seconds or so.
2. Add in the onion and celery and continue to sauté for 3 minutes more until they've softened.
3. Add in the garlic and continue to sauté for 1 minute longer.
4. Stir the remaining ingredients into the saucepan and turn the heat to a simmer. Continue to cook for 10 to 12 minutes or until thoroughly cooked. Serve warm and enjoy!

NUTRITION: Calories: 443, Fat: 19.2g, Carbs: 52.2g, Protein: 18.1g

160. RED KIDNEY BEAN SALAD

COOKING: 10' **PREPARATION: 10'** **SERVES: 4**

INGREDIENTS

- 3/4-pound red kidney beans, soaked overnight
- 2 bell peppers, chopped
- 1 carrot, trimmed and grated
- 3 oz. frozen or canned corn kernels, drained
- 3 heaping tablespoons scallions, chopped
- 2 cloves garlic, minced
- 1 red chile pepper, sliced
- 1/2 cup extra-virgin olive oil
- 2 tablespoons apple cider vinegar
- 2 tablespoons fresh lemon juice
- Sea salt and ground black pepper, to taste
- 2 tablespoons fresh cilantro, chopped
- 2 tablespoons fresh parsley, chopped
- 2 tablespoons fresh basil, chopped

DIRECTIONS

1. Cover the soaked beans with a fresh change of cold water and bring to a boil. Let it boil for about 10 minutes. Turn the heat to a simmer and continue to cook for 50 to 55 minutes or until tender.
2. Allow your beans to cool completely, then, transfer them to a salad bowl.
3. Add in the remaining ingredients and toss to combine well.

NUTRITION: Calories: 443 Fat: 19.2g Carbs: 52.2g Protein: 18.1g

161. ANASAZI BEAN AND VEGETABLE STEW

COOKING: 10'   **PREPARATION: 10'**   **SERVES: 4**

INGREDIENTS

- 1 cup Anasazi beans, soaked overnight and drained
- 3 cups roasted vegetable broth
- 1 bay laurel
- 1 thyme sprig, chopped
- 1 rosemary sprig, chopped
- 3 tablespoons olive oil
- 1 large onion, chopped
- 2 celery stalks, chopped
- 2 carrots, chopped
- 2 bell peppers, seeded and chopped
- 1 green chili pepper, seeded and chopped
- 2 garlic cloves, minced
- Sea salt and ground black pepper, to taste
- 1 teaspoon cayenne pepper
- 1 teaspoon paprika

DIRECTIONS

1. In a saucepan, bring the Anasazi beans and broth to a boil. Once boiling, turn the heat to a simmer. Add in the bay laurel, thyme and rosemary; let it cook for about 50 minutes or until tender.
2. Meanwhile, in a heavy-bottomed pot, heat the olive oil over medium-high heat. Now, sauté the onion, celery, carrots and peppers for about 4 minutes until tender.
3. Add in the garlic and continue to sauté for 30 seconds more or until aromatic.
4. Add the sautéed mixture to the cooked beans. Season with salt, black pepper, cayenne pepper and paprika.
5. Continue to simmer, stirring periodically, for 10 minutes more or until everything is cooked through.

NUTRITION: Calories: 444, Fat: 15.8g, Carbs: 58.2g, Protein: 20.2g

162. EASY AND HEARTY SHAKSHUKA

COOKING: 10'   **PREPARATION: 10'**   **SERVES: 4**

INGREDIENTS

- 2 tablespoons olive oil
- 1 onion, chopped
- 2 bell peppers, chopped
- 1 poblano pepper, chopped
- 2 cloves garlic, minced
- 2 tomatoes, pureed
- Sea salt and black pepper, to taste
- 1 teaspoon dried basil
- 1 teaspoon red pepper flakes
- 1 teaspoon paprika
- 2 bay leaves
- 1 cup chickpeas, soaked overnight, rinsed and drained
- 3 cups vegetable broth
- 2 tablespoons fresh cilantro, roughly chopped

DIRECTIONS

1. Heat the olive oil in a saucepan over medium heat. Once hot, cook the onion, peppers and garlic for about 4 minutes, until tender and aromatic.
2. Add in the pureed tomato tomatoes, sea salt, black pepper, basil, red pepper, paprika and bay leaves.
3. Turn the heat to a simmer and add in the chickpeas and vegetable broth. Cook for 45 minutes or until tender.
4. Taste and adjust seasonings. Spoon your Shakshuka into individual bowls and serve garnished with the fresh cilantro.

NUTRITION: Calories: 324, Fat: 11.2g, Carbs: 42.2g, Protein: 15.8g

THE PLANT BASED DIET COOKBOOK

163. OLD-FASHIONED CHILI

COOKING: 10'   **PREPARATION: 10'**   **SERVES: 4**

INGREDIENTS

- 3/4-pound red kidney beans, soaked overnight
- 2 tablespoons olive oil
- 1 onion, chopped
- 2 bell peppers, chopped
- 1 red chili pepper, chopped
- 2 ribs celery, chopped
- 2 cloves garlic, minced
- 2 bay leaves
- 1 teaspoon ground cumin
- 1 teaspoon thyme, chopped
- 1 teaspoon black peppercorns
- 20 oz. tomatoes, crushed
- 2 cups vegetable broth
- 1 teaspoon smoked paprika
- Sea salt, to taste
- 2 tablespoons fresh cilantro, chopped
- 1 avocado, pitted, peeled and sliced

DIRECTIONS

1. Cover the soaked beans with a fresh change of cold water and bring to a boil. Let it boil for about 10 minutes. Turn the heat to a simmer and continue to cook for 50 to 55 minutes or until tender.
2. In a heavy-bottomed pot, heat the olive oil over medium heat. Once hot, sauté the onion, bell pepper and celery.
3. Sauté the garlic, bay leaves, ground cumin, thyme and black peppercorns for about 1 minute or so.
4. Add in the diced tomatoes, vegetable broth, paprika, salt and cooked beans. Let it simmer, stirring periodically, for 25 to 30 minutes or until cooked through.
5. Serve garnished with fresh cilantro and avocado.

NUTRITION: Calories: 514, Fat: 16.4g, Carbs: 72g, Protein: 25.8g

164. EASY RED LENTIL SALAD

COOKING: 10'   **PREPARATION: 10'**   **SERVES: 4**

INGREDIENTS

- 1/2 cup red lentils, soaked overnight and drained
- 1 ½ cups water
- 1 sprig rosemary
- 1 bay leaf
- 1 cup grape tomatoes, halved
- 1 cucumber, thinly sliced
- 1 bell pepper, thinly sliced
- 1 clove garlic, minced
- 1 onion, thinly sliced
- 2 tablespoons fresh lime juice
- 4 tablespoons olive oil
- Sea salt and ground black pepper, to taste

DIRECTIONS

1. Add the red lentils, water, rosemary and bay leaf to a saucepan and bring to a boil over high heat. Then, turn the heat to a simmer and continue to cook for 20 minutes or until tender.
2. Place the lentils in a salad bowl and let them cool completely.
3. Add in the remaining ingredients and toss to combine well. Serve at room temperature or well-chilled.

NUTRITION: Calories: 295, Fat: 18.8g, Carbs: 25.2g, Protein: 8.5g

165. MEDITERRANEAN-STYLE CHICKPEA SALAD

COOKING: 10'   **PREPARATION: 10'**   **SERVES: 4**

INGREDIENTS

- 2 cups chickpeas, soaked overnight and drained
- 1 Persian cucumber, sliced
- 1 cup cherry tomatoes, halved
- 1 red bell peppers, seeded and sliced
- 1 green bell pepper, seeded and sliced
- 1 teaspoon deli mustard
- 1 teaspoon coriander seeds
- 1 teaspoon jalapeno pepper, minced
- 1 tablespoon fresh lemon juice
- 1 tablespoon balsamic vinegar
- 1/4 cup extra-virgin olive oil
- Sea salt and ground black pepper, to taste
- 2 tablespoons fresh cilantro, chopped
- 2 tablespoons Kalamata olives, pitted and sliced

DIRECTIONS

1. Place the chickpeas in a stockpot; cover the chickpeas with water by 2 inches. Bring it to a boil.
2. Immediately turn the heat to a simmer and continue to cook for about 40 minutes or until tender.
3. Transfer your chickpeas to a salad bowl. Add in the remaining ingredients and toss to combine well.

NUTRITION: Calories: 444, Fat: 15.8g, Carbs: 58.2g, Protein: 20.2g

166. TRADITIONAL TUSCAN BEAN STEW (RIBOLLITA)

COOKING: 10'   **PREPARATION: 10'**   **SERVES: 4**

INGREDIENTS

- 3 tablespoons olive oil
- 1 medium leek, chopped
- 1 celery with leaves, chopped
- 1 zucchini, diced
- 1 Italian pepper, sliced
- 3 garlic cloves, crushed
- 2 bay leaves
- Kosher salt and ground black pepper, to taste
- 1 teaspoon cayenne pepper
- 1 (28-oz.) can tomatoes, crushed
- 2 cups vegetable broth
- 2 (15-oz.) cans Great Northern beans, drained
- 2 cups Lacinato kale, torn into pieces
- 1 cup crostini

DIRECTIONS

1. In a heavy-bottomed pot, heat the olive oil over medium heat. Once hot, sauté the leek, celery, zucchini and pepper for about 4 minutes.
2. Sauté the garlic and bay leaves for about 1 minute or so.
3. Add in the spices, tomatoes, broth and canned beans. Let it simmer, stirring occasionally, for about 15 minutes or until cooked through.
4. Add in the Lacinato kale and continue simmering, stirring occasionally, for 4 minutes.
5. Serve garnished with crostini.

NUTRITION: Calories: 324, Fat: 11.2g, Carbs: 42.2g, Protein: 15.8g

THE PLANT BASED DIET COOKBOOK

167. BELUGA LENTIL AND VEGETABLE MÉLANGE

COOKING: 10'   **PREPARATION: 10'**   **SERVES: 4**

INGREDIENTS

- 3 tablespoons olive oil
- 1 onion, minced
- 2 bell peppers, seeded and chopped
- 1 carrot, trimmed and chopped
- 1 parsnip, trimmed and chopped
- 1 teaspoon ginger, minced
- 2 cloves garlic, minced
- Sea salt and ground black pepper, to taste
- 1 large-sized zucchini, diced
- 1 cup tomato sauce
- 1 cup vegetable broth
- 1 ½ cups beluga lentils, soaked overnight and drained
- 2 cups Swiss chard

DIRECTIONS

1. In a Dutch oven, heat the olive oil until sizzling. Now, sauté the onion, bell pepper, carrot and parsnip, until they've softened.
2. Add in the ginger and garlic and continue sautéing an additional 30 seconds.
3. Now, add in the salt, black pepper, zucchini, tomato sauce, vegetable broth and lentils; let it simmer for about 20 minutes until everything is thoroughly cooked.
4. Add in the Swiss chard; cover and let it simmer for 5 minutes more.

NUTRITION: Calories: 382, Fat: 9.3g, Carbs: 59g, Protein: 17.2g

168. MEXICAN CHICKPEA TACO BOWLS

COOKING: 10'   **PREPARATION: 10'**   **SERVES: 4**

INGREDIENTS

- 2 tablespoons sesame oil
- 1 red onion, chopped
- 1 habanero pepper, minced
- 2 garlic cloves, crushed
- 2 bell peppers, seeded and diced
- Sea salt and ground black pepper
- 1/2 teaspoon Mexican oregano
- 1 teaspoon ground cumin
- 2 ripe tomatoes, pureed
- 1 teaspoon brown sugar
- 16 oz. canned chickpeas, drained
- 4 (8-inch) flour tortillas
- 2 tablespoons fresh coriander, roughly chopped

DIRECTIONS

1. In a large skillet, heat the sesame oil over a moderately high heat. Then, sauté the onions for 2 to 3 minutes or until tender.
2. Add in the peppers and garlic and continue to sauté for 1 minute or until fragrant.
3. Add in the spices, tomatoes and brown sugar and bring to a boil. Immediately turn the heat to a simmer, add in the canned chickpeas and let it cook for 8 minutes longer or until heated through.
4. Toast your tortillas and arrange them with the prepared chickpea mixture.
5. Top with fresh coriander and serve immediately.

NUTRITION: Calories: 409, Fat: 13.5g, Carbs: 61.3g, Protein: 13.8g

169. INDIAN DAL MAKHANI

COOKING: 10' **PREPARATION: 10'** **SERVES: 4**

INGREDIENTS

- 3 tablespoons sesame oil
- 1 large onion, chopped
- 1 bell pepper, seeded and chopped
- 2 garlic cloves, minced
- 1 tablespoon ginger, grated
- 2 green chilies, seeded and chopped
- 1 teaspoon cumin seeds
- 1 bay laurel
- 1 teaspoon turmeric powder
- 1/4 teaspoon red peppers
- 1/4 teaspoon ground allspice
- 1/2 teaspoon garam masala
- 1 cup tomato sauce
- 4 cups vegetable broth
- 1 ½ cups black lentils, soaked overnight and drained
- 4-5 curry leaves, for garnish

DIRECTIONS

1. In a saucepan, heat the sesame oil over medium-high heat; now, sauté the onion and bell pepper for 3 minutes more until they've softened.
2. Add in the garlic, ginger, green chilies, cumin seeds and bay laurel; continue to sauté, stirring frequently, for 1 minute or until fragrant.
3. Stir in the remaining ingredients, except for the curry leaves. Now, turn the heat to a simmer. Continue to cook for 15 minutes more or until thoroughly cooked.
4. Garnish with curry leaves and serve hot!

NUTRITION: Calories: 329, Fat: 8.5g, Carbs: 44.1g, Protein: 16.8g

170. MEXICAN-STYLE BEAN BOWL

COOKING: 10' **PREPARATION: 10'** **SERVES: 4**

INGREDIENTS

- 1 pound red beans, soaked overnight and drained
- 1 cup canned corn kernels, drained
- 2 roasted bell peppers, sliced
- 1 chili pepper, finely chopped
- 1 cup cherry tomatoes, halved
- 1 red onion, chopped
- 1/4 cup fresh cilantro, chopped
- 1/4 cup fresh parsley, chopped
- 1 teaspoon Mexican oregano
- 1/4 cup red wine vinegar
- 2 tablespoons fresh lemon juice
- 1/3 cup extra-virgin olive oil
- Sea salt and ground black, to taste
- 1 avocado, peeled, pitted and sliced

DIRECTIONS

1. Cover the soaked beans with a fresh change of cold water and bring to a boil. Let it boil for about 10 minutes. Turn the heat to a simmer and continue to cook for 50 to 55 minutes or until tender.
2. Allow your beans to cool completely, then, transfer them to a salad bowl.
3. Add in the remaining ingredients and toss to combine well. Serve at room temperature.

NUTRITION: Calories: 465, Fat: 17.9g, Carbs: 60.4g, Protein: 20.2g

THE PLANT BASED DIET COOKBOOK

171. CLASSIC ITALIAN MINESTRONE

COOKING: 10'   **PREPARATION: 10'**   **SERVES: 4**

INGREDIENTS

- 2 tablespoons olive oil
- 1 large onion, diced
- 2 carrots, sliced
- 4 cloves garlic, minced
- 1 cup elbow pasta
- 5 cups vegetable broth
- 1 (15-oz.) can white beans, drained
- 1 large zucchini, diced
- 1 (28-oz.) can tomatoes, crushed
- 1 tablespoon fresh oregano leaves, chopped
- 1 tablespoon fresh basil leaves, chopped
- 1 tablespoon fresh Italian parsley, chopped

DIRECTIONS

1. In a Dutch oven, heat the olive oil until sizzling. Now, sauté the onion and carrots until they've softened.
2. Add in the garlic, uncooked pasta and broth; let it simmer for about 15 minutes.
3. Stir in the beans, zucchini, tomatoes and herbs. Continue to cook, covered, for about 10 minutes until everything is thoroughly cooked.
4. Garnish with some extra herbs, if desired.

NUTRITION: Calories: 305, Fat: 8.6g, Carbs: 45.1g, Protein: 14.2g

172. GREEN LENTIL STEW WITH COLLARD GREENS

COOKING: 10'   **PREPARATION: 10'**   **SERVES: 4**

INGREDIENTS

- 2 tablespoons olive oil
- 1 onion, chopped
- 2 sweet potatoes, peeled and diced
- 1 bell pepper, chopped
- 2 carrots, chopped
- 1 parsnip, chopped
- 1 celery, chopped
- 2 cloves garlic
- 1 ½ cups green lentils
- 1 tablespoon Italian herb mix
- 1 cup tomato sauce
- 5 cups vegetable broth
- 1 cup frozen corn
- 1 cup collard greens, torn into pieces

DIRECTIONS

1. In a Dutch oven, heat the olive oil until sizzling. Now, sauté the onion, sweet potatoes, bell pepper, carrots, parsnip and celery until they've softened.
2. Add in the garlic and continue sautéing an additional 30 seconds.
3. Now, add in the green lentils, Italian herb mix, tomato sauce and vegetable broth; let it simmer for about 20 minutes until everything is thoroughly cooked.
4. Add in the frozen corn and collard greens; cover and let it simmer for 5 minutes more.

NUTRITION: Calories: 415, Fat: 6.6g, Carbs: 71g, Protein: 18.4g

173. CHICKPEA GARDEN VEGETABLE MEDLEY

COOKING: 10' | **PREPARATION: 10'** | **SERVES: 4**

INGREDIENTS

- 2 tablespoons olive oil
- 1 onion, finely chopped
- 1 bell pepper, chopped
- 1 fennel bulb, chopped
- 3 cloves garlic, minced
- 2 ripe tomatoes, pureed
- 2 tablespoons fresh parsley, roughly chopped
- 2 tablespoons fresh basil, roughly chopped
- 2 tablespoons fresh coriander, roughly chopped
- 2 cups vegetable broth
- 14 oz. canned chickpeas, drained
- Kosher salt and ground black pepper, to taste
- 1/2 teaspoon cayenne pepper
- 1 teaspoon paprika
- 1 avocado, peeled and sliced

DIRECTIONS

1. In a heavy-bottomed pot, heat the olive oil over medium heat. Once hot, sauté the onion, bell pepper and fennel bulb for about 4 minutes.
2. Sauté the garlic for about 1 minute or until aromatic.
3. Add in the tomatoes, fresh herbs, broth, chickpeas, salt, black pepper, cayenne pepper and paprika. Let it simmer, stirring occasionally, for about 20 minutes or until cooked through.
4. Taste and adjust the seasonings. Serve garnished with the slices of the fresh avocado.

NUTRITION: Calories: 369, Fat: 18.1g, Carbs: 43.5g, Protein: 13.2g

174. HOT BEAN DIPPING SAUCE

COOKING: 10' | **PREPARATION: 10'** | **SERVES: 4**

INGREDIENTS

- 2 (15-oz.) cans Great Northern beans, drained
- 2 tablespoons olive oil
- 2 tablespoons Sriracha sauce
- 2 tablespoons nutritional yeast
- 4 oz. vegan cream cheese
- 1/2 teaspoon paprika
- 1/2 teaspoon cayenne pepper
- 1/2 teaspoon ground cumin
- Sea salt and ground black pepper, to taste
- 4 oz. tortilla chips

DIRECTIONS

1. Start by preheating your oven to 360°F.
2. Pulse all the ingredients, except for the tortilla chips, in your food processor until your desired consistency is reached.
3. Bake your dip in the preheated oven for about 25 minutes or until hot.
4. Serve with tortilla chips and enjoy!

NUTRITION: Calories: 175, Fat: 4.7g, Carbs: 24.9g, Protein: 8.8g

THE PLANT BASED DIET COOKBOOK

175. CHINESE-STYLE SOYBEAN SALAD

COOKING: 10' **PREPARATION: 10'** **SERVES: 4**

INGREDIENTS

- 1 (15-oz.) can soybeans, drained
- 1 cup arugula
- 1 cup baby spinach
- 1 cup green cabbage, shredded
- 1 onion, thinly sliced
- 1/2 teaspoon garlic, minced
- 1 teaspoon ginger, minced
- 1/2 teaspoon deli mustard
- 2 tablespoons soy sauce
- 1 tablespoon rice vinegar
- 1 tablespoon lime juice
- 2 tablespoons tahini
- 1 teaspoon agave syrup

DIRECTIONS

1. In a salad bowl, place the soybeans, arugula, spinach, cabbage and onion; toss to combine.
2. In a small mixing dish, whisk the remaining ingredients for the dressing.
3. Dress your salad and serve immediately.

NUTRITION: Calories: 265, Fat: 13.7g, Carbs: 21g, Protein: 18g

176. OLD-FASHIONED LENTIL AND VEGETABLE STEW

COOKING: 10' **PREPARATION: 10'** **SERVES: 4**

INGREDIENTS

- 3 tablespoons olive oil
- 1 large onion, chopped
- 1 carrot, chopped
- 1 bell pepper, diced
- 1 habanero pepper, chopped
- 3 cloves garlic, minced
- Kosher salt and black pepper, to taste
- 1 teaspoon ground cumin
- 1 teaspoon smoked paprika
- 1 (28-oz.) can tomatoes, crushed
- 2 tablespoons tomato ketchup
- 4 cups vegetable broth
- 3/4 pound dry red lentils, soaked overnight and drained
- 1 avocado, sliced

DIRECTIONS

1. In a heavy-bottomed pot, heat the olive oil over medium heat. Once hot, sauté the onion, carrot and peppers for about 4 minutes.
2. Sauté the garlic for about 1 minute or so.
3. Add in the spices, tomatoes, ketchup, broth and canned lentils. Let it simmer, stirring occasionally, for about 20 minutes or until cooked through.
4. Serve garnished with the slices of avocado.

NUTRITION: Calories: 475, Fat: 17.3g, Carbs: 61.4g, Protein: 23.7g

177. INDIAN CHANA MASALA

COOKING: 10'　　**PREPARATION: 10'**　　**SERVES: 4**

INGREDIENTS

- 1 cup tomatoes, pureed
- 1 Kashmiri chile pepper, chopped
- 1 large shallot, chopped
- 1 teaspoon fresh ginger, peeled and grated
- 4 tablespoons olive oil
- 2 cloves garlic, minced
- 1 teaspoon coriander seeds
- 1 teaspoon garam masala
- 1/2 teaspoon turmeric powder
- Sea salt and ground black pepper, to taste
- 1/2 cup vegetable broth
- 16 oz. canned chickpeas
- 1 tablespoon fresh lime juice

DIRECTIONS

1. In your blender or food processor, blend the tomatoes, Kashmiri chile pepper, shallot and ginger into a paste.
2. In a saucepan, heat the olive oil over medium heat. Once hot, cook the prepared paste and garlic for about 2 minutes.
3. Add in the remaining spices, broth and chickpeas. Turn the heat to a simmer. Continue to simmer for 8 minutes more or until cooked through.
4. Remove from the heat. Drizzle fresh lime juice over the top of each serving.

NUTRITION: Calories: 305, Fat: 17.1g, Carbs: 30.1g, Protein: 9.4g

178. RED KIDNEY BEAN PÂTÉ

COOKING: 10'　　**PREPARATION: 10'**　　**SERVES: 4**

INGREDIENTS

- 2 tablespoons olive oil
- 1 onion, chopped
- 1 bell pepper, chopped
- 2 cloves garlic, minced
- 2 cups red kidney beans, boiled and drained
- 1/4 cup olive oil
- 1 teaspoon stone-ground mustard
- 2 tablespoons fresh parsley, chopped
- 2 tablespoons fresh basil, chopped
- Sea salt and ground black pepper, to taste

DIRECTIONS

1. In a saucepan, heat the olive oil over medium-high heat. Now, cook the onion, pepper and garlic until just tender or about 3 minutes.
2. Add the sautéed mixture to your blender; add in the remaining ingredients. Puree the ingredients in your blender or food processor until smooth and creamy.

NUTRITION: Calories: 135, Fat: 12.1g, Carbs: 4.4g, Protein: 1.6g

THE PLANT BASED DIET COOKBOOK

179. BROWN LENTIL BOWL

COOKING: 10'   **PREPARATION: 10'**   **SERVES: 4**

INGREDIENTS

- 1 cup brown lentils, soaked overnight and drained
- 3 cups water
- 2 cups brown rice, cooked
- 1 zucchini, diced
- 1 red onion, chopped
- 1 teaspoon garlic, minced
- 1 cucumber, sliced
- 1 bell pepper, sliced
- 4 tablespoons olive oil
- 1 tablespoon rice vinegar
- 2 tablespoons lemon juice
- 2 tablespoons soy sauce
- 1/2 teaspoon dried oregano
- 1/2 teaspoon ground cumin
- Sea salt and ground black pepper, to taste
- 2 cups arugula
- 2 cups Romaine lettuce, torn into pieces

DIRECTIONS

1. Add the brown lentils and water to a saucepan and bring to a boil over high heat. Then, turn the heat to a simmer and continue to cook for 20 minutes or until tender.
2. Place the lentils in a salad bowl and let them cool completely.
3. Add in the remaining ingredients and toss to combine well. Serve at room temperature or well-chilled

NUTRITION: Calories: 452, Fat: 16.6g, Carbs: 61.7g, Protein: 16.4g

180. HOT AND SPICY ANASAZI BEAN SOUP

COOKING: 10'   **PREPARATION: 10'**   **SERVES: 4**

INGREDIENTS

- 2 cups Anasazi beans, soaked overnight, drained and rinsed
- 8 cups water
- 2 bay leaves
- 3 tablespoons olive oil
- 2 medium onions, chopped
- 2 bell peppers, chopped
- 1 habanero pepper, chopped
- 3 cloves garlic, pressed or minced
- Sea salt and ground black pepper, to taste

DIRECTIONS

1. In a soup pot, bring the Anasazi beans and water to a boil. Once boiling, turn the heat to a simmer. Add in the bay leaves and let it cook for about 1 hour or until tender.
2. Meanwhile, in a heavy-bottomed pot, heat the olive oil over medium-high heat. Now, sauté the onion, peppers and garlic for about 4 minutes until tender.
3. Add the sautéed mixture to the cooked beans. Season with salt and black pepper.
4. Continue to simmer, stirring periodically, for 10 minutes more or until everything is cooked through.

NUTRITION: Calories: 352, Fat: 8.5g, Carbs: 50.1g, Protein: 19.7g

181. BLACK-EYED PEA SALAD (ÑEBBE)

COOKING: 10' **PREPARATION: 10'** **SERVES: 4**

INGREDIENTS

- 2 cups dried black-eyed peas, soaked overnight and drained
- 2 tablespoons basil leaves, chopped
- 2 tablespoons parsley leaves, chopped
- 1 shallot, chopped
- 1 cucumber, sliced
- 2 bell peppers, seeded and diced
- 1 Scotch bonnet chili pepper, seeded and finely chopped
- 1 cup cherry tomatoes, quartered
- Sea salt and ground black pepper, to taste
- 2 tablespoons fresh lime juice
- 1 tablespoon apple cider vinegar
- 1/4 cup extra-virgin olive oil
- 1 avocado, peeled, pitted and sliced

DIRECTIONS

1. Cover the black-eyed peas with water by 2 inches and bring to a gentle boil. Let it boil for about 15 minutes.
2. Then, turn the heat to a simmer for about 45 minutes. Let it cool completely.
3. Place the black-eyed peas in a salad bowl. Add in the basil, parsley, shallot, cucumber, bell peppers, cherry tomatoes, salt and black pepper.
4. In a mixing bowl, whisk the lime juice, vinegar and olive oil.
5. Dress the salad, garnish with fresh avocado and serve immediately.

NUTRITION: Calories: 471, Fat: 17.5g, Carbs: 61.5g, Protein: 20.6g

182. MOM'S FAMOUS CHILI

COOKING: 10' **PREPARATION: 10'** **SERVES: 4**

INGREDIENTS

- 1 pound red black beans, soaked overnight and drained
- 3 tablespoons olive oil
- 1 large red onion, diced
- 2 bell peppers, diced
- 1 poblano pepper, minced
- 1 large carrot, trimmed and diced
- 2 cloves garlic, minced
- 2 bay leaves
- 1 teaspoon mixed peppercorns
- Kosher salt and cayenne pepper, to taste
- 1 tablespoon paprika
- 2 ripe tomatoes, pureed
- 2 tablespoons tomato ketchup
- 3 cups vegetable broth

DIRECTIONS

1. Cover the soaked beans with a fresh change of cold water and bring to a boil. Let it boil for about 10 minutes. Turn the heat to a simmer and continue to cook for 50 to 55 minutes or until tender.
2. In a heavy-bottomed pot, heat the olive oil over medium heat. Once hot, sauté the onion, peppers and carrot.
3. Sauté the garlic for about 30 seconds or until aromatic.
4. Add in the remaining ingredients along with the cooked beans. Let it simmer, stirring periodically, for 25 to 30 minutes or until cooked through.
5. Discard the bay leaves, ladle into individual bowls and serve hot!

NUTRITION: Calories: 455, Fat: 10.5g, Carbs: 68.6g, Protein: 24.7g

183. CREAMED CHICKPEA SALAD WITH PINE NUTS

COOKING: 10' **PREPARATION: 10'** **SERVES: 4**

INGREDIENTS

- 16 oz. canned chickpeas, drained
- 1 teaspoon garlic, minced
- 1 shallot, chopped
- 1 cup cherry tomatoes, halved
- 1 bell pepper, seeded and sliced
- 1/4 cup fresh basil, chopped
- 1/4 cup fresh parsley, chopped
- 1/2 cup vegan mayonnaise
- 1 tablespoon lemon juice
- 1 teaspoon capers, drained
- Sea salt and ground black pepper, to taste
- 2 oz. pine nuts

DIRECTIONS

1. Place the chickpeas, vegetables and herbs in a salad bowl.
2. Add in the mayonnaise, lemon juice, capers, salt and black pepper. Stir to combine.
3. Top with pine nuts and serve immediately.

NUTRITION: Calories: 386, Fat: 22.5g, Carbs: 37.2g, Protein: 12.9g

184. BLACK BEAN BUDA BOWL

COOKING: 10' **PREPARATION: 10'** **SERVES: 4**

INGREDIENTS

- 1/2 pound black beans, soaked overnight and drained
- 2 cups brown rice, cooked
- 1 medium-sized onion, thinly sliced
- 1 cup bell pepper, seeded and sliced
- 1 jalapeno pepper, seeded and sliced
- 2 cloves garlic, minced
- 1 cup arugula
- 1 cup baby spinach
- 1 teaspoon lime zest
- 1 tablespoon Dijon mustard
- 1/4 cup red wine vinegar
- 1/4 cup extra-virgin olive oil
- 2 tablespoons agave syrup
- Flaky sea salt and ground black pepper, to taste
- 1/4 cup fresh Italian parsley, roughly chopped

DIRECTIONS

1. Cover the soaked beans with a fresh change of cold water and bring to a boil. Let it boil for about 10 minutes. Turn the heat to a simmer and continue to cook for 50 to 55 minutes or until tender.
2. To serve, divide the beans and rice between serving bowls; top with the vegetables.
3. A small mixing dish thoroughly combines the lime zest, mustard, vinegar, olive oil, agave syrup, salt and pepper. Drizzle the vinaigrette over the salad.
4. Garnish with fresh Italian parsley.

NUTRITION: Calories: 365, Fat: 14.1g, Carbs: 45.6g, Protein: 15.5g

185. MIDDLE EASTERN CHICKPEA STEW

COOKING: 10'   **PREPARATION: 10'**   **SERVES: 4**

INGREDIENTS

- 1 onion, chopped
- 1 chili pepper, chopped
- 2 garlic cloves, chopped
- 1 teaspoon mustard seeds
- 1 teaspoon coriander seeds
- 1 bay leaf
- 1/2 cup tomato puree
- 2 tablespoons olive oil
- 1 celery with leaves, chopped
- 2 medium carrots, trimmed and chopped
- 2 cups vegetable broth
- 1 teaspoon ground cumin
- 1 small-sized cinnamon stick
- 16 oz. canned chickpeas, drained
- 2 cups Swiss chard, torn into pieces

DIRECTIONS

1. In your blender or food processor, blend the onion, chili pepper, garlic, mustard seeds, coriander seeds, bay leaf and tomato puree into a paste.
2. In a stockpot, heat the olive oil until sizzling. Now, cook the celery and carrots for about 3 minutes or until they've softened. Add in the paste and continue to cook for a further 2 minutes.
3. Then, add vegetable broth, cumin, cinnamon and chickpeas; bring it to a gentle boil.
4. Turn the heat to simmer and let it cook for 6 minutes; fold in Swiss chard and continue to cook for 4 to 5 minutes more or until the leaves wilt. Serve hot and enjoy!

NUTRITION: Calories: 305, Fat: 11.2g, Carbs: 38.6g, Protein: 12.7g

186. LENTIL AND TOMATO DIP

COOKING: 10'   **PREPARATION: 10'**   **SERVES: 4**

INGREDIENTS

- 16 oz. lentils, boiled and drained
- 4 tablespoons sun-dried tomatoes, chopped
- 1 cup tomato paste
- 4 tablespoons tahini
- 1 teaspoon stone-ground mustard
- 1 teaspoon ground cumin
- 1/4 teaspoon ground bay leaf
- 1 teaspoon red pepper flakes
- Sea salt and ground black pepper, to taste

DIRECTIONS

1. Blitz all the ingredients in your blender or food processor until your desired consistency is reached.
2. Place in your refrigerator until ready to serve.
3. Serve with toasted pita wedges or vegetable sticks. Enjoy!

NUTRITION: Calories: 144, Fat: 4.5g, Carbs: 20.2g, Protein: 8.1g

THE PLANT BASED DIET COOKBOOK

187. CREAMED GREEN PEA SALAD

COOKING: 10' **PREPARATION: 10'** **SERVES: 4**

INGREDIENTS

- 2 (14.5 oz.) cans green peas, drained
- 1/2 cup vegan mayonnaise
- 1 teaspoon Dijon mustard
- 2 tablespoons scallions, chopped
- 2 pickles, chopped
- 1/2 cup marinated mushrooms, chopped and drained
- 1/2 teaspoon garlic, minced
- Sea salt and ground black pepper, to taste

DIRECTIONS

1. Place all the ingredients in a salad bowl. Gently stir to combine.
2. Place the salad in your refrigerator until ready to serve.

NUTRITION: Calories: 154, Fat: 6.7g, Carbs: 17.3g, Protein: 6.9g

---

188. MIDDLE EASTERN ZA'ATAR HUMMUS

COOKING: 10' **PREPARATION: 10'** **SERVES: 4**

INGREDIENTS

- 10 oz. chickpeas, boiled and drained
- 1/4 cup tahini
- 2 tablespoons extra-virgin olive oil
- 2 tablespoons sun-dried tomatoes, chopped
- 1 lemon, freshly squeezed
- 2 garlic cloves, minced
- Kosher salt and ground black pepper, to taste
- 1/2 teaspoon smoked paprika
- 1 teaspoon Za'atar

DIRECTIONS

1. Blitz all the ingredients in your food processor until creamy and uniform.
2. Place in your refrigerator until ready to serve.

NUTRITION: Calories: 140, Fat: 8.5g, Carbs: 12.4g, Protein: 4.6g

CHAPTER 12: SOUPS AND STEWS

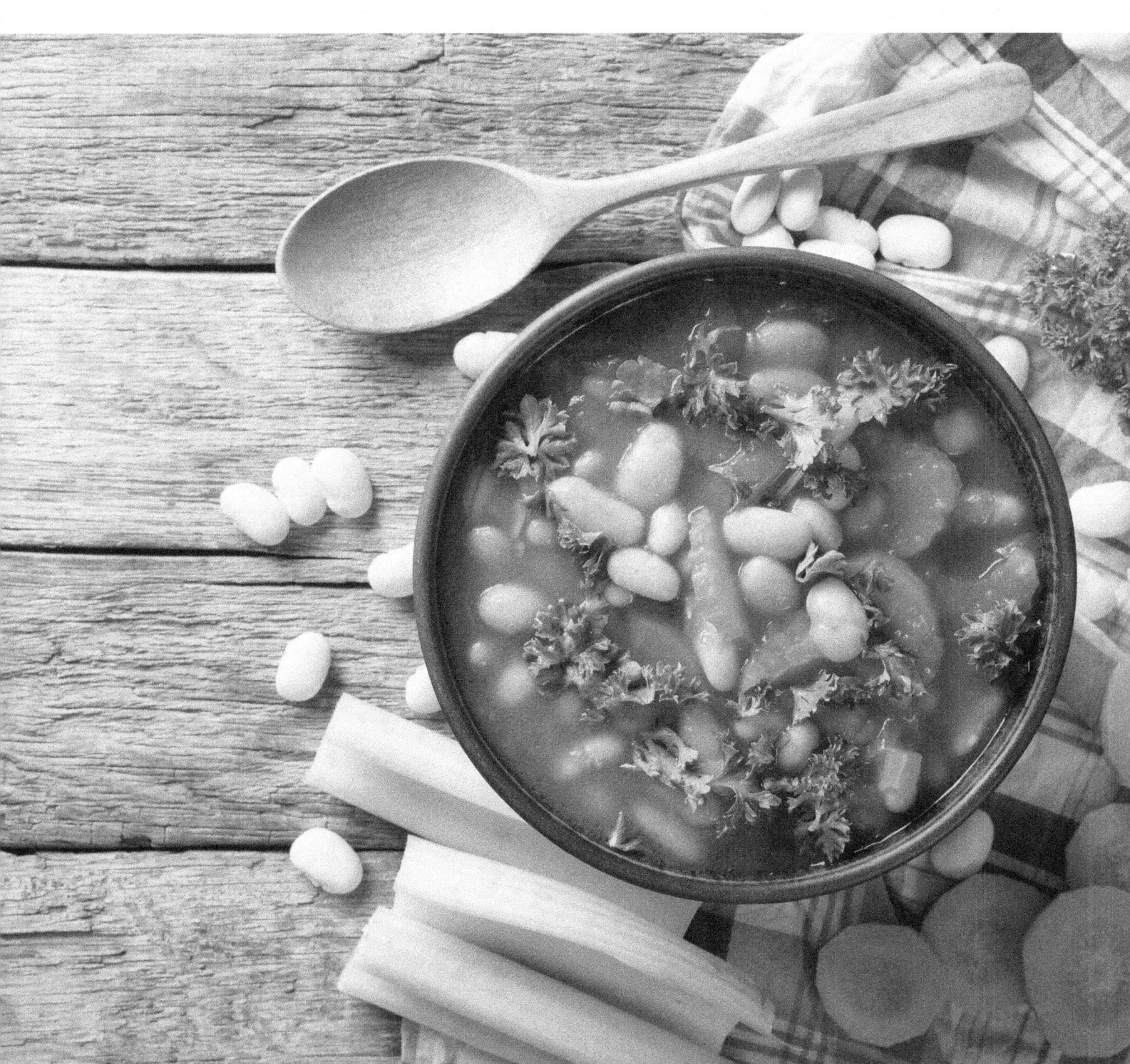

189. TOMATO GAZPACHO

COOKING: 55'   **PREPARATION: 30'**   **SERVES: 6**

INGREDIENTS

- 2 Tablespoons + 1 Teaspoon Red Wine Vinegar, Divided
- ½ Teaspoon Pepper
- 1 Teaspoon Sea Salt
- 1 Avocado,
- ¼ Cup Basil, Fresh & Chopped
- 3 Tablespoons + 2 Teaspoons Olive Oil, Divided
- 1 Clove Garlic, crushed
- 1 Red Bell Pepper, Sliced & Seeded
- 1 Cucumber, Chunked
- 2 ½ lbs. Large Tomatoes, Cored & Chopped

DIRECTIONS

1. Place half of your cucumber, bell pepper, and ¼ cup of each tomato in a bowl, covering. Set it in the fried.
2. Puree your remaining tomatoes, cucumber and bell pepper with garlic, three tablespoons oil, two tablespoons of vinegar, sea salt and black pepper into a blender, blending until smooth. Transfer it to a bowl, and chill for two hours.
3. Chop the avocado, adding it to your chopped vegetables, adding your remaining oil, vinegar, salt, pepper and basil.
4. Ladle your tomato puree mixture into bowls, and serve with chopped vegetables as a salad.

NUTRITION: Calories: 201 Protein: 23g Fat: 4g Carbs: 2g

190. TOMATO PUMPKIN SOUP

COOKING: 25'   **PREPARATION: 25'**   **SERVES: 4**

INGREDIENTS

- 2 cups pumpkin, diced
- 1/2 cup tomato, chopped
- 1/2 cup onion, chopped
- 1 1/2 tsp curry powder
- 1/2 tsp paprika
- 2 cups vegetable stock
- 1 tsp olive oil
- 1/2 tsp garlic, minced

DIRECTIONS

1. In a saucepan, add oil, garlic, and onion and sauté for 3 minutes over medium heat.
2. Add remaining ingredients into the saucepan and bring to boil.
3. Reduce heat and cover and simmer for 10 minutes.
4. Puree the soup using a blender until smooth.
5. Stir well and serve warm.

NUTRITION: Calories: 340 Protein: 50g Carbs: 14g Fat: 10g

191. CREAMY GARLIC ONION SOUP

COOKING: 25'   **PREPARATION: 45'**   **SERVES: 4**

INGREDIENTS

- 1 onion, sliced
- 4 cups vegetable stock
- 1 1/2 tbsp olive oil
- 1 shallot, sliced
- 2 garlic clove, chopped
- 1 leek, sliced
- Salt

DIRECTIONS

1. Add stock and olive oil in a saucepan and bring to boil.
2. Add remaining ingredients and stir well.
3. Cover and simmer for 25 minutes.
4. Puree the soup using an immersion blender until smooth.
5. Stir well and serve warm.

NUTRITION: Calories: 115 Protein: 30g Fat: 0g Carbs: 3g

192. AVOCADO BROCCOLI SOUP

COOKING: 5'   **PREPARATION: 20'**   **SERVES: 4**

INGREDIENTS

- 2 cups broccoli florets, chopped
- 5 cups vegetable broth
- 2 avocados, chopped
- Pepper
- Salt

DIRECTIONS

1. Cook broccoli in boiling water for 5 minutes. Drain well.
2. Add broccoli, vegetable broth, avocados, pepper, and salt to the blender and blend until smooth.
3. Stir well and serve warm.

NUTRITION: Calories: 265 Protein: 35g Fat: 13 Carbs: 5

193. GREEN SPINACH KALE SOUP

COOKING: 5'   **PREPARATION: 10'**   **SERVES: 6**

INGREDIENTS

- 2 avocados
- 8 oz. spinach
- 8 oz. kale
- 1 fresh lime juice
- 1 cup water
- 3 1/3 cup coconut milk
- 3 oz. olive oil
- 1/4 tsp pepper
- 1 tsp salt

DIRECTIONS

1. Heat olive oil in a saucepan over medium heat.
2. Add kale and spinach to the saucepan and sauté for 2-3 minutes. Remove saucepan from heat. Add coconut milk, spices, avocado, and water. Stir well.
3. Puree the soup using an immersion blender until smooth and creamy. Add fresh lime juice and stir well.
4. Serve and enjoy.
5.

NUTRITION: Calories: 312 Protein: 9g Fat: 10 Carbs: 22

THE PLANT BASED DIET COOKBOOK

194. CAULIFLOWER ASPARAGUS SOUP

COOKING: 30' **PREPARATION: 10'** **SERVES: 4**

INGREDIENTS

- 20 asparagus spears, chopped
- 4 cups vegetable stock
- ½ cauliflower head, chopped
- 2 garlic cloves, chopped
- 1 tbsp coconut oil
- Pepper
- Salt

DIRECTIONS

1. Heat coconut oil in a large saucepan over medium heat.
2. Add garlic and sauté until softened.
3. Add cauliflower, vegetable stock, pepper, and salt. Stir well and bring to boil.
4. Reduce heat to low and simmer for 20 minutes.
5. Add chopped asparagus and cook until softened.
6. Puree the soup using an immersion blender until smooth and creamy.
7. Stir well and serve warm.

NUTRITION: Calories: 298 Carbs: 26g Protein: 21g Fat: 9g

195. AFRICAN PINEAPPLE PEANUT STEW

COOKING: 20' **PREPARATION: 10'** **SERVES: 4**

INGREDIENTS

- 4 cups sliced kale
- 1 cup chopped onion
- 1/2 cup peanut butter
- 1 tbsp. hot pepper sauce or 1 tbsp. Tabasco sauce
- 2 minced garlic cloves
- 1/2 cup chopped cilantro
- 2 cups pineapple, undrained, canned & crushed
- 1 tbsp. vegetable oil

DIRECTIONS

1. In a saucepan (preferably covered), sauté the garlic and onions in the oil until the onions are lightly browned, approximately 10 minutes, stirring often.
2. Wash the kale, till the time the onions are sauté.
3. Get rid of the stems. Mound the leaves on a cutting surface & slice crosswise into slices (preferably 1" thick).
4. Now put the pineapple and juice to the onions & bring to a simmer. Stir the kale in, cover and simmer until just tender, stirring frequently, approximately 5 minutes.
5. Mix in the hot pepper sauce, peanut butter & simmer for more 5 minutes.
6. Add salt according to your taste.

NUTRITION: Calories: 265 Protein: 35g Fat: 13 Carbs: 5

193. GREEN SPINACH KALE SOUP

COOKING: 5' **PREPARATION: 10'** **SERVES: 6**

INGREDIENTS

- 2 avocados
- 8 oz. spinach
- 8 oz. kale
- 1 fresh lime juice
- 1 cup water
- 3 1/3 cup coconut milk
- 3 oz. olive oil
- 1/4 tsp pepper
- 1 tsp salt

DIRECTIONS

1. Heat olive oil in a saucepan over medium heat.
2. Add kale and spinach to the saucepan and sauté for 2-3 minutes. Remove saucepan from heat. Add coconut milk, spices, avocado, and water. Stir well.
3. Puree the soup using an immersion blender until smooth and creamy. Add fresh lime juice and stir well.
4. Serve and enjoy.

NUTRITION: Calories: 402 Carbs: 7g Protein: 21g Fat: 34g

196. CABBAGE & BEET STEW

COOKING: 10'   **PREPARATION: 20'**   **SERVES: 4**

INGREDIENTS

- 2 Tablespoons Olive Oil
- 3 Cups Vegetable Broth
- 2 Tablespoons Lemon Juice, Fresh
- ½ Teaspoon Garlic Powder
- ½ Cup Carrots, Shredded
- 2 Cups Cabbage, Shredded
- 1 Cup Beets, Shredded
- Dill for Garnish
- ½ Teaspoon Onion Powder
- Sea Salt & Black Pepper to Taste

DIRECTIONS

1. Heat oil in a pot, and then sauté your vegetables.
2. Pour your broth in, mixing in your seasoning. Simmer until it's cooked through, and then top with dill.

NUTRITION: Calories: 263 Carbs: 8g Protein: 20.3g Fat: 24g

197. BASIL TOMATO SOUP

COOKING: 10'   **PREPARATION: 10'**   **SERVES: 6**

INGREDIENTS

- 28 oz. can tomatoes
- ¼ cup basil pesto
- ¼ tsp dried basil leaves
- 1 tsp apple cider vinegar
- 2 tbsp erythritol
- ¼ tsp garlic powder
- ½ tsp onion powder
- 2 cups water
- 1 ½ tsp kosher salt

DIRECTIONS

1. Add tomatoes, garlic powder, onion powder, water, and salt in a saucepan.
2. Bring to boil over medium heat. Reduce heat and simmer for 2 minutes.
3. Remove saucepan from heat and puree the soup using a blender until smooth.
4. Stir in pesto, dried basil, vinegar, and erythritol.
5. Stir well and serve warm.

NUTRITION: Calories: 662 Carbs: 18g Protein: 8g Fat: 55g

198. MUSHROOM & BROCCOLI SOUP

COOKING: 45'   **PREPARATION: 20'**   **SERVES: 8**

INGREDIENTS

- 1 bundle broccoli (around 1-1/2 lb.)
- 1 tablespoon canola oil
- 1/2 pound cut crisp mushrooms
- 1 tablespoon diminished sodium soy sauce
- 2 medium carrots, finely slashed
- 2 celery ribs, finely slashed
- 1/4 cup finely slashed onion
- 1 garlic clove, minced
- 1 container (32 oz.) vegetable juices
- 2 cups of water
- 2 tablespoons lemon juice

DIRECTIONS

1. Cut broccoli florets into reduced down pieces. Strip and hack stalks.
2. In an enormous pot, heat oil over medium-high warmth; saute mushrooms until delicate, 4-6 minutes. Mix in soy sauce; expel from skillet.
3. In the same container, join broccoli stalks, carrots, celery, onion, garlic, soup, and water; heat to the point of boiling. Diminish heat; stew, revealed, until vegetables are relaxed, 25-30 minutes.
4. Puree soup utilizing a drenching blender. Or then again, cool marginally, puree the soup in a blender; come back to the dish.
5. Mix in florets and mushrooms; heat to the point of boiling. Lessen warmth to medium; cook until broccoli is delicate, 8-10 minutes, blending infrequently. Mix in lemon juice.

NUTRITION: Calories: 830 Carbs: 8g Protein: 45g Fat: 64g

THE PLANT BASED DIET COOKBOOK

199. CREAMY CAULIFLOWER PAKORA SOUP

COOKING: 20' **PREPARATION: 20'** **SERVES: 8**

INGREDIENTS

- 1 huge head cauliflower, cut into little florets
- 5 medium potatoes, stripped and diced
- 1 huge onion, diced
- 4 medium carrots, stripped and diced
- 2 celery ribs, diced
- 1 container (32 oz.) vegetable stock
- 1 teaspoon garam masala
- 1 teaspoon garlic powder
- 1 teaspoon ground coriander
- 1 teaspoon ground turmeric
- 1 teaspoon ground cumin
- 1 teaspoon pepper
- 1 teaspoon salt
- 1/2 teaspoon squashed red pepper chips
- Water or extra vegetable stock
- New cilantro leaves
- Lime wedges, discretionary

DIRECTIONS

1. In a Dutch stove over medium-high warmth, heat initial 14 fixings to the point of boiling. Cook and mix until vegetables are delicate, around 20 minutes. Expel from heat; cool marginally. Procedure in groups in a blender or nourishment processor until smooth. Modify consistency as wanted with water (or extra stock). Sprinkle with new cilantro. Serve hot, with lime wedges whenever wanted.
2. Stop alternative: Before including cilantro, solidify cooled soup in cooler compartments. To utilize, in part defrost in cooler medium-term.
3. Warmth through in a pan, blending every so often and including a little water if fundamental. Sprinkle with cilantro. Whenever wanted, present with lime wedges.

NUTRITION: Calories: 248 Carbs: 7g Protein: 1g Fat: 19g

200. GARDEN VEGETABLE AND HERB SOUP

COOKING: 30' **PREPARATION: 20'** **SERVES: 8**

INGREDIENTS

- 2 tablespoons olive oil
- 2 medium onions, hacked
- 2 huge carrots, cut
- 1 pound red potatoes (around 3 medium), cubed
- 2 cups of water
- 1 can (14-1/2 oz.) diced tomatoes in sauce
- 1-1/2 cups vegetable soup
- 1-1/2 teaspoons garlic powder
- 1 teaspoon dried basil
- 1/2 teaspoon salt
- 1/2 teaspoon paprika
- 1/4 teaspoon dill weed
- 1/4 teaspoon pepper
- 1 medium yellow summer squash, split and cut
- 1 medium zucchini, split and cut

DIRECTIONS

1. In a huge pan, heat oil over medium warmth. Include onions and carrots; cook and mix until onions are delicate, 4-6 minutes. Include potatoes and cook 2 minutes. Mix in water, tomatoes, juices, and seasonings.
2. Heat to the point of boiling. Diminish heat; stew, revealed, until potatoes and carrots are delicate, 9 minutes.
3. Include yellow squash and zucchini; cook until vegetables are delicate, 9 minutes longer. Serve or, whenever wanted, puree blend in clusters, including extra stock until desired consistency is accomplished.

NUTRITION: Calories: 252 Carbs: 12g Protein: 1g Fat: 11g

201. THE MEDITERRANEAN DELIGHT WITH FRESH VINAIGRETTE

COOKING: 10' **PREPARATION: 5'** **SERVES: 2**

INGREDIENTS

Herbed citrus vinaigrette:
- 1 tablespoon of lemon juice
- 2 tablespoons of orange juice
- ½ teaspoon of lemon zest
- ½ teaspoon of orange zest
- 2 tablespoons of olive oil
- 1 tablespoon of finely chopped fresh oregano leaves
- Salt to taste
- Black pepper to taste
- 2-3 tablespoons of freshly julienned mint leaves

Salad:
- 1 freshly diced medium-sized cucumber
- 2 cups of cooked and rinsed chickpeas
- ½ cup of freshly diced red onion
- 2 freshly diced medium-sized tomatoes
- 1 freshly diced red bell pepper
- ¼ cup of green olives
- ½ cup of pomegranates

DIRECTIONS

1. In a large salad bowl, add the juice and zest of both the lemon and the orange and oregano and olive oil. Whisk together so that they are mixed well. Season the vinaigrette with salt and pepper to taste.
2. After draining the chickpeas, add them to the dressing. Then, add the onions. Give them a thorough mix, so that the onion and chickpeas absorb the flavors.
3. Now, chop the rest of the veggies and start adding them to the salad bowl. Give them a good toss.
4. Lastly, add the olives and fresh mint. Adjust the salt and pepper as required.
5. Serve this Mediterranean delight chilled — a cool summer salad that is good for the tummy and the soul.

NUTRITION: Calories: 286 Carbs: 29g Protein: 1g Fat: 11g

202. VEGETABLE BROTH SANS SODIUM

COOKING: 60' **PREPARATION: 5'** **SERVES: 1 CUP**

INGREDIENTS

- 5 sprigs of dill
- 2 freshly sliced yellow onions
- 4 chives
- 6 freshly peeled and sliced carrots
- 10 cups of water
- 4 freshly sliced celery stalks
- 3 cloves of freshly minced garlic
- 4 sprigs of parsley

DIRECTIONS

1. Put a large pot on medium heat and stir the onions. Fry the onions for 1 minute until they become fragrant. Add the garlic, celery, carrots, and dill along with the chives and parsley and cook everything. You will know that the mix is ready when it becomes fragrant.
2. Add the water and allow the mixture to boil. Reduce the heat and allow everything to cook for 45 minutes.
3. Turn off the heat. The broth will cool in about 15 minutes.
4. Strain the broth with the help of a sieve so that you have a clear vegetable broth.
5. If you are not using the broth right away, store it as ice cubes. You can store the ice cubes for a week.

NUTRITION: Calories: 362 Carbs: 12g Protein: 12g Fat: 12g

203. AMAZING CHICKPEA AND NOODLE SOUP

COOKING: 20'   **PREPARATION: 10'**   **SERVES: 1**

INGREDIENTS

- 1 freshly diced celery stalk
- ¼ cup of 'chicken' seasoning
- 1 cup of freshly diced onion
- 3 cloves of freshly crushed garlic
- 2 cups of cooked chickpeas
- 4 cups of vegetable broth
- Freshly chopped cilantro
- 2 freshly cubed medium-size potatoes
- Salt
- 2 freshly sliced carrots
- ½ teaspoon of dried thyme
- Pepper
- 2 cups of water
- 6 oz. of gluten-free spaghetti
- 'Chicken' seasoning
- 1 tablespoon of garlic powder
- 2 teaspoons of sea salt
- 1 1/3 cup of nutritional yeast
- 3 tablespoons of onion powder
- 1 teaspoon of oregano
- ½ teaspoon of turmeric
- 1 ½ tablespoons of dried basil

DIRECTIONS

1. Put a pot on medium heat and sauté the onion. It will soften within 3 minutes.
2. Add celery, potato, and carrots and sauté for another 3 minutes
3. Add the 'chicken' seasoning to the garlic, thyme, water, and vegetable broth.
4. Simmer the mix on medium-high heat. Cook the veggies for about 20 minutes until they soften.
5. Add the cooked pasta and chickpeas.
6. Add salt and pepper to taste.
7. Put the fresh cilantro on top and enjoy the fresh soup!

NUTRITION: Calories: 405 Carbs: 21g Protein: 19g Fat: 18g

204. LENTIL SOUP THE VEGAN WAY

COOKING: 20'   **PREPARATION: 5'**   **SERVES: 1 CUP**

INGREDIENTS

- 2 tablespoons of water
- 4 stalks of thinly sliced celery
- 2 cloves of freshly minced garlic
- 4 thinly sliced large carrots
- Sea salt
- 2 freshly diced small shallots
- Pepper
- 3 cups of red/yellow baby potatoes
- 2 cups of chopped sturdy greens
- 4 cups of vegetable broth
- 1 cup of uncooked brown or green lentils
- Fresh rosemary/thyme

DIRECTIONS

1. Put a large pot over medium heat. Once the pot is hot enough, add the shallots, garlic, celery, and carrots in water. Season the veggies with a little bit of pepper and salt.
2. Sauté the veggies for 5 minutes until they are tender. You will know that the veggies are ready when they have turned golden brown. Be careful with the garlic, because it can easily burn.
3. Add the potatoes and some more seasoning. Cook for 2 minutes.
4. Mix the vegetable broth with the rosemary. Now Increase the heat to medium-high. Allow the veggies to be in a rolling simmer. Add the lentils and give everything a thorough stir.
5. Once it starts to simmer again, decrease the heat and simmer for about 20 minutes without a cover. You will know that the veggies are ready when both the lentils and potatoes are soft
6. Add the greens. Cook for 4 minutes until they wilt. You can adjust the flavor with seasonings.
7. Enjoy this with rice or flatbread. The leftovers are equally tasty, so store them well to enjoy on a day when you are not in the mood to cook.

NUTRITION: Calories: 284 Carbs: 21g Protein: 11g Fat: 19g

205. BEET AND KALE SALAD

COOKING: 5'   **PREPARATION: 5'**   **SERVES: 1**

INGREDIENTS

- 8 oz. of beet and kale blend
- 1 tablespoon of olive oil
- 1 cucumber
- 6 oz. of chickpeas
- Salt
- 2 tablespoons of red wine vinegar
- Pepper
- ¼ cup of walnuts
- 2 oz. of dried cranberries
- Cashew cheese

DIRECTIONS

1. Cut the veggies and combine everything in a big salad bowl.
2. Serve the fresh salad and enjoy a hearty meal.

NUTRITION: Calories: 490 Carbs: 31g Protein: 19g Fat: 21g

206. KALE AND CAULIFLOWER SALAD

COOKING: 15'   **PREPARATION: 10'**   **SERVES: 1**

INGREDIENTS

- 6 oz. of Lacinato kale
- 8 oz. of cauliflower florets
- 1 lemon
- 1 tablespoon of Italian spice
- 2 radishes
- oz. of butter beans
- Olive oil
- ¼ cup of walnuts
- ¼ cup of vegan Caesar dressing
- Pepper
- Salt

DIRECTIONS

1. Preheat the oven to 400°F. Put the cauliflower florets on a baking sheet, toss them with olive oil and spices, and add salt. Roast the cauliflower until it is brown. It will be done within 15-20 minutes.
2. De-stem the kale and slice the leaves. Slice the radishes. Both kale and radish should be sliced thinly. Cut the lemon in half.
3. Put the kale in a large bowl and add the lemon juice and salt along with the pepper. Massage the kale so that it is properly covered with seasoning. The leaves will soon turn dark green. Mix the radishes.
4. Rinse the butter beans and pat them dry with a towel. On medium-high heat, put a large skillet, add some olive oil, and sauté the butter beans in a layer. Sprinkle some salt on top and shake the pan. The butter beans will be brown in places within 7 minutes.
5. Take two large plates and divide both the kale and beans equally. Put the walnuts and roasted cauliflower on top. Add the Caesar dressing on top and enjoy the amazing salad.

NUTRITION: Calories: 378 Carbs: 11g Protein: 18g Fat: 27g

207. ASIAN DELIGHT WITH CRUNCHY DRESSING

COOKING: 10' — **PREPARATION: 20'** — **SERVES: 1 BOWL**

INGREDIENTS

Salad Dressing:
- ½ teaspoon of powdered ginger or 1 teaspoon of freshly chopped ginger
- 1 tablespoon of honey
- ¼ cup of rice wine vinegar
- 2 tablespoons of soy sauce
- 3 tablespoons of sesame oil
- 3 tablespoons of creamy peanut butter
- ¼ cup of vegetable oil
- 2 tablespoons of toasted sesame seeds

Salad:
- 1 finely shredded carrot
- 1 thinly sliced red bell pepper
- 6 cups of washed and dried spinach
- ¼ thinly sliced red onion
- 1 thinly sliced cucumber
- ½ pound of snap peas
- ½ cup of roasted peanuts
- 1 tablespoon of toasted sesame seeds

DIRECTIONS

1. In a medium bowl, mix the dressing ingredients and whisk them well. Do not put the sesame seeds in this dressing mixture.
2. Put some water in the pot and bring it to a boil. Add the sugar snap peas and cook them for about 5 minutes until they are crisp and tender. Drain and rinse them repeatedly in cold water so that the peas retain their crispy nature.
3. In a large bowl, add all the other ingredients for the salad. Put the salad dressing on top so that the veggies are well-coated. Add the toasted sesame seeds. Enjoy this salad when you are not in the mood for anything heavy.

NUTRITION: Calories: 378 Carbs: 11g Protein: 18g Fat: 27g

---

208. BROCCOLI SALAD THE THAI WAY

COOKING: 25' — **PREPARATION: 10'** — **SERVES: 1**

INGREDIENTS

- 1 tablespoon of tamari
- ¾ cup of mung beans
- 1 lime
- 2 garlic cloves
- 3 tablespoons of cashew butter
- 1 cucumber
- ¼ oz. of fresh mint
- 1 tablespoon of chili-garlic sauce
- 1 head of artisan lettuce
- 3 Thai chilis
- 6 oz. of broccoli florets
- 2 tablespoons of olive oil
- Salt
- Pepper

DIRECTIONS

1. On high heat, add the mung beans to 3 cups of cold water. After they start boiling, reduce the heat to medium. Allow the beans to simmer, but stir them from time to time. The mung beans will be tender within 20 minutes. Drain the excess water and add some salt.
2. Mince the garlic and cut the lime in half. In a medium bowl, mix the lime juice, minced garlic, tamari, and cashew butter with chili-garlic sauce. Add 3 tablespoons of warm water. Whisk the mixture well.
3. Slice the cucumber, cut the broccoli into bite-size pieces, and chop the lettuce. Pick the mint leaves as well. Lastly, slice the Thai chilis.
4. On a non-stick skillet, put 2 tablespoons of olive oil. Turn the heat to medium-high. Once the oil is hot, add the broccoli florets and cook until they are brown. They will be crisp-tender. Add some pepper and salt to the broccoli and add the lime juice and Thai chilis.
5. In a shallow bowl, spread some cashew sauce. Add some chopped lettuce, mung beans, broccoli, and cucumber. Add mint leaves and mix the Thai chilies. Add some more cashew sauce and enjoy the salad!

NUTRITION: Calories: 203 Fat: 1.4g Carbs: 41.6g Proteins: 4.8g

209. SWEET POTATO, CORN AND JALAPENO BISQUE

COOKING: 15'   **PREPARATION: 10'**   **SERVES: 4**

INGREDIENTS

- 4 ears corn
- 1 seeded and chopped jalapeno
- 4 cups vegetable broth
- 1 tablespoon olive oil
- 3 peeled and cubed sweet potatoes
- 1 chopped onion
- ½ tablespoon salt
- ¼ teaspoon black pepper
- 1 minced garlic clove

DIRECTIONS

1. In a pan, heat the oil over medium flame and sauté onion and garlic in it and cook for around 3 minutes. Put broth and sweet potatoes in it and bring it to boil. Reduce the flame and cook it for an additional 10 minutes.
2. Remove it from the stove and blend it with a blender. Again, put it on the stove and add corn, jalapeno, salt, and black pepper and serve it.

NUTRITION: Calories 332 Carbs: 31g Protein: 6g Fat: 4g

210. CREAMY PEA SOUP WITH OLIVE PESTO

COOKING: 20'   **PREPARATION: 20'**   **SERVES: 4**

INGREDIENTS

- 1 grated carrot
- 1 rinsed chopped leek
- 1 minced garlic clove
- 2 tablespoons olive oil
- 1 stem fresh thyme leaves
- 15 oz. rinsed and drained peas
- ½ tablespoon salt
- ¼ teaspoon ground black pepper
- 2 ½ cups vegetable broth
- ¼ cup parsley leaves
- 1 ¼ cups pitted green olives
- 1 teaspoon drained capers
- 1 garlic clove

DIRECTIONS

1. Take a pan with oil and put it over medium flame and whisk garlic, leek, thyme, and carrot in it. Cook it for around 4 minutes.
2. Add broth, peas, salt, and pepper and increase the heat. When it starts boiling, lower down the heat and cook it with a lid on for around 15 minutes and remove from heat and blend it.
3. For making pesto whisk parsley, olives, capers, and garlic and blend it in a way that it has little chunks. Top the soup with the scoop of olive pesto.

NUTRITION: Calories: 230 Carbs: 23g Protein: 6g Fat: 15g

THE PLANT BASED DIET COOKBOOK

211. SPINACH SOUP WITH DILL AND BASIL

COOKING: 25'   **PREPARATION: 10'**   **SERVES: 8**

INGREDIENTS

- 1 pound peeled and diced potatoes
- 1 tablespoon minced garlic
- 1 teaspoon dry mustard
- 6 cups vegetable broth
- 20 oz. chopped frozen spinach
- 2 cups chopped onion
- 1 ½ tablespoons salt
- ½ cup minced dill
- 1 cup basil
- ½ teaspoon ground black pepper

DIRECTIONS

1. Whisk onion, garlic, potatoes, broth, mustard, and salt in a pan and cook it over medium flame. When it starts boiling, low down the heat and cover it with the lid and cook for 20 minutes.
2. Add the remaining ingredients in it and blend it and cook it for few more minutes and serve it.

NUTRITION: Calories: 165 Carbs: 12g Protein: 13g Fat: 1g

212. COCONUT WATERCRESS SOUP

COOKING: 20'   **PREPARATION: 10'**   **SERVES: 4**

INGREDIENTS

- 1 teaspoon coconut oil
- 1 onion, diced
- ¾ cup coconut milk

DIRECTIONS

1. Melt the coconut oil in a large pot over medium-high heat. Add the onion and cook until soft, about 5 minutes, then add the peas and the water. Bring to a boil, lower the heat and add the watercress, mint, salt, and pepper.
2. Cover and simmer for 5 minutes. Stir in the coconut milk, and purée the soup until smooth in a blender or with an immersion blender.
3. Try this soup with any other fresh, leafy green—anything from spinach to collard greens to arugula to swiss chard.

NUTRITION: Calories: 160 Fat: 5g Carbs: 25g Proteins: 2g

213. ROASTED RED PEPPER AND BUTTERNUT SQUASH SOUP

COOKING: 45' **PREPARATION: 10'** **SERVES: 6**

INGREDIENTS

- 1 small butternut squash
- 1 tablespoon olive oil
- 1 teaspoon sea salt
- 2 red bell peppers
- 1 yellow onion
- 1 head garlic
- 2 cups water, or vegetable broth
- Zest and juice of 1 lime
- 1 to 2 tablespoons tahini
- Pinch cayenne pepper
- ½ teaspoon ground coriander
- ½ teaspoon ground cumin
- Toasted squash seeds (optional)

DIRECTIONS

1. Preheat the oven to 350°F.
2. Prepare the squash for roasting by cutting it in half lengthwise, scooping out the seeds, and poking holes in the flesh with a fork. Reserve the seeds if desired.
3. Rub a small amount of oil over the flesh and skin, rub with a bit of sea salt and put the halves skin-side down in a large baking dish. Put it in the oven while you prepare the rest of the vegetables.
4. Prepare the peppers the same way, except they do not need to be poked.
5. Slice the onion in half and rub oil on the exposed faces. Slice the top off the head of garlic and rub oil on the exposed flesh.
6. After the squash has cooked for 20 minutes, add the peppers, onion, and garlic, and roast for another 20 minutes. Optionally, you can toast the squash seeds by putting them in the oven in a separate baking dish 10 to 15 minutes before the vegetables are finished.
7. Keep a close eye on them. When the vegetables are cooked, take them out and let them cool before handling them. The squash will be very soft when poked with a fork.
8. Scoop the flesh out of the squash skin into a large pot (if you have an immersion blender) or into a blender.
9. Chop the pepper roughly, remove the onion skin and chop the onion roughly, and squeeze the garlic cloves out of the head, all into the pot or blender. Add the water, the lime zest and juice, and the tahini. Purée the soup, adding more water if you like, to your desired consistency. Season with the salt, cayenne, coriander, and cumin. Serve garnished with toasted squash seeds (if using).

NUTRITION: Calories: 156 Protein: 4g Fat: 11g Carbs: 22g

214. CAULIFLOWER SPINACH SOUP

COOKING: 25' **PREPARATION: 30'** **SERVES: 5**

INGREDIENTS

- 1/2 cup unsweetened coconut milk
- 5 oz. fresh spinach, chopped
- 5 watercress, chopped
- 8 cups vegetable stock
- 1 lb cauliflower, chopped
- Salt

DIRECTIONS

1. Add stock and cauliflower in a large saucepan and bring to boil over medium heat for 15 minutes.
2. Add spinach and watercress and cook for another 10 minutes.
3. Remove from heat and puree the soup using a blender until smooth.
4. Add coconut milk and stir well. Season with salt.
5. Stir well and serve hot.

NUTRITION: Calories: 271 Fat: 3.7g Carbs: 54g Proteins: 6.5g

THE PLANT BASED DIET COOKBOOK

215. AVOCADO MINT SOUP

COOKING: 10' **PREPARATION: 10'** **SERVES: 2**

INGREDIENTS

- 1 medium avocado, peeled, pitted, and cut into pieces
- 1 cup coconut milk
- 2 romaine lettuce leaves
- 20 fresh mint leaves
- 1 tbsp fresh lime juice
- 1/8 tsp salt

DIRECTIONS

1. Add all ingredients into the blender and blend until smooth. Soup should be thick not as a puree.
2. Pour into the serving bowls and place in the refrigerator for 10 minutes.
3. Stir well and serve chilled.

NUTRITION: Calories: 377 Fat: 14.9g Carbs: 20.7g Protein: 6.4g

216. CREAMY SQUASH SOUP

COOKING: 25' **PREPARATION: 10'** **SERVES: 8**

INGREDIENTS

- 3 cups butternut squash, chopped
- 1 ½ cups unsweetened coconut milk
- 1 tbsp coconut oil
- 1 tsp dried onion flakes
- 1 tbsp curry powder
- 4 cups water
- 1 garlic clove
- 1 tsp kosher salt

DIRECTIONS

1. Add squash, coconut oil, onion flakes, curry powder, water, garlic, and salt into a large saucepan. Bring to boil over high heat.
2. Turn heat to medium and simmer for 20 minutes.
3. Puree the soup using a blender until smooth. Return soup to the saucepan and stir in coconut milk and cook for 2 minutes.
4. Stir well and serve hot.

NUTRITION: Calories: 271 Fat: 3.7g Carbs: 54g Protein: 6.5g

217. ZUCCHINI SOUP

COOKING: 15' **PREPARATION: 10'** **SERVES: 8**

INGREDIENTS

- 2 ½ lbs zucchini, peeled and sliced
- 1/3 cup basil leaves
- 4 cups vegetable stock
- 4 garlic cloves, chopped
- 2 tbsp olive oil
- 1 medium onion, diced
- Pepper
- Salt

DIRECTIONS

1. Heat olive oil in a pan over medium-low heat.
2. Add zucchini and onion and sauté until softened. Add garlic and sauté for a minute.
3. Add vegetable stock and simmer for 15 minutes.
4. Remove from heat. Stir in basil and puree the soup using a blender until smooth and creamy. Season with pepper and salt.
5. Stir well and serve.

NUTRITION: Calories: 434 Fat: 35g Carbs: 27g Protein: 6.7g

218. CREAMY CELERY SOUP

COOKING: 20'   **PREPARATION: 20'**   **SERVES: 4**

INGREDIENTS

- 6 cups celery
- ½ tsp dill
- 2 cups water
- 1 cup coconut milk
- 1 onion, chopped
- Pinch of salt

DIRECTIONS

1. Add all ingredients into the electric pot and stir well.
2. Cover electric pot with the lid and select soup setting.
3. Release pressure using a quick release method than open the lid.
4. Puree the soup using an immersion blender until smooth and creamy.
5. Stir well and serve warm.

NUTRITION: Calories: 159 Fat: 8.4g Carbs: 19.8g Proteins: 4.6g

219. AVOCADO CUCUMBER SOUP

COOKING: 0'   **PREPARATION: 20'**   **SERVES: 3**

INGREDIENTS

- 1 large cucumber, peeled and sliced
- ¾ cup water
- ¼ cup lemon juice
- 2 garlic cloves
- 6 green onion
- 2 avocados, pitted
- ½ tsp black pepper
- ½ tsp pink salt

DIRECTIONS

1. Add all ingredients into the blender and blend until smooth and creamy.
2. Place in refrigerator for 30 minutes.
3. Stir well and serve chilled.

NUTRITION: Calories: 127 Fat: 6.6g Carbs: 13g Protein: 0.7g

220. GARDEN VEGETABLE STEW

COOKING: 60'   **PREPARATION: 5'**   **SERVES: 4**

INGREDIENTS

- 2 tablespoons olive oil
- 1 medium red onion, chopped
- 1 medium carrot, cut into 1/4-inch slices
- 1/2 cup dry white wine
- 3 medium new potatoes, unpeeled and cut into 1-inch pieces
- 1 medium red bell pepper, cut into 1/2-inch dice
- 11/2 cups vegetable broth
- 1 tablespoon minced fresh savory or 1 teaspoon dried

DIRECTIONS

1. In a large saucepan, heat the oil over medium heat. Add the onion and carrot, cover, and cook until softened, 7 minutes. Add the wine and cook, uncovered, for 5 minutes. Stir in the potatoes, bell pepper, and broth and bring to a boil. Reduce the heat to medium and simmer for 15 minutes.
2. Add the zucchini, yellow squash, and tomatoes. Season with salt and black pepper to taste, cover, and simmer until the vegetables are tender, 20 to 30 minutes. Stir in the corn, peas, basil, parsley, and savory. Taste, adjusting seasonings if necessary. Simmer to blend flavors, about 10 minutes more. Serve immediately.

NUTRITION: Calories: 219 Fat: 4.5g Carbs: 38.2g Protein: 6.4g

THE PLANT BASED DIET COOKBOOK

221. MOROCCAN VERMICELLI VEGETABLE SOUP

COOKING: 35' **PREPARATION: 5'** **SERVES: 4-6**

INGREDIENTS

- 1 tablespoon olive oil
- 1 small onion, chopped
- 1 large carrot, chopped
- 1 celery rib, chopped
- 3 small zucchinis, cut into 1/4-inch dice
- 1 (28-oz.) can diced tomatoes, drained
- 2 tablespoons tomato paste
- 1 1/2 cups cooked or 1 (15.5-oz.) can chickpeas, drained and rinsed
- 2 teaspoons smoked paprika
- 1 teaspoon ground cumin
- 1 teaspoon za'atar spice (optional)
- 1/4 teaspoon ground cayenne
- 6 cups vegetable broth, homemade (see light vegetable broth) or store-bought, or water
- Salt
- 4 oz. vermicelli
- 2 tablespoons minced fresh cilantro, for garnish

DIRECTIONS

1. In a large soup pot, heat the oil over medium heat. Add the onion, carrot, and celery. Cover and cook until softened, about 5 minutes. Stir in the zucchini, tomatoes, tomato paste, chickpeas, paprika, cumin, za'atar, and cayenne.
2. Add the broth and salt to taste. Bring to a boil, then reduce heat to low and simmer, uncovered, until the vegetables are tender, about 30 minutes.
3. Shortly before serving, stir in the vermicelli and cook until the noodles are tender, about 5 minutes. Ladle the soup into bowls, garnish with cilantro, and serve.

NUTRITION: Calories: 236 Fat: 1.8g Carbs: 48.3g Protein: 7g

---

222. MOROCCAN VEGETABLE STEW

COOKING: 35' **PREPARATION: 5'** **SERVES: 4**

INGREDIENTS

- 1 tablespoon olive oil
- 2 medium yellow onions, chopped
- 2 medium carrots, cut into 1/2-inch dice
- 1/2 teaspoon ground cumin
- 1/2 teaspoon ground cinnamon or allspice
- 1/2 teaspoon ground ginger
- 1/2 teaspoon sweet or smoked paprika
- 1/2 teaspoon saffron or turmeric
- 1 (14.5-oz.) can diced tomatoes, undrained
- 8 oz. green beans, trimmed and cut into 1-inch pieces
- 2 cups peeled, seeded, and diced winter squash
- 1 large russet or other baking potato, peeled and cut into 1/2-inch dice
- 1 1/2 cups vegetable broth
- 1 1/2 cups cooked or 1 (15.5-oz.) can chickpeas, drained and rinsed
- 3/4 cup frozen peas
- 1/2 cup pitted dried plums (prunes)
- 1 teaspoon lemon zest
- Salt and freshly ground black pepper
- 1/2 cup pitted green olives
- 1 tablespoon minced fresh cilantro or parsley, for garnish
- 1/2 cup toasted slivered almonds, for garnish

DIRECTIONS

1. In a large saucepan, heat the oil over medium heat. Add the onions and carrots, cover, and cook for 5 minutes. Stir in the cumin, cinnamon, ginger, paprika, and saffron. Cook, uncovered, stirring, for 30 seconds.
2. Add the tomatoes, green beans, squash, potato, and broth and bring to a boil. Reduce heat to low, cover, and simmer until the vegetables are tender, about 20 minutes.
3. Add the chickpeas, peas, dried plums, and lemon zest. Season with salt and pepper to taste. Stir in the olives and simmer, uncovered, until the flavors are blended, about 10 minutes. Sprinkle with cilantro and almonds and serve immediately.

NUTRITION: Calories: 71 Fat: 2.8g Carbs: 9.8g Protein: 3.7g

223. BASIC RECIPE FOR VEGETABLE BROTH

COOKING: 60' **PREPARATION: 10'** **SERVES: 2 QUARTS**

INGREDIENTS

- 8 cups Water
- 1 Onion, chopped
- 4 Garlic cloves, crushed
- 2 Celery Stalks, chopped
- Pinch of Salt
- 1 Carrot, chopped
- Dash of Pepper
- 1 Potato, medium & chopped
- 1 tbsp. Soy Sauce
- 3 Bay Leaves

DIRECTIONS

1. To make the vegetable broth, you need to place all of the ingredients in a deep saucepan.
2. Heat the pan over a medium-high heat. Bring the vegetable mixture to a boil.
3. Once it starts boiling, lower the heat to medium-low and allow it to simmer for at least an hour or so. Cover it with a lid.
4. When the time is up, pass it through a filter and strain the vegetables, garlic, and bay leaves.
5. Allow the stock to cool completely and store in an air-tight container.

NUTRITION: Calories: 44 Fat: 0.6g Carbs: 9.7g Protein: 0.9g

224. CUCUMBER DILL GAZPACHO

COOKING: 2H **PREPARATION: 10'** **SERVES: 4**

INGREDIENTS

- 4 large cucumbers, peeled, deseeded, and chopped
- 1/8 tsp salt
- 1 tsp chopped fresh dill + more for garnishing
- 2 tbsp freshly squeezed lemon juice
- 1 ½ cups green grape, seeds removed
- 3 tbsp extra virgin olive oil
- 1 garlic clove, minced

DIRECTIONS

1. Add all the ingredients to a food processor and blend until smooth.
2. Pour the soup into serving bowls and chill for 1 to 2 hours.
3. Garnish with dill and serve chilled.

NUTRITION: Calories: 236 Fat: 1.8g Carbs: 48.3g Protein: 7g

225. RED LENTIL SOUP

COOKING: 25' **PREPARATION: 5'** **SERVES: 6 QUARTS**

INGREDIENTS

- 2 tbsp. Nutritional Yeast
- 1 cup Red Lentil, washed
- ½ tbsp. Garlic, minced
- 4 cups Vegetable Stock
- 1 tsp. Salt
- 2 cups Kale, shredded
- 3 cups Mixed Vegetables

DIRECTIONS

1. To start with, place all ingredients needed to make the soup in a large pot.
2. Heat the pot over medium-high heat and bring the mixture to a boil.
3. Once it starts boiling, lower the heat to low. Allow the soup to simmer.
4. Simmer it for 10 to 15 minutes or until cooked.
5. Serve and enjoy.

NUTRITION: Calories: 212 Fat: 11.9g Carbs: 31.7g Protein: 7.3g

226. SPINACH AND KALE SOUP

COOKING: 5' **PREPARATION: 5'** **SERVES: 2**

INGREDIENTS

- 3 oz. vegan butter
- 1 cup fresh spinach, chopped coarsely
- 1 cup fresh kale, chopped coarsely
- 1 large avocado
- 3 tbsp chopped fresh mint leaves
- 3 ½ cups coconut cream
- 1 cup vegetable broth
- Salt and black pepper to taste
- 1 lime, juiced

DIRECTIONS

1. Melt the vegan butter in a medium pot over medium heat and sauté the kale and spinach until wilted, 3 minutes. Turn the heat off.
2. Stir in the remaining ingredients and using an immersion blender, puree the soup until smooth.
3. Dish the soup and serve warm.

NUTRITION: Calories: 380 Fat: 10g Protein: 20g Carbs: 30g

227. COCONUT AND GRILLED VEGETABLE SOUP

COOKING: 45'   **PREPARATION: 5'**   **SERVES: 4**

INGREDIENTS

- 2 small red onions cut into wedges
- 2 garlic cloves
- 10 oz. butternut squash, peeled and chopped
- 10 oz. pumpkins, peeled and chopped
- 4 tbsp melted vegan butter
- Salt and black pepper to taste
- 1 cup of water
- 1 cup unsweetened coconut milk
- 1 lime juiced
- ¾ cup vegan mayonnaise
- Toasted pumpkin seeds for garnishing

DIRECTIONS

1. Preheat the oven to 400°F.
2. On a baking sheet, spread the onions, garlic, butternut squash, and pumpkins and drizzle half of the butter on top. Season with salt, black pepper, and rub the seasoning well onto the vegetables. Roast in the oven for 45 minutes or until the vegetables are golden brown and softened.
3. Transfer the vegetables to a pot; add the remaining ingredients except for the pumpkin seeds and using an immersion blender puree the ingredients until smooth.
4. Dish the soup, garnish with the pumpkin seeds and serve warm.

NUTRITION: Calories: 290 Fat: 10g Protein: 30g Carbs: 10g

228. CELERY DILL SOUP

COOKING: 25'   **PREPARATION: 5'**   **SERVES: 4**

INGREDIENTS

- 2 tbsp coconut oil
- ½ lb celery root, trimmed
- 1 garlic clove
- 1 medium white onion
- ¼ cup fresh dill, roughly chopped
- 1 tsp cumin powder
- ¼ tsp nutmeg powder
- 1 small head cauliflower, cut into florets
- 3½ cups seasoned vegetable stock
- 5 oz. vegan butter
- Juice from 1 lemon
- ¼ cup coconut cream
- Salt and black pepper to taste

DIRECTIONS

1. Melt the coconut oil in a large pot and sauté the celery root, garlic, and onion until softened and fragrant, 5 minutes.
2. Stir in the dill, cumin, and nutmeg, and stir-fry for 1 minute. Mix in the cauliflower and vegetable stock. Allow the soup to boil for 15 minutes and turn the heat off.
3. Add the vegan butter and lemon juice, and puree the soup using an immersion blender.
4. Stir in the coconut cream, salt, black pepper, and dish the soup.
5. Serve warm.

NUTRITION: Calories: 320 Fat: 10g Protein: 20g Carbs: 9g

229. BROCCOLI FENNEL SOUP

COOKING: 10'   **PREPARATION: 15'**   **SERVES: 4**

INGREDIENTS

- 1 fennel bulb, white and green parts coarsely chopped
- 10 oz. broccoli, cut into florets
- 3 cups vegetable stock
- Salt and freshly ground black pepper
- 1 garlic clove
- 1 cup dairy-free cream cheese
- 3 oz. vegan butter
- ½ cup chopped fresh oregano

DIRECTIONS

1. In a medium pot, combine the fennel, broccoli, vegetable stock, salt, and black pepper. Bring to a boil until the vegetables soften, 10 to 15 minutes.
2. Stir in the remaining ingredients and simmer the soup for 3 to 5 minutes.
3. Adjust the taste with salt and black pepper, and dish the soup.
4. Serve warm.

NUTRITION: Calories: 240 Fat: 8g Protein: 5g Carbs: 12g

230. TOFU GOULASH SOUP

COOKING: 20'   **PREPARATION: 35'**   **SERVES: 4**

INGREDIENTS

- 4¼ oz. vegan butter
- 1 white onion, chopped
- 2 garlic cloves, minced
- 1 ½ cups butternut squash
- 1 red bell pepper, deseeded and chopped
- 1 tbsp paprika powder
- ¼ tsp red chili flakes
- 1 tbsp dried basil
- ½ tbsp crushed cardamom seeds
- Salt and black pepper to taste
- 1 ½ cups crushed tomatoes
- 3 cups vegetable broth
- 1½ tsp red wine vinegar
- Chopped parsley to serve

DIRECTIONS

1. Place the tofu between two paper towels and allow draining of water for 30 minutes. After, crumble the tofu and set aside.
2. Melt the vegan butter in a large pot over medium heat and sauté the onion and garlic until the veggies are fragrant and soft, 3 minutes.
3. Stir in the tofu and cook until golden brown, 3 minutes.
4. Add the butternut squash, bell pepper, paprika, red chili flakes, basil, cardamom seeds, salt, and black pepper. Cook for 2 minutes to release some flavor and mix in the tomatoes and 2 cups of vegetable broth.
5. Close the lid, bring the soup to a boil, and then simmer for 10 minutes.
6. Stir in the remaining vegetable broth, the red wine vinegar, and adjust the taste with salt and black pepper.
7. Dish the soup, garnish with the parsley and serve warm.

NUTRITION: Calories: 320 Fat: 10g Protein: 10g Carbs: 20g

231. PESTO PEA SOUP

COOKING: 20'   **PREPARATION: 10'**   **SERVES: 4**

INGREDIENTS

- 2 cups Water
- 8 oz. Tortellini
- ¼ cup Pesto
- 1 Onion, small & finely chopped
- 1 lb. Peas, frozen
- 1 Carrot, medium & finely chopped
- 1 ¾ cup Vegetable Broth, less sodium
- 1 Celery Rib, medium & finely chopped

DIRECTIONS

1. To start with, boil the water in a large pot over a medium-high heat.
2. Next, stir in the tortellini to the pot and cook it following the packet's instructions.
3. In the meantime, cook the onion, celery, and carrot in a deep saucepan along with the water and broth.
4. Cook the celery-onion mixture for 6 minutes or until softened.
5. Now, spoon in the peas and allow it to simmer while keeping it uncovered.
6. Cook the peas for few minutes or until they are bright green and soft.
7. Then, spoon in the pesto to the peas mixture. Combine well.
8. Pour the mixture into a high-speed blender and blend for 2 to 3 minutes or until you get a rich, smooth soup.
9. Return the soup to the pan. Spoon in the cooked tortellini.
10. Finally, pour into a serving bowl and top with more cooked peas if desired.
11. Tip: If desired, you can season it with Maldon salt at the end.

NUTRITION: Calories: 356 Fat: 12g Protein: 13g Carbs: 25g

232. TOFU AND MUSHROOM SOUP

COOKING: 10'   **PREPARATION: 15'**   **SERVES: 4**

INGREDIENTS

- 2 tbsp olive oil
- 1 garlic clove, minced
- 1 large yellow onion, finely chopped
- 1 tsp freshly grated ginger
- 1 cup vegetable stock
- 2 small potatoes, peeled and chopped
- ¼ tsp salt
- ¼ tsp black pepper
- 2 (14 oz) silken tofu, drained and rinsed
- 2/3 cup baby Bella mushrooms, sliced
- 1 tbsp chopped fresh oregano
- 2 tbsp chopped fresh parsley to garnish

DIRECTIONS

1. Heat the olive oil in a medium pot over medium heat and sauté the garlic, onion, and ginger until soft and fragrant.
2. Pour in the vegetable stock, potatoes, salt, and black pepper. Cook until the potatoes soften, 12 minutes.
3. Stir in the tofu and using an immersion blender, puree the ingredients until smooth.
4. Mix in the mushrooms and simmer with the pot covered until the mushrooms warm up while occasionally stirring to ensure that the tofu doesn't curdle, 7 minutes.
5. Stir oregano, and dish the soup.
6. Garnish with the parsley and serve warm.

NUTRITION: Calories: 310 Fat: 10g Protein: 40g Carbs: 18g

THE PLANT BASED DIET COOKBOOK

CHAPTER 13: SALADS AND SIDE DISHES

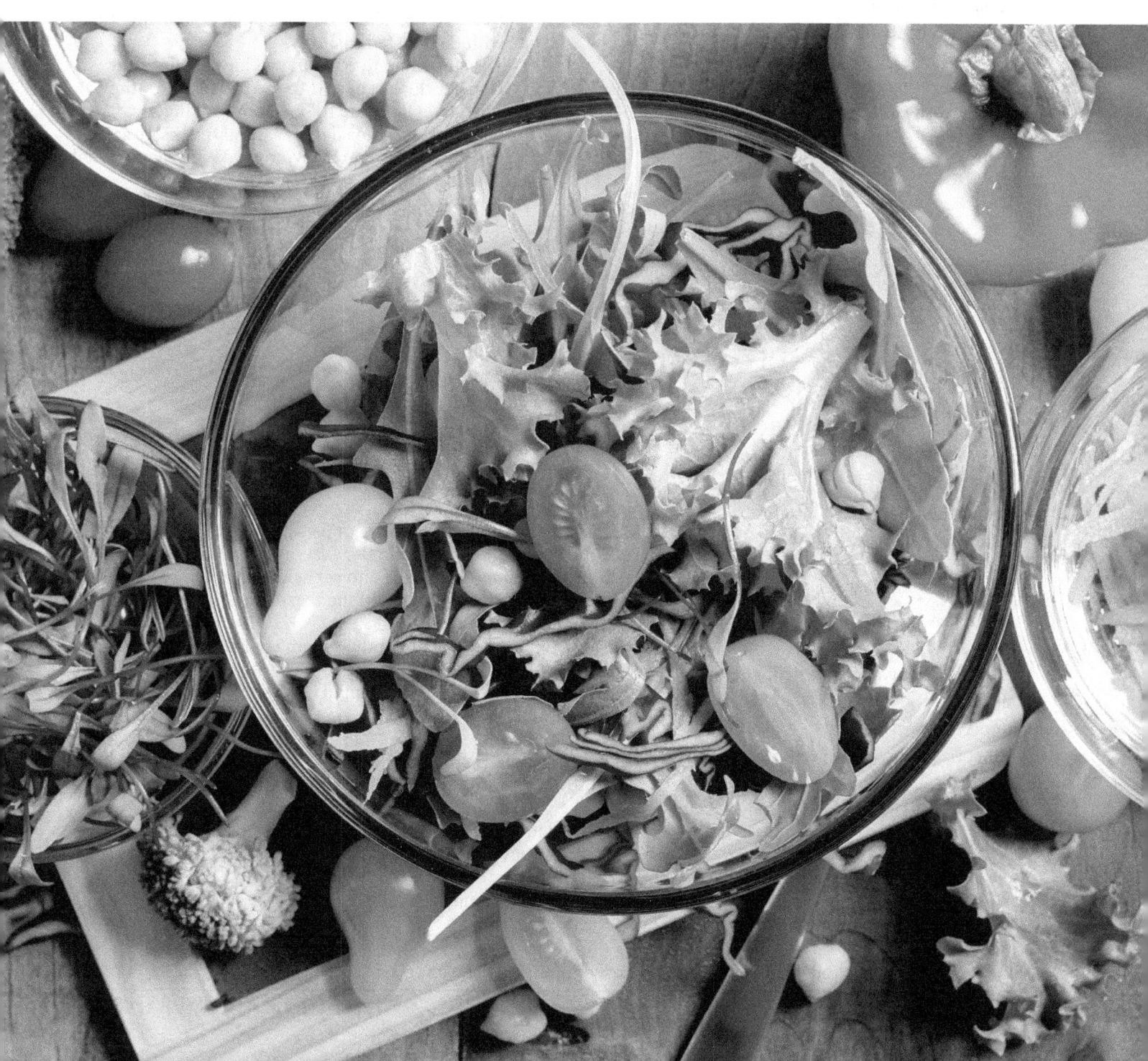

233. CASHEW SIAM SALAD

COOKING: 3'   **PREPARATION: 10'**   **SERVES: 4**

INGREDIENTS

Salad:
- 4 cups baby spinach, rinsed, drained
- ½ cup pickled red cabbage
- Dressing:
- 1-inch piece ginger, finely chopped
- 1 tsp. chili garlic paste
- 1 tbsp. soy sauce
- ½ tbsp. rice vinegar
- 1 tbsp. sesame oil
- 3 tbsp. avocado oil

Toppings:
- ½ cup raw cashews, unsalted
- ¼ cup fresh cilantro, chopped

DIRECTIONS

1. Put the spinach and red cabbage in a large bowl. Toss to combine and set the salad aside.
2. Toast the cashews in a frying pan over medium-high heat, stirring occasionally until the cashews are golden brown. This should take about 3 minutes. Turn off the heat and set the frying pan aside.
3. Mix all the dressing ingredients in medium-sized bowl and use a spoon to mix them into a smooth dressing.
4. Pour the dressing over the spinach salad and top with the toasted cashews.
5. Toss the salad to combine all ingredients and transfer the large bowl to the fridge. Allow the salad to chill for up to one hour – doing so will guarantee a better flavor. Alternatively, the salad can be served right away, topped with the optional cilantro. Enjoy!

NUTRITION: Calories: 160 Fat: 12.9g Carbs: 9.1g Protein: 4.1g

234. CUCUMBER EDAMAME SALAD

COOKING: 8'   **PREPARATION: 5'**   **SERVES: 2**

INGREDIENTS

- 3 tbsp. avocado oil
- 1 cup cucumber, sliced into thin rounds
- ½ cup fresh sugar snap peas, sliced or whole
- ½ cup fresh edamame
- ¼ cup radish, sliced
- 1 large Hass avocado, peeled, pitted, sliced
- 1 nori sheet, crumbled
- 2 tsp. roasted sesame seeds
- 1 tsp. salt

DIRECTIONS

1. Bring a medium-sized pot filled half way with water to a boil over medium-high heat.
2. Add the sugar snaps and cook them for about 2 minutes.
3. Take the pot off the heat, drain the excess water, transfer the sugar snaps to a medium-sized bowl and set aside for now.
4. Fill the pot with water again, add the teaspoon of salt and bring to a boil over medium-high heat.
5. Add the edamame to the pot and let them cook for about 6 minutes.
6. Take the pot off the heat, drain the excess water, transfer the soybeans to the bowl with sugar snaps and let them cool down for about 5 minutes.
7. Combine all ingredients, except the nori crumbs and roasted sesame seeds, in a medium-sized bowl.
8. Carefully stir, using a spoon, until all ingredients are evenly coated in oil.
9. Top the salad with the nori crumbs and roasted sesame seeds.
10. Transfer the bowl to the fridge and allow the salad to cool for at least 30 minutes.
11. Serve chilled and enjoy!

NUTRITION: Calories: 182 Fat: 10.9g Carbs: 14.2g Protein: 10.7g

235. SPINACH AND MASHED TOFU SALAD

COOKING: 0'   **PREPARATION: 20'**   **SERVES: 4**

INGREDIENTS

- 2 8-oz. blocks firm tofu, drained
- 4 cups baby spinach leaves
- 4 tbsp. cashew butter
- 1½ tbsp. soy sauce
- 1 tbsp ginger, chopped
- 1 tsp. red miso paste
- 2 tbsp. sesame seeds
- 1 tsp. organic orange zest
- 1 tsp. nori flakes
- 2 tbsp. water

DIRECTIONS

1. Use paper towels to absorb any excess water left in the tofu before crumbling both blocks into small pieces.
2. In a large bowl, combine the mashed tofu with the spinach leaves.
3. Mix the remaining ingredients in another small bowl and, if desired, add the optional water for a smoother dressing.
4. Pour this dressing over the mashed tofu and spinach leaves.
5. Transfer the bowl to the fridge and allow the salad to chill for up to one hour. Doing so will guarantee a better flavor. Or, the salad can be served right away. Enjoy!

NUTRITION: Calories: 623 Fat: 30.5g Carbs: 48g Protein: 48.4g

236. SUPER SUMMER SALAD

COOKING: 0'   **PREPARATION: 10'**   **SERVES: 2**

INGREDIENTS

Dressing:
- 1 tbsp. olive oil
- ¼ cup chopped basil
- 1 tsp. lemon juice
- ¼ tsp Salt
- 1 medium avocado, halved, diced
- ¼ cup water

Salad:
- ¼ cup dry chickpeas
- ¼ cup dry red kidney beans
- 4 cups raw kale, shredded
- 2 cups Brussel sprouts, shredded
- 2 radishes, thinly sliced
- 1 tbsp. walnuts, chopped
- 1 tsp. flax seeds
- Salt and pepper to taste

DIRECTIONS

1. Prepare the chickpeas and kidney beans according to the method.
2. Soak the flax seeds according the method, and then drain excess water.
3. Prepare the dressing by adding the olive oil, basil, lemon juice, salt, and half of the avocado to a food processor or blender, and pulse on low speed.
4. Keep adding small amounts of water until the dressing is creamy and smooth.
5. Transfer the dressing to a small bowl and set it aside.
6. Combine the kale, Brussel sprouts, cooked chickpeas, kidney beans, radishes, walnuts, and remaining avocado in a large bowl and mix thoroughly.
7. Store the mixture, or, serve with the dressing and flax seeds, and enjoy!

NUTRITION: Calories: 266 Fat: 26.6g Carbs: 8.8g Protein: 2g

237. ROASTED ALMOND PROTEIN SALAD

COOKING: 0' **PREPARATION: 30'** **SERVES: 4**

INGREDIENTS

- ½ cup dry quinoa
- ½ cup dry navy beans
- ½ cup dry chickpeas
- ½ cup raw whole almonds
- 1 tsp. extra virgin olive oil
- ½ tsp. salt
- ½ tsp. paprika
- ½ tsp. cayenne
- Dash of chili powder
- 4 cups spinach, fresh or frozen
- ¼ cup purple onion, chopped

DIRECTIONS

1. Prepare the quinoa according to the recipe. Store in the fridge for now.
2. Prepare the beans according to the method. Store in the fridge for now.
3. Toss the almonds, olive oil, salt, and spices in a large bowl, and stir until the ingredients are evenly coated.
4. Put a skillet over medium-high heat, and transfer the almond mixture to the heated skillet.
5. Roast while stirring until the almonds are browned, around 5 minutes. You may hear the ingredients pop and crackle in the pan as they warm up. Stir frequently to prevent burning.
6. Turn off the heat and toss the cooked and chilled quinoa and beans, onions, spinach, or mixed greens in the skillet. Stir well before transferring the roasted almond salad to a bowl.
7. Enjoy the salad with a dressing of choice, or, store for later!

NUTRITION: Calories: 347 Fat: 10.5g Carbs: 49.2g Protein: 17.2g

238. LENTIL, LEMON & MUSHROOM SALAD

COOKING: 0' **PREPARATION: 10'** **SERVES: 2**

INGREDIENTS

- ½ cup dry lentils of choice
- 2 cups vegetable broth
- 3 cups mushrooms, thickly sliced
- 1 cup sweet or purple onion, chopped
- 4 tsp. extra virgin olive oil
- 2 tbsp. garlic powder
- ¼ tsp. chili flakes
- 1 tbsp. lemon juice
- 2 tbsp. cilantro, chopped
- ½ cup arugula
- ¼ tsp Salt
- ¼ tsp pepper

DIRECTIONS

1. Sprout the lentils according the method. (Don't cook them).
2. Place the vegetable stock in a deep saucepan and bring it to a boil.
3. Add the lentils to the boiling broth, cover the pan, and cook for about 5 minutes over low heat until the lentils are a bit tender.
4. Remove the pan from heat and drain the excess water.
5. Put a frying pan over high heat and add 2 tablespoons of olive oil.
6. Add the onions, garlic, and chili flakes, and cook until the onions are almost translucent, around 5 to 10 minutes while stirring.
7. Add the mushrooms to the frying pan and mix in thoroughly. Continue cooking until the onions are completely translucent and the mushrooms have softened; remove the pan from the heat.
8. Mix the lentils, onions, mushrooms, and garlic in a large bowl.
9. Add the lemon juice and the remaining olive oil. Toss or stir to combine everything thoroughly.
10. Serve the mushroom/onion mixture over some arugala in bowl, adding salt and pepper to taste, or, store and enjoy later!

NUTRITION: Calories: 365 Fat: 11.7g Carbs: 45.2g Protein: 22.8g

239. SWEET POTATO & BLACK BEAN PROTEIN SALAD

COOKING: 0' **PREPARATION: 15'** **SERVES: 2**

INGREDIENTS

- 1 cup dry black beans
- 4 cups of spinach
- 1 medium sweet potato
- 1 cup purple onion, chopped
- 2 tbsp. olive oil
- 2 tbsp. lime juice
- 1 tbsp. minced garlic
- ½ tbsp. chili powder
- ¼ tsp. cayenne
- ¼ cup parsley
- ¼ tsp Salt
- ¼ tsp pepper

DIRECTIONS

1. Prepare the black beans according to the method.
2. Preheat the oven to 400°F.
3. Cut the sweet potato into ¼-inch cubes and put these in a medium-sized bowl. Add the onions, 1 tablespoon of olive oil, and salt to taste.
4. Toss the ingredients until the sweet potatoes and onions are completely coated.
5. Transfer the ingredients to a baking sheet lined with parchment paper and spread them out in a single layer.
6. Put the baking sheet in the oven and roast until the sweet potatoes start to turn brown and crispy, around 40 minutes.
7. Meanwhile, combine the remaining olive oil, lime juice, garlic, chili powder, and cayenne thoroughly in a large bowl, until no lumps remain.
8. Remove the sweet potatoes and onions from the oven and transfer them to the large bowl.
9. Add the cooked black beans, parsley, and a pinch of salt.
10. Toss everything until well combined.
11. Then mix in the spinach, and serve in desired portions with additional salt and pepper.
12. Store or enjoy!

NUTRITION: Calories: 558 Fat: 16.2g Carbs: 84g Protein: 25.3g

240. LENTIL RADISH SALAD

COOKING: 0' **PREPARATION: 15'** **SERVES: 3**

INGREDIENTS

Dressing:
- 1 tbsp. extra virgin olive oil
- 1 tbsp. lemon juice
- 1 tbsp. maple syrup
- 1 tbsp. water
- ½ tbsp. sesame oil
- 1 tbsp. miso paste, yellow or white
- ¼ tsp. salt
- ¼ tsp Pepper

Salad:
- ½ cup dry chickpeas
- ¼ cup dry green or brown lentils
- 1 14-oz. pack of silken tofu
- 5 cups mixed greens, fresh or frozen
- 2 radishes, thinly sliced
- ½ cup cherry tomatoes, halved
- ¼ cup roasted sesame seeds

DIRECTIONS

1. Prepare the chickpeas according to the method.
2. Prepare the lentils according to the method.
3. Put all the ingredients for the dressing in a blender or food processor. Mix on low until smooth, while adding water until it reaches the desired consistency.
4. Add salt, pepper (to taste), and optionally more water to the dressing; set aside.
5. Cut the tofu into bite-sized cubes.
6. Combine the mixed greens, tofu, lentils, chickpeas, radishes, and tomatoes in a large bowl.
7. Add the dressing and mix everything until it is coated evenly.
8. Top with the optional roasted sesame seeds, if desired.
9. Refrigerate before serving and enjoy, or, store for later!

NUTRITION: Calories: 621 Fat: 19.6g Carbs: 82.7g Protein: 31.3g

241. JICAMA AND SPINACH SALAD

COOKING: 20'   **PREPARATION: 10'**   **SERVES: 4**

INGREDIENTS

- **Salad:**
- 10 oz. baby spinach, washed and dried
- Grape or cherry tomatoes, cut in half
- 1 jicama, washed, peeled, and cut in strips
- Green or Kalamata olives, chopped
- 8 tsp walnuts, chopped
- 1 tsp raw or roasted sunflower seeds
- Maple Mustard Dressing

Dressing:
- 1 heaping tbsp Dijon mustard
- Dash cayenne pepper
- 2 tbsp maple syrup
- 2 garlic cloves, minced
- 1 to 2 tbsp water
- ¼ tsp sea salt

DIRECTIONS

1. For the salad:
2. Divide the baby spinach onto 4 salad plates. Top each serving with ¼ of the jicama, ¼ of the chopped olives, and 4 tomatoes. Sprinkle 1 tsp of the sunflower seeds and 2 tsp of the walnuts.
3. For the dressing:
4. In a small mixing bowl, whisk all the ingredients together until emulsified. Check the taste and add more maple syrup for sweetness.
5. Drizzle 1½ tbsp of the dressing over each salad and serve.

NUTRITION: Calories: 196 Fat: 2g Protein: 7g Carbs: 28g

243. SOUTHWEST STYLE SALAD

COOKING: 0'   **PREPARATION: 10'**   **SERVES: 3**

INGREDIENTS

- ½ cup dry black beans
- ½ cup dry chickpeas
- 1/3 cup purple onion, diced
- 1 red bell pepper, pitted, sliced
- 4 cups mixed greens, fresh or frozen, chopped
- 1 cup cherry tomatoes, halved or quartered
- 1 medium avocado, peeled, pitted, and cubed
- 1 cup sweet kernel corn, canned, drained
- ½ tsp. chili powder
- ¼ tsp. cumin
- ¼ tsp Salt
- ¼ tsp pepper
- 2 tsp. olive oil
- 1 tbsp. vinegar

DIRECTIONS

1. Prepare the black beans and chickpeas according to the method.
2. Put all of the ingredients into a large bowl.
3. Toss the mix of veggies and spices until combined thoroughly.
4. Store, or serve chilled with some olive oil and vinegar on top!

NUTRITION: Calories: 635 Fat: 19.9g Carbs: 95.4g Protein: 24.3g

244. SHAVED BRUSSEL SPROUT SALAD

COOKING: 0'   **PREPARATION: 5'**   **SERVES: 4**

INGREDIENTS

Dressing:
- 1 tbsp. brown mustard
- 1 tbsp. maple syrup
- 2 tbsp. apple cider vinegar
- 2 tbsp. extra virgin olive oil
- ½ tbsp. garlic minced

Salad:
- ½ cup dry red kidney beans
- ¼ cup dry chickpeas
- 2 cups Brussel sprouts
- 1 cup purple onion
- 1 small sour apple
- ½ cup slivered almonds, crushed
- ½ cup walnuts, crushed
- ½ cup cranberries, dried
- ¼ tsp Salt
- ¼ tsp pepper

DIRECTIONS

1. Prepare the beans according to the method.
2. Combine all dressing ingredients in a bowl and stir well until combined.
3. Refrigerate the dressing for up to one hour before serving.
4. Using a greater, mandolin, or knife to thinly slice each Brussel sprout. Repeat this with the apple and onion.
5. Take a large bowl to mix the chickpeas, beans, sprouts, apples, onions, cranberries, and nuts.
6. Drizzle the cold dressing over the salad to coat.
7. Serve with salt and pepper to taste, or, store for later!

NUTRITION: Calories: 432 Fat: 23.5g Carbs: 45.3g Protein: 15.9g

245. COLORFUL PROTEIN POWER SALAD

COOKING: 0'   **PREPARATION: 20'**   **SERVES: 2**

INGREDIENTS

- ½ cup dry quinoa
- 2 cups dry navy beans
- 1 green onion, chopped
- 2 tsp. garlic, minced
- 3 cups green or purple cabbage, chopped
- 4 cups kale, fresh or frozen, chopped
- 1 cup shredded carrot, chopped
- 2 tbsp. extra virgin olive oil
- 1 tsp. lemon juice
- ¼ tsp Salt
- ¼ tsp pepper

DIRECTIONS

1. Prepare the quinoa according to the recipe.
2. Prepare the beans according to the method.
3. Heat 1 tablespoon of the olive oil in a frying pan over medium heat.
4. Add the chopped green onion, garlic, and cabbage, and sauté for 2-3 minutes.
5. Add the kale, the remaining 1 tablespoon of olive oil, and salt. Lower the heat and cover until the greens have wilted, around 5 minutes. Remove the pan from the stove and set aside.
6. Take a large bowl and mix the remaining ingredients with the kale and cabbage mixture once it has cooled down. Add more salt and pepper to taste.
7. Mix until everything is distributed evenly.
8. Serve topped with a dressing, or, store for later!

NUTRITION: Calories: 1100 Fat: 19.9g Carbs: 180.8g Protein: 58.6g

246. EDAMAME & GINGER CITRUS SALAD

COOKING: 0'   **PREPARATION: 15'**   **SERVES: 3**

INGREDIENTS

Dressing:
- ¼ cup orange juice
- 1 tsp. lime juice
- ½ tbsp. maple syrup
- ½ tsp. ginger, finely minced
- ½ tbsp. sesame oil

Salad:
- ½ cup dry green lentils
- 2 cups carrots, shredded
- 4 cups kale, fresh or frozen, chopped
- 1 cup edamame, shelled
- 1 tablespoon roasted sesame seeds
- 2 tsp. mint, chopped
- Salt and pepper to taste
- 1 small avocado, peeled, pitted, diced

DIRECTIONS

1. Prepare the lentils according to the method.
2. Combine the orange and lime juices, maple syrup, and ginger in a small bowl. Mix with a whisk while slowly adding the sesame oil.
3. Add the cooked lentils, carrots, kale, edamame, sesame seeds, and mint to a large bowl.
4. Add the dressing and stir well until all the ingredients are coated evenly.
5. Store or serve topped with avocado and an additional sprinkle of mint.

NUTRITION: Calories: 507 Fat: 23.1g Carbs: 56.8g Protein: 24.6g

247. TACO TEMPEH SALAD

COOKING: 0'   **PREPARATION: 25'**   **SERVES: 3**

INGREDIENTS

- 1 cup dry black beans
- 1 8-oz. package tempeh
- 1 tbsp. lime or lemon juice
- 2 tbsp. extra virgin olive oil
- 1 tsp. maple syrup
- ½ tsp. chili powder
- ¼ tsp. cumin
- ¼ tsp. paprika
- 1 large bunch of kale, fresh or frozen, chopped
- 1 large avocado, peeled, pitted, diced
- ½ cup salsa
- ¼ tsp Salt
- ¼ tsp pepper

DIRECTIONS

1. Prepare the beans according to the method.
2. Cut the tempeh into ¼-inch cubes, place in a bowl, and then add the lime or lemon juice, 1 tablespoon of olive oil, maple syrup, chili powder, cumin, and paprika.
3. Stir well and let the tempeh marinate in the fridge for at least 1 hour, up to 12 hours.
4. Heat the remaining 1 tablespoon of olive oil in a frying pan over medium heat.
5. Add the marinated tempeh mixture and cook until brown and crispy on both sides, around 10 minutes.
6. Put the chopped kale in a bowl with the cooked beans and prepared tempeh.
7. Store, or serve the salad immediately, topped with salsa, avocado, and salt and pepper to taste.

NUTRITION: Calories: 627 Fat: 31.7g Carbs: 62.7g Protein: 31.4g

248. LEBANESE POTATO SALAD

COOKING: 10' — **PREPARATION: 5'** — **SERVES: 4**

INGREDIENTS

- 1-pound Russet potatoes
- 1 ½ tablespoons extra virgin olive oil
- 2 scallions, thinly sliced
- Freshly ground pepper to taste
- 2 tablespoons lemon juice
- ¼ teaspoon salt or to taste
- 2 tablespoons fresh mint leaves, chopped

DIRECTIONS

1. Place a saucepan half filled with water over medium heat. Add salt and potatoes and cook for 10 minutes until tender. Drain the potatoes and place in a bowl of cold water. When cool enough to handle, peel and cube the potatoes. Place in a bowl.

To make dressing:

2. Add oil, lemon juice, salt and pepper in a bowl and whisk well. Drizzle dressing over the potatoes. Toss well.
3. Add scallions and mint and toss well.
4. Divide into 4 plates and serve.

NUTRITION: Calories: 129 Fat: 5.5g Carbs: 18.8g Protein: 2.2g

249. CHICKPEA AND SPINACH SALAD

COOKING: 0' — **PREPARATION: 5'** — **SERVES: 4**

INGREDIENTS

- 2 cans (14.5 oz. each) chickpeas, drained, rinsed
- 7 oz. vegan feta cheese, crumbled or chopped
- 1 tablespoon lemon juice
- 1/3 -½ cup olive oil
- ½ teaspoon salt or to taste
- 4-6 cups spinach, torn
- ½ cup raisins
- 2 tablespoons honey
- 1-2 teaspoons ground cumin
- 1 teaspoon chili flakes

DIRECTIONS

1. Add cheese, chickpeas and spinach into a large bowl.
2. To make dressing: Add rest of the ingredients into another bowl and mix well.
3. Pour dressing over the salad. Toss well and serve.

NUTRITION: Calories: 822 Fat: 42.5g Carbs: 89.6g Protein: 29g

THE PLANT BASED DIET COOKBOOK

250. TEMPEH "CHICKEN" SALAD

COOKING: 0' **PREPARATION: 10'** **SERVES: 2**

INGREDIENTS

- 4 tablespoons light mayonnaise
- 2 scallions, sliced
- Pepper to taste
- 4 cups mixed salad greens
- 4 teaspoons white miso
- 2 tablespoons chopped fresh dill
- 1 ½ cups crumbled tempeh
- 1 cup sliced grape tomatoes

DIRECTIONS

To make dressing:
1. Add mayonnaise, scallions, miso, dill and pepper into a bowl and whisk well.
2. Add tempeh and fold gently.

To serve:
3. Divide the greens into 4 plates. Divide the tempeh among the plates. Top with tomatoes and serve.

NUTRITION: Calories: 452 Fat: 24.5g Carbs: 37.2g Protein: 29.9g

---

251. SPINACH & DILL PASTA SALAD

COOKING: 0' **PREPARATION: 5'** **SERVES: 4**

INGREDIENTS

For salad:
- 3 cups cooked whole-wheat fusilli
- 2 cups cherry tomatoes, halved
- ½ cup vegan cheese, shredded
- 4 cups spinach, chopped
- 2 cups edamame, thawed
- 1 large red onion, finely chopped

For dressing:
- 2 tablespoons white wine vinegar
- ½ teaspoon dried dill
- 2 tablespoons extra-virgin olive oil
- Salt to taste
- Pepper to taste

DIRECTIONS

To make dressing:
1. Add all the ingredients for dressing into a bowl and whisk well. Set aside for a while for the flavors to set in.

To make salad:
2. Add all the ingredients of the salad in a bowl. Toss well.
3. Drizzle dressing on top. Toss well.
4. Divide into 4 plates and serve.

NUTRITION: Calories: 684 Fat: 33.6g Carbs: 69.5g Protein: 31.7g

252. ITALIAN VEGGIE SALAD

COOKING: 0'   **PREPARATION: 10'**   **SERVES: 8**

INGREDIENTS

For salad:
- 1 cup fresh baby carrots, quartered lengthwise
- 1 celery rib, sliced
- 3 large mushrooms, thinly sliced
- 1 cup cauliflower florets, bite sized, blanched
- 1 cup broccoli florets, blanched
- 1 cup thinly sliced radish
- 4-5 oz. hearts of romaine salad mix to serve

For dressing:
- ½ package Italian salad dressing mix
- 3 tablespoons white vinegar
- 3 tablespoons water
- 3 tablespoons olive oil
- 3-4 pepperoncino, chopped

DIRECTIONS

To make salad:
1. Add all the ingredients of the salad except hearts of romaine to a bowl and toss.
2. To make dressing:
3. Add all the ingredients of the dressing in a small bowl. Whisk well.
4. Pour dressing over salad and toss well. Refrigerate for a couple of hours.
5. Place romaine in a large bowl. Place the chilled salad over it and serve.

NUTRITION: Calories: 84 Fat: 6.7g Carbs: 5g Protein: 2g

253. GLAZED CARROTS

COOKING: 8'   **PREPARATION: 15'**   **SERVES: 4**

INGREDIENTS

- 1-pound baby carrots, peeled
- 1 tablespoon Maple syrup
- 1 tablespoon olive oil
- 1 teaspoon coriander, ground
- 1/2 teaspoon minced garlic
- 1 teaspoon turmeric powder
- 1 tablespoon apple cider vinegar
- 1 tablespoon sesame seeds
- 1/2 cup of water

DIRECTIONS

1. In a bowl, mix the carrots with the maple syrup and the other Ingredients, toss and leave aside for 10 minutes.
2. Transfer the mix in the instant pot. Add water and cook on Manual mode (High pressure) for 8 minutes.
3. Then make quick pressure release.
4. Transfer the mix in the serving bowls and serve.

NUTRITION: Calories: 172, Fat: 4.9g, Fiber: 1.5g, Carbs: 6.1g, Protein: 4.3g

254. BROCCOLI PUREE

COOKING: 15' **PREPARATION: 15'** **SERVES: 6**

INGREDIENTS

- 1-pound broccoli florets
- 1/3 cup almond milk
- 1 cup of water
- 1 teaspoon dried oregano
- 1/2 teaspoon coriander, ground

DIRECTIONS

1. Put the broccoli and the water in the instant pot and close the lid.
2. Cook on Manual mode (High pressure) for 15 minutes. Use natural pressure release for 10 minutes.
3. Strain, transfer to the food processor, add the rest of the Ingredients and pulse.
4. Divide between plates and serve.

NUTRITION: Calories: 182, Fat: 3.8g, Fiber: 4.8g, Carbs: 11.1g, Protein: 2g

255. LEMON CAULIFLOWER

COOKING: 8' **PREPARATION: 7'** **SERVES: 4**

INGREDIENTS

- 1-pound cauliflower florets
- 1 teaspoon lemon zest
- 1 tablespoon lemon juice
- 1 teaspoon turmeric powder
- 1 teaspoon black pepper
- 1 teaspoon Pink salt
- 1 tablespoon fresh dill, chopped
- 1/4 cup vegetable broth
- 1 tablespoon olive oil

DIRECTIONS

1. In the instant pot, mix the cauliflower with the lemon juice, zest and the other Ingredients, close the lid and cook on Manual mode for 8 minutes.
2. Allow natural pressure release.

NUTRITION: Calories: 205, Fat: 4.5g, Fiber: 3.3g, Carbs: 14.5g, Protein: 4.2g

256. LEMONGRASS RICE

COOKING: 15'   **PREPARATION: 15'**   **SERVES: 3**

INGREDIENTS

- 1 cup wild rice
- 1 cup vegetable broth
- 1 tablespoon lemongrass, chopped
- 1 teaspoon turmeric powder
- 1 teaspoon oregano, dried
- 1 tablespoon almond butter
- 3/4 teaspoon ground nutmeg
- 1/3 teaspoon Pink salt

DIRECTIONS

1. Put quinoa in an instant pot.
2. Add the rest of the Ingredients and toss. Close the lid, seal it, and set Manual mode (high pressure).
3. Cook for 15 minutes and allow natural pressure release for 10 minutes.
4. Divide between plates and serve.

NUTRITION: Calories: 225, Fat: 7.1g, Fiber: 4.6g, Carbs: 22.3g, Protein: 10.8g

257. CHIVES COUSCOUS

COOKING: 5'   **PREPARATION: 15'**   **SERVES: 4**

INGREDIENTS

- 1 1/2 cup yellow couscous
- 2 cups of water
- 1 tablespoon chives, chopped
- 1 teaspoon cumin, ground
- 1 teaspoon coriander, ground
- 1 teaspoon cayenne pepper
- 1 tablespoon olive oil
- 1 teaspoon salt

DIRECTIONS

1. Preheat instant pot on Saute mode for 3 minutes.
2. Pour olive oil inside it and add couscous.
3. Stir it gently and saute for 2 minutes.
4. Add the rest of the Ingredients and toss. Close the lid. Set manual mode (High pressure).
5. Cook the side dish for 2 minutes.
6. Release the pressure manually for 10 minutes

NUTRITION: Calories: 96, Fat: 3.6g, Fiber: 0.8g, Carbs: 11.5g, Protein: 4.5g

258. COCONUT CAULIFLOWER MIX

COOKING: 10' **PREPARATION: 10'** **SERVES: 6**

INGREDIENTS

- 1-pound cauliflower florets
- 1 cup of water
- 1/4 cup of coconut milk
- 1 tablespoon coconut yogurt
- 1 teaspoon salt
- 1 teaspoon hot paprika
- 1 teaspoon Italian seasoning
- 1 tablespoon chives, chopped

DIRECTIONS

1. Place cauliflower and water in the instant pot. Add salt and close the lid.
2. Cook the vegetables on Manual mode for 10 minutes.
3. Then use quick pressure release.
4. Open the lid, drain water and mash the cauliflower.
5. Add the rest of the Ingredients, stir well and serve.

NUTRITION: Calories: 211, Fat: 4.6g, Fiber: 5.3g, Carbs: 24.2g, Protein: 3.9g

259. PEPPERS BOWL

COOKING: 10' **PREPARATION: 10'** **SERVES: 2**

INGREDIENTS

- 2 1/2 cup cauliflower florets, grated
- 1 teaspoon black pepper
- 1 teaspoon oregano, dried
- 1 teaspoon turmeric powder
- 1 teaspoon salt
- 1/2 cup of water
- 1 teaspoon olive oil
- 1 tablespoon chives, chopped

DIRECTIONS

1. In an instant pot, mix the cauliflower rice with black pepper and the other Ingredients and close the lid.
2. Set manual mode and cook on High for 6 minute. Make a quick pressure release.
3. Chill the cauliflower rice for 2-5 minutes before serving.

NUTRITION: Calories: 32, Fat: 1.4g, Fiber: 1.6g, Carbs: 3.5g, Protein: 1.7g

261. POTATO MASH

COOKING: 9'   **PREPARATION: 10'**   **SERVES: 6**

INGREDIENTS

- 1 and 1/2 lb.' white potatoes, peeled, chopped
- 1 teaspoon salt
- 1/2 teaspoon hot paprika
- 1 teaspoon dill, dried
- 1 tablespoon coconut butter
- 1 teaspoon ground black pepper
- 1 cup vegetable broth
- 1 tablespoon fresh parsley, chopped

DIRECTIONS

1. Put potatoes, salt, and vegetable broth in the instant pot.
2. Close the lid and set manual mode. Cook on High for 9 minutes.
3. Then make quick pressure release, strain the sweet potatoes and mash until smooth.
4. Add the rest of the Ingredients, stir well and serve.

NUTRITION: Calories: 123, Fat: 4.3g, Fiber: 2.2g, Carbs: 11.4g, Protein: 4.3g

262. RED CABBAGE AND CARROTS

COOKING: 7'   **PREPARATION: 10'**   **SERVES: 3**

INGREDIENTS

- 1-pound red cabbage, shredded
- 2 carrots, peeled and grated
- 1 teaspoon turmeric powder
- 1 teaspoon coriander, ground
- 1 teaspoon black pepper
- 1 teaspoon salt
- 1/4 cup of coconut milk
- 3/4 cup almond milk
- 1/2 tablespoon chives, chopped

DIRECTIONS

1. In an instant pot, mix the cabbage with the carrots and the other ingredients, toss and set manual mode (High pressure).
2. Cook the cabbage for 7 minutes. Then allow natural pressure release.
3. Transfer the meal into the serving bowls and cool down before serving.

NUTRITION: Calories: 182, Fat: 5.1g, Fiber: 3.4g, Carbs: 12.3g, Protein: 2.6g

263. SPAGHETTI SQUASH AND LEEKS

COOKING: 10' **PREPARATION: 15'** **SERVES: 4**

INGREDIENTS

- 2 leeks, sliced
- 1 teaspoon chili powder
- 1 teaspoon cumin, ground
- 1 teaspoon onion powder
- 1 teaspoon apple cider vinegar
- 1-pound spaghetti squash, halved, seeds removed
- 1 tablespoon Italian seasoning
- 1 cup water, for cooking

DIRECTIONS

1. Pour water in the instant pot and insert steamer rack.
2. Arrange spaghetti squash on the rack and close the lid.
3. Cook it on High for 10 minutes. Then allow natural pressure release for 5 minutes.
4. Check if the spaghetti squash is soft, shred the flesh with a fork's help, and transfer to a bowl.
5. Add the rest of the Ingredients, toss and serve.

NUTRITION: Calories: 110, Fat: 1.7g, Fiber: 9g, Carbs: 4.3g, Protein: 2.8g

264. PAPRIKA SWEET POTATO

COOKING: 10' **PREPARATION: 11'** **SERVES: 2**

INGREDIENTS

- 2 sweet potatoes
- 2 teaspoons sweet paprika
- 1/2 teaspoon oregano, dried
- 1 teaspoon chili powder
- 1 teaspoon chives, chopped
- 1/2 cup of water

DIRECTIONS

1. Pour water in the instant pot and insert steamer rack.
2. Put potatoes on the rack and close the lid.
3. Set Manual mode (High pressure) and cook for 11 minutes. Then use quick pressure release.
4. Transfer the potatoes on the plate, cut into halves, sprinkle the rest of the Ingredients on top and serve.

NUTRITION: Calories: 159, Fat: 3.4g, Fiber: 2.8g, Carbs: 33.8g, Protein: 3.6g

265. CINNAMON CARROTS

COOKING: 15' **PREPARATION: 10'** **SERVES: 4**

INGREDIENTS

- 1-pound baby carrots, scrubbed
- 1/3 cup water
- 1 teaspoon ground cinnamon
- 1/4 teaspoon chili powder
- 1 teaspoon black pepper

DIRECTIONS

1. In the instant pot, mix the carrots with the water and the other Ingredients, close the lid and Manual mode (High pressure) for 15 minutes.
2. After this, use quick pressure release.
3. Divide between plates and serve.

NUTRITION: Calories: 147, Fat: 0.5g, Fiber: 7.1g, Carbs: 9.9g, Protein: 4.3g

266. WILD RICE AND CORN

COOKING: 8' **PREPARATION: 10'** **SERVES: 4**

INGREDIENTS

- 1 cup wild rice
- 1 tablespoon Italian seasoning
- 1/4 cup corn kernels, canned
- 1 teaspoon chili powder
- 1 teaspoon salt
- 2 cups vegetable broth
- 1 tablespoon chives, chopped
- 2 tablespoons olive oil

DIRECTIONS

1. Pour olive oil in the instant pot and set Saute mode.
2. Add rice and seasoning and cook for 2 minutes.
3. Add the rest of the Ingredients and toss.
4. Set Manual mode (High pressure) and close the lid. Seal it.
5. Cook rice for 6 minutes. Use quick pressure release.

NUTRITION: Calories: 254, Fat: 4.3g, Carbs: 25.4, Protein: 5.4g

267. KALE POLENTA

COOKING: 8' **PREPARATION: 5'** **SERVES: 5**

INGREDIENTS

- 1 cup polenta
- 1/2 cup kale, chopped
- 1 teaspoon turmeric powder
- 1 teaspoon smoked paprika
- 4 cups vegetable broth
- 2 tablespoons coconut milk
- 1/2 teaspoon ground black pepper
- 1 teaspoon salt

DIRECTIONS

1. Whisk together polenta and vegetable broth.
2. Pour mixture in the instant pot, add the rest of the ingredients and toss.
3. Close the lid and cook it on Manual mode (High pressure) for 8 minutes. Use quick pressure release/
4. Transfer cooked polenta in the bowl, stir and serve

NUTRITION: Calories: 182, Fat: 2.8g, Fiber: 1g, Carbs: 20.5g, Protein: 6.3g

268. BROCCOLI SALAD

COOKING: 25' **PREPARATION: 5'** **SERVES: 6**

INGREDIENTS

- 2 tablespoons sherry vinegar
- ¼ cup olive oil
- 2 teaspoons fresh thyme, chopped
- 1 teaspoon Dijon mustard
- 1 teaspoon honey
- Salt to taste
- 8 cups broccoli florets, steamed or roasted
- 2 red onions, sliced thinly
- ½ cup Parmesan cheese, shaved
- ¼ cup pecans, toasted and chopped

DIRECTIONS

1. Mix the sherry vinegar, olive oil, thyme, mustard, honey and salt in a bowl.
2. In a serving bowl, combine the broccoli florets and onions.
3. Drizzle the dressing on top.
4. Sprinkle with the pecans and Parmesan cheese before serving.

NUTRITION: Calories: 199 Fat: 17.4g Carbs: 7.5g Protein: 5.2g

269. POTATO CARROT SALAD

COOKING: 10' **PREPARATION: 15'** **SERVES: 6**

INGREDIENTS

- Water
- 6 potatoes, sliced into cubes
- 3 carrots, sliced into cubes
- 1 tablespoon milk
- 1 tablespoon Dijon mustard
- ¼ cup mayonnaise
- Pepper to taste
- 2 teaspoons fresh thyme, chopped
- 1 stalk celery, chopped
- 2 scallions, chopped
- 1 slice turkey bacon, cooked crispy and crumbled

DIRECTIONS

1. Fill your pot with water.
2. Place it over medium high heat.
3. Boil the potatoes and carrots for 10 minutes or until tender.
4. Drain and let cool.
5. In a bowl, mix the milk mustard, mayo, pepper and thyme.
6. Stir in the potatoes, carrots and celery.
7. Coat evenly with the sauce.
8. Cover and refrigerate for 4 hours.
9. Top with the scallions and turkey bacon bits before serving.

NUTRITION: Calories: 106 Fat: 5.3 Carbs: 12.6g Protein: 2g

270. PEA SALAD

COOKING: 0' **PREPARATION: 40'** **SERVES: 6**

INGREDIENTS

- 1 cup chickpeas, rinsed and drained
- 1 ½ cups peas, divided
- Salt to taste
- 3 tablespoons olive oil
- ½ cup buttermilk
- Pepper to taste
- 8 cups pea greens
- 3 carrots, shaved
- 1 cup snow peas, trimmed

DIRECTIONS

1. Add the chickpeas and half of the peas to your food processor.
2. Season with the salt.
3. Pulse until smooth. Set aside.
4. In a bowl, toss the remaining peas in oil, milk, salt and pepper.
5. Transfer the mixture to your food processor.
6. Process until pureed.
7. Transfer this mixture to a bowl.
8. Arrange the pea greens in a serving plate.
9. Top with the shaved carrots and snow peas.
10. Stir in the pea and milk dressing.
11. Serve with the reserved chickpea hummus.

NUTRITION: Calories: 214 Fat: 8.6g Carbs: 27.3g Protein: 8g

271. SNAP PEA SALAD

COOKING: 0' **PREPARATION:** 1 H **SERVES:** 6

INGREDIENTS

- 2 tablespoons mayonnaise
- ¾ teaspoon celery seed
- ¼ cup cider vinegar
- 1 teaspoon yellow mustard
- 1 tablespoon sugar
- Salt and pepper to taste
- 4 oz. radishes, sliced thinly
- 12 oz. sugar snap peas, sliced thinly

DIRECTIONS

1. In a bowl, combine the mayonnaise, celery seeds, vinegar, mustard, sugar, salt and pepper.
2. Stir in the radishes and snap peas.
3. Refrigerate for 30 minutes.

NUTRITION: Calories: 69 Fat: 3.7g Carbs: 7.1g Protein: 2g

272. CUCUMBER TOMATO CHOPPED SALAD

COOKING: 0' **PREPARATION:** 15' **SERVES:** 6

INGREDIENTS

- ½ cup light mayonnaise
- 1 tablespoon lemon juice
- 1 tablespoon fresh dill, chopped
- 1 tablespoon chives, chopped
- ½ cup feta cheese, crumbled
- Salt and pepper to taste
- 1 red onion, chopped
- 1 cucumber, diced
- 1 radish, diced
- 3 tomatoes, diced
- Chives, chopped

DIRECTIONS

1. Combine the mayo, lemon juice, fresh dill, chives, feta cheese, salt and pepper in a bowl. Mix well.
2. Stir in the onion, cucumber, radish and tomatoes. Coat evenly.
3. Garnish with the chopped chives.

NUTRITION: Calories: 187 Fat: 16.7g Carbs: 6.7g Protein: 3.3g

273. ZUCCHINI PASTA SALAD

COOKING: 0'   **PREPARATION: 4'**   **SERVES: 15**

INGREDIENTS

- 5 tablespoons olive oil
- 2 teaspoons Dijon mustard
- 3 tablespoons red-wine vinegar
- 1 clove garlic, grated
- 2 tablespoons fresh oregano, chopped
- 1 shallot, chopped
- ¼ teaspoon red pepper flakes
- 16 oz. zucchini noodles
- ¼ cup Kalamata olives, pitted
- 3 cups cherry tomatoes, sliced in half
- ¾ cup Parmesan cheese, shaved

DIRECTIONS

1. Mix the olive oil, Dijon mustard, red-wine vinegar, garlic, oregano, shallot and red pepper flakes in a bowl.
2. Stir in the zucchini noodles.
3. Sprinkle on top the olives, tomatoes and Parmesan cheese.

NUTRITION: Calories: 299 Fat: 24.7g Carbs: 11.6g Protein: 7g

274. EGG AVOCADO SALAD

COOKING: 0'   **PREPARATION: 10'**   **SERVES: 4**

INGREDIENTS

- 1 avocado
- 6 hard-boiled eggs, peeled and chopped
- 1 tablespoon mayonnaise
- 2 tablespoons freshly squeezed lemon juice
- ¼ cup celery, chopped
- 2 tablespoons chives, chopped
- Salt and pepper to taste

DIRECTIONS

1. Add the avocado to a large bowl.
2. Mash the avocado using a fork.
3. Stir in the egg and mash the eggs.
4. Add the mayo, lemon juice, celery, chives, salt and pepper.
5. Chill in the refrigerator for at least 30 minutes before serving.

NUTRITION: Calories: 224 Fat: 18g Carbs: 6.1g Protein: 10.6g

275. PEPPER TOMATO SALAD

COOKING: 0' **PREPARATION: 1H 25'** **SERVES: 8**

INGREDIENTS

- 2 tablespoons balsamic vinegar
- 2 tablespoons olive oil
- ½ teaspoon Dijon mustard
- 2 teaspoons fresh basil leaves, chopped
- 1 tablespoon fresh chives, chopped
- 1 teaspoon sugar
- Pepper to taste
- 2 cups yellow bell peppers, sliced into rings
- 1 cups orange bell pepper, sliced into rings
- 4 tomatoes, sliced into rounds
- ¼ cup blue cheese, crumbled

DIRECTIONS

1. Mix the vinegar, olive oil, mustard, basil, chives, sugar and pepper in a bowl.
2. Arrange the tomatoes and pepper rings in a serving plate.
3. Sprinkle the crumbled blue cheese on top.
4. Drizzle with the dressing.
5. Chill in the refrigerator for 1 hour before serving.

NUTRITION: Calories: 116 Fat: 7g Carbs: 11g Protein: 3g

276. PENNE WITH VEGGIES

COOKING: 25' **PREPARATION: 5'** **SERVES: 6**

INGREDIENTS

- 2 teaspoons olive oil
- 2 cloves garlic, crushed and minced
- ½ cup shallots, chopped
- 2 tablespoons dry white wine
- 1 cup Brussels sprouts, trimmed and chopped
- 6 cups bok choy, chopped
- 6 cups cooked penne pasta
- 1 tablespoons vegetable oil spread
- Salt and pepper to taste
- 2 teaspoons dried Italian seasoning
- 3 tablespoons Parmesan cheese, grated

DIRECTIONS

1. Pour the oil into a pan over medium heat.
2. Cook the garlic and shallots for 3 minutes.
3. Pour in the wine.
4. Scrape the browned bits using a wooden spoon.
5. Stir in the Brussels sprouts.
6. Cook for 3 minutes.
7. Stir in the bok choy and cook for 2 to 3 minutes.
8. Toss the pasta in the veggies.
9. Add the vegetable oil into the mix.
10. Season with the salt, pepper and Italian seasoning.
11. Sprinkle the Parmesan cheese on top.

NUTRITION: Calories: 27 Fat: 4g Carbs: 17g Protein: 6g

277. MARINATED VEGGIE SALAD

COOKING: 0' | **PREPARATION: 4H 30'** | **SERVES: 6**

INGREDIENTS

- 1 zucchini, sliced
- 4 tomatoes, sliced into wedges
- ¼ cup red onion, sliced thinly
- 1 green bell pepper, sliced
- 2 tablespoons fresh parsley, chopped
- 2 tablespoons red-wine vinegar
- 2 tablespoons olive oil
- 1 clove garlic, minced
- 1 teaspoon dried basil
- 2 tablespoons water
- Pine nuts, toasted and chopped

DIRECTIONS

1. In a bowl, combine the zucchini, tomatoes, red onion, green bell pepper and parsley.
2. Pour the vinegar and oil into a glass jar with lid.
3. Add the garlic, basil and water.
4. Seal the jar and shake well to combine.
5. Pour the dressing into the vegetable mixture.
6. Cover the bowl.
7. Marinate in the refrigerator for 4 hours.
8. Garnish with the pine nuts before serving.

NUTRITION: Calories: 65 Fat: 4.7g Carbs: 5.3g Protein: 0.9g

278. ARUGULA SALAD

COOKING: 0' | **PREPARATION: 15'** | **SERVES: 4**

INGREDIENTS

- 6 cups fresh arugula leaves
- 2 cups radicchio, chopped
- ¼ cup low-Fat: balsamic vinaigrette
- ¼ cup pine nuts, toasted and chopped

DIRECTIONS

1. Arrange the arugula leaves in a serving bowl. Sprinkle the radicchio on top.
2. Drizzle with the vinaigrette. Sprinkle the pine nuts on top.

NUTRITION: Calories: 85 Fat: 6.6g Carbs: 5.1g Protein: 2.2g

279. MEDITERRANEAN SALAD

COOKING: 5'   **PREPARATION: 20'**   **SERVES: 2**

INGREDIENTS

- 2 teaspoons balsamic vinegar
- 1 tablespoon basil pesto
- 1 cup lettuce
- ¼ cup broccoli florets, chopped
- ½ cup zucchini, chopped
- ¼ cup tomato, chopped
- ¼ cup yellow bell pepper, chopped
- 2 tablespoons feta cheese, crumbled

DIRECTIONS

1. Arrange the lettuce on a serving platter.
2. Top with the broccoli, zucchini, tomato and bell pepper.
3. In a bowl, mix the vinegar and pesto.
4. Drizzle the dressing on top.
5. Sprinkle the feta cheese and serve.

NUTRITION: Calories: 100 Fat: 6g Carbs: 7g Protein: 4g

280. POTATO TUNA SALAD

COOKING: 10'   **PREPARATION: 4H 20'**   **SERVES: 6**

INGREDIENTS

- Water
- 3 potatoes, peeled and sliced into cubes
- ½ cup plain yogurt
- ½ cup mayonnaise
- 1 clove garlic, crushed and minced
- 1 tablespoon almond milk
- 1 tablespoon fresh dill, chopped
- ½ teaspoon lemon zest
- Salt to taste
- 1 cup cucumber, chopped
- ¼ cup scallions, chopped
- ¼ cup radishes, chopped
- 9 oz. canned tuna flakes
- 2 hard-boiled eggs, chopped
- 6 cups lettuce, chopped

DIRECTIONS

1. Fill your pot with water. Add the potatoes and boil.
2. Cook for 10 minutes or until slightly tender.
3. Drain and let cool.
4. In a bowl, mix the yogurt, mayo, garlic, almond milk, fresh dill, lemon zest and salt.
5. Stir in the potatoes, tuna flakes and eggs. Mix well.
6. Chill in the refrigerator for 4 hours.
7. Stir in the shredded lettuce before serving.

NUTRITION: Calories: 243 Fat: 9.9g Carbs: 22.2g Protein: 17.5g

281. SHRIMP VEGGIE PASTA SALAD

COOKING: 10' **PREPARATION: 50'** **SERVES: 6**

INGREDIENTS

- 1 lb. shrimp, peeled and deveined
- 8 oz. asparagus, sliced
- Salt and pepper to taste
- 12 oz. farfalle, penne or macaroni pasta, cooked
- 2 tablespoons parsley, chopped
- ½ cup shallots, sliced thinly
- ¼ cup Parmesan cheese, grated
- 2 tablespoons freshly squeezed lemon juice
- ½ cup mayonnaise
- 2 teaspoons garlic, minced
- 1 teaspoon Worcestershire sauce
- 1 teaspoon Dijon mustard
- 1 lemon, sliced into wedges

DIRECTIONS

1. Preheat your oven to 400°F.
2. Arrange the shrimp and asparagus in a baking pan.
3. Season with the salt and pepper.
4. Roast in the oven for 10 minutes.
5. Let cool. Transfer to a bowl.
6. Stir in the cooked pasta, parsley and shallots.
7. Sprinkle the Parmesan cheese on top.
8. In another bowl, combine the lemon juice, mayonnaise, garlic, Worcestershire sauce and Dijon mustard.
9. Add this mixture to the pasta salad. Toss to coat evenly.
10. Refrigerate for at least 30 minutes before serving.
11. Garnish with the lemon wedges.

NUTRITION: Calories: 429 Fat: 17.1g Carbs: 45.6g Protein: 25g

282. SAUTÉED CABBAGE

COOKING: 12' **PREPARATION: 8'** **SERVES: 8**

INGREDIENTS

- ¼ cup butter
- 1 onion, sliced thinly
- 1 head cabbage, sliced into wedges
- Salt and pepper to taste
- Crumbled crispy bacon bits

DIRECTIONS

1. Add the butter to a pan over medium-high heat.
2. Cook the onion for 1 minute, stirring frequently.
3. Season with the salt and pepper.
4. Add the cabbage and cook while stirring for 12 minutes.
5. Sprinkle with the crispy bacon bits.

NUTRITION: Calories: 77 Fat: 5.9g Carbs: 6.1g Protein: 1.3g

CHAPTER 14: SNACK AND SIDES

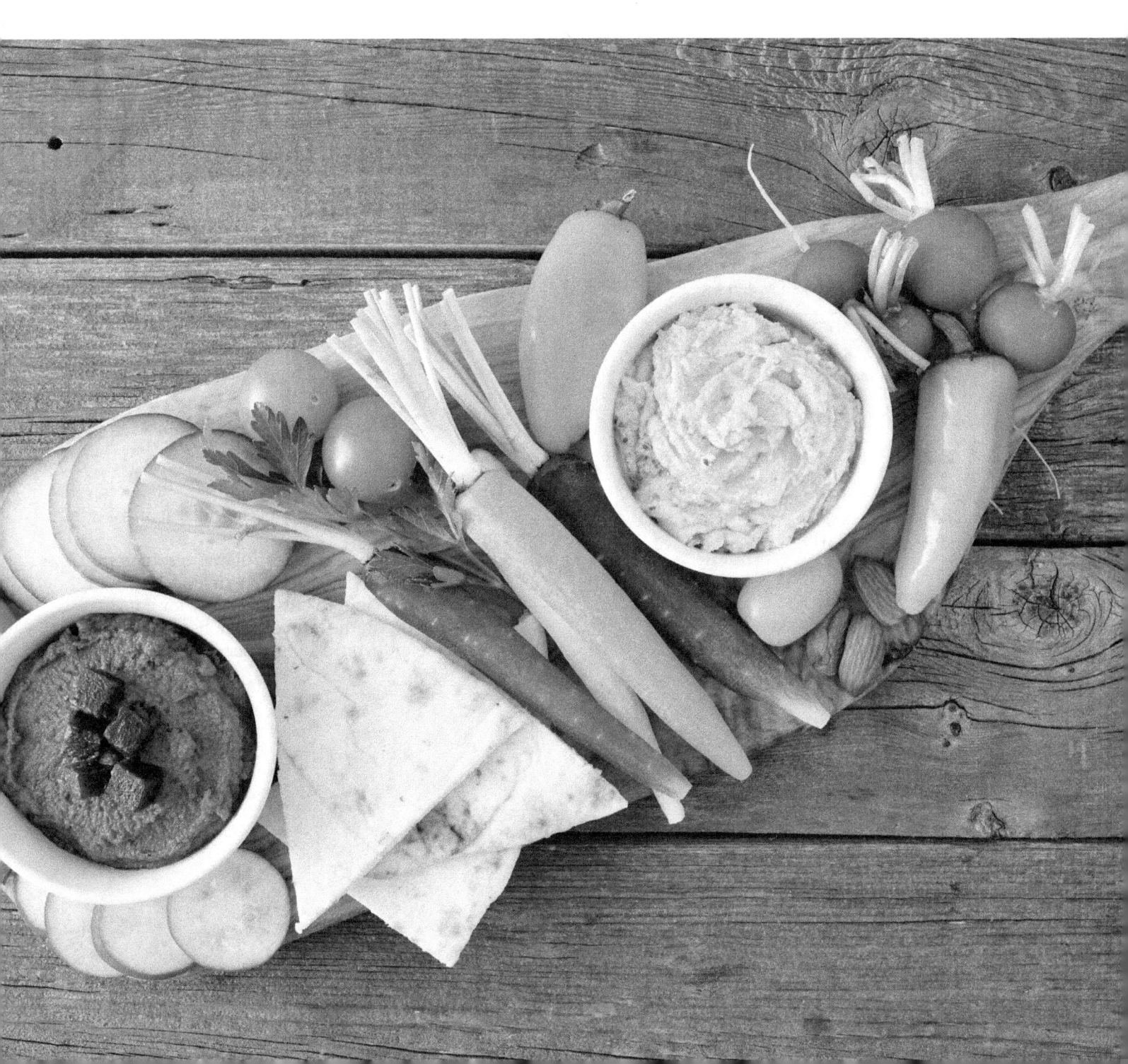

283. BLACK BEAN LIME DIP

COOKING: 6'   **PREPARATION: 5'**   **SERVES: 4**

INGREDIENTS

- 15.5 oz. cooked black beans
- 1 teaspoon minced garlic
- ½ of a lime, juiced
- 1 inch of ginger, grated
- 1/3 teaspoon salt
- 1/3 teaspoon ground black pepper
- 1 tablespoon olive oil

DIRECTIONS

1. Take a frying pan, add oil and when hot, add garlic and ginger and cook for 1 minute until fragrant.
2. Then add beans, splash with some water and fry for 3 minutes until hot.
3. Season beans with salt and black pepper, drizzle with lime juice, remove the pan from heat and mash the beans until smooth pasta comes together.
4. Serve the dip with whole-grain bread sticks or vegetables.

NUTRITION: Calories: 374 Fat: 14g Carbs: 46g Protein: 15g

284. BEETROOT HUMMUS

COOKING: 60'   **PREPARATION: 10'**   **SERVES: 4**

INGREDIENTS

- 15 oz. cooked chickpeas
- 3 small beets
- 1 teaspoon minced garlic
- 1/2 teaspoon smoked paprika
- 1 teaspoon of sea salt
- 1/4 teaspoon red chili flakes
- 2 tablespoons olive oil
- 1 lemon, juiced
- 2 tablespoon tahini
- 1 tablespoon chopped almonds
- 1 tablespoon chopped cilantro

DIRECTIONS

1. Drizzle oil over beets, season with salt, then wrap beets in a foil and bake for 60 minutes at 425°F until tender.
2. When done, let beet cool for 10 minutes, then peel and dice them and place them in a food processor.
3. Add remaining ingredients and pulse for 2 minutes until smooth, tip the hummus in a bowl, drizzle with some more oil, and then serve straight away.

NUTRITION: Calories: 50.1 Fat: 2.5g Carbs: 5g Protein: 2g

285. ZUCCHINI HUMMUS

COOKING: 0'   **PREPARATION: 5'**   **SERVES: 8**

INGREDIENTS

- 1 cup diced zucchini
- 1/2 teaspoon sea salt
- 1 teaspoon minced garlic
- 2 teaspoons ground cumin
- 3 tablespoons lemon juice
- 1/3 cup tahini

DIRECTIONS

1. Place all the ingredients in a food processor and pulse for 2 minutes until smooth.
2. Tip the hummus in a bowl, drizzle with oil and serve.

NUTRITION: Calories: 65 Fat: 5g Carbs: 3g Protein: 2g

286. CHIPOTLE AND LIME TORTILLA CHIPS

COOKING: 15'   **PREPARATION: 10'**   **SERVES: 4**

INGREDIENTS

- 12 oz. whole-wheat tortillas
- 4 tablespoons chipotle seasoning
- 1 tablespoon olive oil
- 4 limes, juiced

DIRECTIONS

1. Whisk together oil and lime juice, brush it well on tortillas, then sprinkle with chipotle seasoning and bake for 15 minutes at 350°F until crispy, turning halfway.
2. When done, let the tortilla cool for 10 minutes, then break it into chips and serve.

NUTRITION: Calories: 150 Fat: 7g Carbs: 18g Protein: 2g

THE PLANT BASED DIET COOKBOOK

287. CARROT AND SWEET POTATO FRITTERS

COOKING: 8' | **PREPARATION: 10'** | **SERVES: 10**

INGREDIENTS

- 1/3 cup quinoa flour
- 1½ cups shredded sweet potato
- 1 cup grated carrot
- 1/3 teaspoon ground black pepper
- 2/3 teaspoon salt
- 2 teaspoons curry powder
- 2 flax eggs
- 2 tablespoons coconut oil

DIRECTIONS

1. Place all the ingredients in a bowl, except for oil, stir well until combined and then shape the mixture into ten small patties
2. Take a large pan, place it over medium-high heat, add oil and when it melts, add patties in it and cook for 3 minutes per side until browned.
3. Serve straight away

NUTRITION: Calories: 70 Fat: 3g Carbs: 8g Protein: 1g

288. BUFFALO QUINOA BITES

COOKING: 30' | **PREPARATION: 15'** | **SERVES: 20**

INGREDIENTS

For the Bites:
- 1 cup cooked quinoa
- 15 oz. cooked white beans
- 3 tablespoons chickpea flour
- 1 medium shallot, peeled, chopped
- 3 cloves of garlic, peeled
- ½ teaspoon ground black pepper
- 1/2 teaspoon salt
- 1 teaspoon smoked paprika
- 1/4 cup vegan buffalo sauce

For the Dressing:
- 1/4 cup chives
- 2 tablespoons hemp hearts
- 1 tablespoon nutritional yeast
- 1 teaspoon garlic powder
- 1 teaspoon onion powder
- 1/2 teaspoon salt
- ½ teaspoon ground black pepper
- 2 teaspoons dried dill
- 1 lemon, juiced
- 1/4 cup tahini
- 3/4 cup water

DIRECTIONS

1. Prepare the bites, and for this, place half of the beans in a food processor, add garlic and shallots, and pulse for 2 minutes until mixture comes together.
2. Then add all the spices of the bites and buffalo sauce and pulse for 2 minutes until smooth. Add remaining beans along with chickpea flour and quinoa and pulse until just combined.
3. Tip the mixture in a dish, shape it in the dough, shape it into twenty balls, about the golf-ball size, and bake for 30 minutes at 350°F until crispy and browned, turning halfway.
4. Meanwhile, prepare the dressing and place all of its ingredients in a food processor and pulse for 2 minutes until smooth.
5. Serve bites with prepared dressing.

NUTRITION: Calories: 78 Fat: 3g Carbs: 9g Protein: 4g

289. TOMATO AND PESTO TOAST

COOKING: 0'   **PREPARATION: 5'**   **SERVES: 4**

INGREDIENTS

- 1 small tomato, sliced
- ¼ teaspoon ground black pepper
- 1 tablespoon vegan pesto
- 2 tablespoons hummus
- 1 slice of whole-grain bread, toasted
- Hemp seeds as needed for garnishing

DIRECTIONS

1. Spread hummus on one side of the toast, top with tomato slices and then drizzle with pesto.
2. Sprinkle black pepper on the toast along with hemp seeds and then serve straight away.

NUTRITION: Calories: 214 Fat: 7.2g Carbs: 32g Protein: 6.5g

290. AVOCADO AND SPROUT TOAST

COOKING: 0   **PREPARATION: 5'**   **SERVES: 4**

INGREDIENTS

- 1/2 of a medium avocado, sliced
- 1 slice of whole-grain bread, toasted
- 2 tablespoons sprouts
- 2 tablespoons hummus
- ¼ teaspoon lemon zest
- ½ teaspoon hemp seeds
- ¼ teaspoon red pepper flakes

DIRECTIONS

1. Spread hummus on one side of the toast and then top with avocado slices and sprouts.
2. Sprinkle with lemon zest, hemp seeds, and red pepper flakes and then serve straight away.

NUTRITION: Calories: 200 Fat: 10.5g Carbs: 22g Protein: 7g

291. APPLE AND HONEY TOAST

COOKING: 0   **PREPARATION: 5'**   **SERVES: 4**

INGREDIENTS

- ½ of a small apple, cored, sliced
- 1 slice of whole-grain bread, toasted
- 1 tablespoon honey
- 2 tablespoons hummus
- 1/8 teaspoon cinnamon

DIRECTIONS

1. Spread hummus on one side of the toast, top with apple slices and then drizzle with honey.
2. Sprinkle cinnamon on it and then serve straight away.

NUTRITION: Calories: 212 Fat: 7g Carbs: 35g Protein: 4g

THE PLANT BASED DIET COOKBOOK

292. THAI SNACK MIX

COOKING: 90' **PREPARATION: 15'** **SERVES: 4**

INGREDIENTS

- 5 cups mixed nuts
- 1 cup chopped dried pineapple
- 1 cup pumpkin seed
- 1 teaspoon onion powder
- 1 teaspoon garlic powder
- 2 teaspoons paprika
- 1/2 teaspoon ground black pepper
- 1 teaspoon of sea salt
- 1/4 cup coconut sugar
- 1/2 teaspoon red chili powder
- 1 tablespoon red pepper flakes
- 1/2 tablespoon red curry powder
- 2 tablespoons soy sauce
- 2 tablespoons coconut oil

DIRECTIONS

1. Switch on the slow cooker, add all the ingredients except for dried pineapple and red pepper flakes, stir until combined and cook for 90 minutes at high heat setting, stirring every 30 minutes.
2. When done, spread the nut mixture on a baking sheet lined with parchment paper and let it cool.
3. Then spread dried pineapple on top, sprinkle with red pepper flakes and serve.

NUTRITION: Calories: 230 Fat: 17.5g Carbs: 11.5g Protein: 6.5g

293. ZUCCHINI FRITTERS

COOKING: 6' **PREPARATION: 10'** **SERVES: 12**

INGREDIENTS

- 1/2 cup quinoa flour
- 3 1/2 cups shredded zucchini
- 1/2 cup chopped scallions
- 1/3 teaspoon ground black pepper
- 1 teaspoon salt
- 2 tablespoons coconut oil
- 2 flax eggs

DIRECTIONS

1. Squeeze moisture from the zucchini by wrapping it in a cheesecloth and then transfer it to a bowl.
2. Add remaining ingredients, except for oil, stir until combined and then shape the mixture into twelve patties.
3. Take a skillet pan, place it over medium-high heat, add oil and when hot, add patties and cook for 3 minutes per side until brown.
4. Serve the patties with your favorite vegan sauce.

NUTRITION: Calories: 37 Fat: 1g Carbs: 4g Protein: 2g

294. ZUCCHINI CHIPS

COOKING: 120' **PREPARATION: 10'** **SERVES: 4**

INGREDIENTS

- 1 large zucchini, thinly sliced
- 1 teaspoon salt
- 2 tablespoons olive oil

DIRECTIONS

1. Pat dry zucchini slices and then spread them in an even layer on a baking sheet lined with parchment sheet.
2. Whisk together salt and oil, brush this mixture over zucchini slices on both sides and then bake for 2 hours or more until brown and crispy.
3. When done, let the chips cool for 10 minutes and then serve straight away.

NUTRITION: Calories: 54 Fat: 5g Carbs: 1g Protein: 0g

295. ROSEMARY BEET CHIPS

COOKING: 20' **PREPARATION:** 10' **SERVES:** 3

INGREDIENTS

- 3 large beets, scrubbed, thinly sliced
- 1/8 teaspoon ground black pepper
- ¼ teaspoon of sea salt
- 3 sprigs of rosemary, leaves chopped
- 4 tablespoons olive oil

DIRECTIONS

1. Spread beet slices in a single layer between two large baking sheets, brush the slices with oil, then season with spices and rosemary, toss until well coated, and bake for 20 minutes at 375°F until crispy, turning halfway.
2. When done, let the chips cool for 10 minutes and then serve.

NUTRITION: Calories: 79 Fat: 4.7g Carbs: 8.6g Protein: 1.5g

296. QUINOA BROCCOLI TOTS

COOKING: 20' **PREPARATION:** 10' **SERVES:** 6

INGREDIENTS

- 2 tablespoons quinoa flour
- 2 cups steamed and chopped broccoli florets
- 1/2 cup nutritional yeast
- 1 teaspoon garlic powder
- 1 teaspoon miso paste
- 2 flax eggs
- 2 tablespoons hummus

DIRECTIONS

1. Place all the ingredients in a bowl, stir until well combined, and then shape the mixture into sixteen small balls.
2. Arrange the balls on a baking sheet lined with parchment paper, spray with foil and bake at 400°F for 20 minutes until brown, turning halfway.
3. When done, let the tots cool for 10 minutes and then serve straight away.

NUTRITION: Calories: 19 Fat: 0g Carbs: 2g Protein: 1g

297. SPICY ROASTED CHICKPEAS

COOKING: 20' **PREPARATION:** 10' **SERVES:** 6

INGREDIENTS

- 30 oz. cooked chickpeas
- ½ teaspoon salt
- 2 teaspoons mustard powder
- ½ teaspoon cayenne pepper
- 2 tablespoons olive oil

DIRECTIONS

1. Place all the ingredients in a bowl and stir until well coated and then spread the chickpeas in an even layer on a baking sheet greased with oil.
2. Bake the chickpeas for 20 minutes at 400°F until golden brown and crispy and then serve straight away.

NUTRITION: Calories: 187.1 Fat: 7.4g Carbs: 24.2g Protein: 7.3g

298. CINNAMON BAKED APPLE CHIPS

COOKING: 2H — **PREPARATION: 5'** — **SERVES: 2**

INGREDIENTS

- 1 teaspoon cinnamon
- 1-2 apples

DIRECTIONS

1. Preheat your oven to 200°F
2. Take a sharp knife and slice apples into thin slices. Discard seeds
3. Line a baking sheet with parchment paper and arrange apples on it
4. Make sure they do not overlap
5. Once done, sprinkle cinnamon over apples
6. Bake in the oven for 1 hour
7. Flip and bake for an hour more until no longer moist
8. Serve and enjoy!

NUTRITION: Calories: 147 Fat: 0g Carbs: 39g Protein: 1g

299. ACORN SQUASH WITH MANGO CHUTNEY

COOKING: 3H 10' — **PREPARATION: 10'** — **SERVES: 4**

INGREDIENTS

- 1 large acorn squash
- ¼ cup mango chutney
- ¼ cup flaked coconut
- Salt and pepper as needed

DIRECTIONS

1. Cut the squash into quarters and remove the seeds, discard the stringy pulp.
2. Spray your cooker with olive oil.
3. Transfer the squash to the slow cooker
4. Take a bowl, add coconut and chutney, mix well, and divide it into the center of the Squash. Season well.
5. Place lid on top and cook on LOW for 2-3 hours. Enjoy!

NUTRITION: Calories: 226 Fat: 6g Carbs: 24g Protein: 17g

300. HEALTHY CARROT CHIPS

COOKING: 10' — **PREPARATION: 10'** — **SERVES: 4**

INGREDIENTS

- 3 cups carrots, sliced into paper-thin rounds
- 2 tablespoons olive oil
- 2 teaspoons ground cumin
- ½ teaspoon smoked paprika
- Pinch of salt

DIRECTIONS

1. Preheat your oven to 400°F
2. Slice carrot into paper-thin shaped coins using a peeler
3. Place slices in a bowl and toss with oil and spices
4. Layout the slices onto a parchment paper-lined baking sheet in a single layer
5. Sprinkle salt. Transfer to oven and bake for 8-10 minutes
6. Remove and serve. Enjoy!

NUTRITION: Calories: 434 Fat: 35g Carbs: 31g Protein: 2g

301. HEARTY BRUSSELS AND PISTACHIO

COOKING: 15'   **PREPARATION: 15'**   **SERVES: 4**

INGREDIENTS

- 1 pound Brussels sprouts, tough bottom trimmed and halved lengthwise
- 4 shallots, peeled and quartered
- 1 tablespoon extra-virgin olive oil
- Sea salt
- Freshly ground black pepper
- ½ cup roasted pistachios, chopped
- Zest of ½ lemon
- Juice of ½ lemon

DIRECTIONS

1. Preheat your oven to 400°F
2. Take a baking sheet and line it with aluminum foil
3. Keep it on the side
4. Take a large bowl and add Brussels and shallots and dress them with olive oil
5. Season with salt and pepper and spread veggies onto a sheet
6. Bake for 15 minutes until slightly caramelized
7. Remove the oven and transfer to a serving bowl
8. Toss with lemon zest, lemon juice, and pistachios
9. Serve and enjoy!

NUTRITION: Calories: 126 Fat: 7g Carbs: 14g Protein: 6g

302. BUFFALO CASHEWS CHUTNEY

COOKING: 55'   **PREPARATION: 10'**   **SERVES: 4**

INGREDIENTS

- 2 cups raw cashews
- ¾ cup red hot sauce
- 1/3 cup avocado oil
- ½ teaspoon garlic powder
- ¼ teaspoon turmeric

DIRECTIONS

1. Mix wet ingredients in a bowl and stir in seasoning
2. Add cashews to the bowl and mix
3. Soak cashews in hot sauce mix for 2-4 hours
4. Preheat your oven to 325°F
5. Spread cashews onto a baking sheet
6. Bake for 35-55 minutes, turn every 10-15 minutes
7. Let them cool and serve!

NUTRITION: Calories: 268 Fat: 16g Carbs: 20g Protein: 14g

303. MORNING PEACH

COOKING: 5'   **PREPARATION: 10'**   **SERVES: 4**

INGREDIENTS

- 6 small peaches, cored and cut into wedges
- ¼ cup of coconut sugar
- 2 tablespoons almond butter
- ¼ teaspoon almond extract

DIRECTIONS

1. Take a small pan and add peaches, sugar, butter and almond extract
2. Toss well
3. Cook over medium-high heat for 5 minutes, divide the mix into bowls and serve
4. Enjoy!
5. Remove and serve. Enjoy!

NUTRITION: Calories: 198 Fat: 2g Carbs: 11g Protein: 8g

THE PLANT BASED DIET COOKBOOK

304. STICKY MANGO RICE

COOKING: 20-30' **PREPARATION: 10'** **SERVES: 4**

INGREDIENTS

- 1/2 cup sugar
- 1 mango, sliced
- 14 oz. coconut milk, canned
- 1/2 cup basmati rice

DIRECTIONS

1. Cook the rice according to package instructions, add half of the sugar while cooking rice. Make sure to substitute half of the required water with coconut milk
2. Take another skillet and boil remaining coconut milk with sugar, once the mixture is thick adding rice and gently stir
3. Add mango slices and serve
4. Enjoy!

NUTRITION: Calories: 550 Fat: 30g Carbs: 70g Protein: 6g

305. PECAN AND BLUEBERRY CRUMBLE

COOKING: 20-30' **PREPARATION: 10'** **SERVES: 4**

INGREDIENTS

- 14 oz. blueberries
- 1 tablespoon lemon juice, fresh
- 1 and ½ teaspoon stevia powder
- 3 tablespoons chia seeds
- 2 cups almond flour, blanched
- ¼ cup pecans, chopped
- 5 tablespoons coconut oil
- 2 tablespoons cinnamon

DIRECTIONS

1. Take a bowl and mix in blueberries, stevia, chia seeds, and lemon juice and stir
2. Take an iron skillet and place it overheat, add mixture and stir
3. Take a bowl and mix in remaining ingredients, spread mixture over blueberries
4. Preheat your oven to 400°F
5. Transfer baking dish to your oven, bake for 30 minutes
6. Serve and enjoy!

NUTRITION: Calories: 380 Fat: 32g Carbs: 20g Protein: 10g

306. HEALTHY RICE PUDDING

COOKING: 20-30' **PREPARATION: 10'** **SERVES: 4**

INGREDIENTS

- 1 cup of brown rice
- 1 teaspoon vanilla extract
- ½ teaspoon salt
- ½ teaspoon cinnamon
- ¼ teaspoon nutmeg
- 3 egg substitute
- 3 cups coconut milk, light
- 2 cups brown rice, cooked

DIRECTIONS

1. Take a bowl and mix in all ingredients, stir well
2. Preheat your oven to 300°F
3. Transfer mixture to a baking dish and transfer dish to the oven
4. Bake for 90 minutes
5. Serve and enjoy!

NUTRITION: Calories: 330 Fat: 10g Carbs: 52g Protein: 5g

307. OATMEAL COOKIES

COOKING: 15'   **PREPARATION: 10'**   **SERVES: 4**

INGREDIENTS

- 1/4 cup applesauce
- 1/2 teaspoon cinnamon
- 1/3 cup raisins
- 1/2 teaspoon vanilla extract, pure
- 1 cup ripe banana, mashed
- 2 cups oatmeal

DIRECTIONS

1. Preheat your oven to 350°F
2. Take a bowl and mix in everything until you have a gooey mixture
3. Pour batter into ungreased baking sheet drop by drop and flatten them using a tablespoon
4. Transfer to your oven, bake for 15 minutes
5. Serve once ready!

NUTRITION: Calories: 80 Fat: 1g Carbs: 16g Protein: 2g

308. APPLE SLICES

COOKING: 10'   **PREPARATION: 10'**   **SERVES: 4**

INGREDIENTS

- 1 cup of coconut oil
- ¼ cup date paste
- 2 tablespoons ground cinnamon
- 4 granny smith apples, peeled and sliced, cored

DIRECTIONS

1. Take a large-sized skillet and place it over medium heat
2. Add oil and allow the oil to heat up
3. Stir cinnamon and date paste into the oil
4. Add cut up apples and cook for 5-8 minutes until crispy
5. Serve and enjoy!

NUTRITION: Calories: 368 Fat: 23g Carbs: 44g Protein: 1g

309. EASY PORTOBELLO MUSHROOMS

COOKING: 10'   **PREPARATION: 10'**   **SERVES: 4**

INGREDIENTS

- 12 cherry tomatoes
- 2 oz. scallions
- 4 Portobello mushrooms
- 4 and ¼ oz. of almond butter
- Sunflower seeds and pepper to taste

DIRECTIONS

1. Take a large skillet and melt almond butter over medium heat
2. Add mushrooms and sauté for 3 minutes
3. Stir in cherry tomatoes and scallions
4. Sauté for 5 minutes
5. Season accordingly
6. Sauté until veggies are tender. Enjoy!

NUTRITION: Calories: 154 Fat: 10g Carbs: 2g Protein: 7g

310. THE GARBANZO BEAN EXTRAVAGANZA

COOKING: 0' **PREPARATION: 10'** **SERVES: 5**

INGREDIENTS

- 1 can garbanzo beans, chickpeas
- 1 tablespoon olive oil
- 1 teaspoon sunflower seeds
- 1 teaspoon garlic powder
- ½ teaspoon paprika

DIRECTIONS

1. Preheat your oven to 375°F
2. Line a baking sheet with silicone baking mat
3. Drain and rinse garbanzo beans, pat garbanzo beans dry and put into a large bowl
4. Toss with olive oil, sunflower seeds, garlic powder, paprika and mix well
5. Spread over a baking sheet
6. Bake for 20 minutes at 375°F
7. Turn chickpeas so they are roasted well
8. Place back in the oven and bake for 25 minutes at 375°F
9. Let them cool and enjoy!

NUTRITION: Calories: 395 Fat: 7g Carbs: 52g Protein: 35g

311. ROASTED ONIONS AND GREEN BEANS

COOKING: 15' **PREPARATION: 10'** **SERVES: 6**

INGREDIENTS

- 1 yellow onion, sliced into rings
- ½ teaspoon onion powder
- 2 tablespoons coconut flour
- 1 and 1/3 lb. fresh green beans, trimmed and chopped

DIRECTIONS

1. Take a large bowl and mix sunflower seeds with onion powder and coconut flour
2. Add onion rings
3. Mix well to coat
4. Spread the rings on the baking sheet, lined with parchment paper
5. Drizzled with some oil
6. Bake for 10 minutes at 400°F
7. Parboil the green beans for 3 to 5 minutes in the boiling water
8. Drain and serve the beans with baked onion rings
9. Eat warm and enjoy!

NUTRITION: Calories: 214 Fat: 19.4g Carbs: 3.7g Protein: 8.3g

312. LEMONY SPROUTS

COOKING: 0' **PREPARATION: 10'** **SERVES: 4**

INGREDIENTS

- 1-pound Brussels, trimmed and shredded
- 8 tablespoons olive oil
- 1 lemon, juiced and tested
- Salt and pepper to taste
- ¾ cup spicy almond and seed mix

DIRECTIONS

1. Take a bowl and mix in lemon juice, salt, pepper and olive oil
2. Mix well
3. Stir in shredded Brussels and toss
4. Let it sit for 10 minutes
5. Add nuts and toss
6. Serve and enjoy!

NUTRITION: Calories: 382 Fat: 36g Carbs: 9g Protein: 7g

313. SAUSAGE ROLLS

COOKING: 35'   **PREPARATION: 6'**   **SERVES: 6**

INGREDIENTS

- 2 slices whole-wheat bread
- .5 cup mixed nuts, halves and pieces
- 1 Onion, small, diced
- 2 tablespoons cranberries, dried
- 1.5 teaspoons sea salt
- 1 teaspoon thyme, fresh, chopped
- 1 teaspoon sage, dried
- .5 teaspoon fennel seeds
- 1 teaspoon paprika, smoked
- 1 teaspoon paprika, sweet
- 3 cloves garlic, minced
- .25 teaspoon black pepper, ground
- 1.5 tablespoons tamari sauce
- 1 teaspoon sriracha
- 2 tablespoons aquafaba egg replacement
- 10 oz. tofu, firm
- Vegan puff pastry – 3 prepared sheets

DIRECTIONS

1. Preheat your large baking oven to a temperature of 375°F and prepare a large sheet for baking with either non-stick silicone or kitchen parchment.
2. In a large food processor, pulse together the sliced bread, mixed nuts, cranberries, and herbs until they form a fine meal or crumb.
3. The food processor, along with the bread and nut mixture, add the tofu, sea salt, tamari sauce, sriracha, aquafaba, ground black pepper, and both the smoked and sweet paprika. Pulse this mixture until it is well combined, stirring the container's sides with a spatula as needed. Set this aside.
4. Lay out the three prepared sheets of puff pastry on a cutting board and slice each sheet into four evenly-sized squares so that you end up with twelve squares in all.
5. Divide the tofu sausage mixture between the twelve squares, placing the mixture in each puff pastry piece's center. Roll the squares up so that the puff pastry completely contains the filling.
6. Using a sharp knife cut each of the twelve rolls in half so that you end up with twenty-four smaller sausage rolls. Place all twenty-four sausage rolls on the prepared baking tray with the puff pastry's seam side facing downward. This will prevent the filling from falling out during the cooking process.
7. Place the sausage rolls in the oven until the puff pastry is golden, about twenty to twenty-five minutes. Serve the rolls alone or with your favorite complimentary chutney.

NUTRITION: Calories: 308 Protein: 13g Fat: 18g Carbs: 25

314. ONION RINGS

COOKING: 20'   **PREPARATION: 10'**   **SERVES: 4**

INGREDIENTS

- 2 sweet onions, large
- .66 cup soy milk, unsweetened
- .66 cup flour
- 1 tablespoon nutritional yeast
- 1 teaspoon garlic powder
- 1 teaspoon paprika, smoked
- 1 teaspoon sea salt
- 1 cup panko bread crumbs (vegan)

DIRECTIONS

1. Preheat the oven to 375°F before lining a large baking sheet with either non-stick silicone or kitchen parchment.
2. A medium-sized bowl to mix whisk the flour, nutritional yeast, garlic powder, smoked paprika, and unsweetened soy milk until no clumps remain. Set this batter aside while you prepare the onions.
3. Peel the large sweet onions and then cut them into rings about one-quarter of an inch thick before carefully separating them from each other, avoiding breaking them.
4. Place the panko bread crumbs in a separate bowl for mixing and then begin to coat the onion rings. To do this, you first dip the rings one to two at a time in the batter. After the rings are coated in the batter, you then coat them in the panko bread crumb mixture.
5. Place the battered and coated onion rings on the prepared baking pans and allow them to cook for twenty minutes, flipping them over halfway through the cooking time to ensure they become evenly crispy.
6. Serve the onion rings immediately either on their own or with your favorite dipping sauce.

NUTRITION: Calories: 256 Protein: 7g Fat: 1g Carbs: 49g

315. AVOCADO PUDDING

COOKING: 0'   **PREPARATION: 10'**   **SERVES: 8**

INGREDIENTS

- 2 ripe avocados, peeled, pitted and cut into pieces
- 1 tbsp fresh lime juice
- 14 oz. can coconut milk
- 80 drops of liquid stevia
- 2 tsp vanilla extract

DIRECTIONS

1. Add all ingredients into the blender and blend until smooth.
2. Serve and enjoy.

NUTRITION: Calories: 317 Fat: 30.1g Carbs: 9.3g Protein: 3.4g

316. ALMOND BUTTER BROWNIES

COOKING: 20'   **PREPARATION: 30'**   **SERVES: 4**

INGREDIENTS

- 1 scoop Protein: powder
- 2 tbsp cocoa powder
- 1/2 cup almond butter, melted
- 1 cup bananas, overripe

DIRECTIONS

1. Preheat the oven to 350°F.
2. Spray brownie tray with cooking spray.
3. Add all ingredients into the blender and blend until smooth.
4. Pour batter into the prepared dish and bake in preheated oven for 20 minutes.
5. Serve and enjoy.

NUTRITION: Calories: 82 Fat: 2.1g Carbs: 11.4g Protein: 6.9g

317. RASPBERRY CHIA PUDDING

COOKING: 0'   **PREPARATION: 3H 10'**   **SERVES: 2**

INGREDIENTS

- 4 tbsp chia seeds
- 1 cup coconut milk
- 1/2 cup raspberries

DIRECTIONS

1. Add raspberry and coconut milk in a blender and blend until smooth.
2. Pour mixture into the mason jar.
3. Add chia seeds in a jar and stir well.
4. Close jar tightly with lid and shake well.
5. Place in refrigerator for 3 hours.
6. Serve chilled and enjoy.

NUTRITION: Calories: 361 Fat: 33.4g Carbs: 13.3g Protein: 6.2g

318. CHOCOLATE FUDGE

COOKING: 0'   **PREPARATION: 10'**   **SERVES: 2**

INGREDIENTS

- 4 oz. unsweetened dark chocolate
- 3/4 cup coconut butter
- 15 drops liquid stevia
- 1 tsp vanilla extract

DIRECTIONS

1. Melt coconut butter and dark chocolate.
2. Add ingredients to the large bowl and combine well.
3. Pour mixture into a silicone loaf pan and place in refrigerator until set.
4. Cut into pieces and serve.

NUTRITION: Calories: 157 Fat: 14.1g Carbs: 6.1g Protein: 2.3g

319. CARROT ENERGY BALLS

COOKING: 0'   **PREPARATION: 10'**   **SERVES: 8**

INGREDIENTS

- 1 large carrot, grated carrot
- 1 ½ cups old-fashioned oats
- 1 cup raisins
- 1 cup dates, pitied
- 1 cup coconut flakes
- 1/4 teaspoon ground cloves
- 1/2 teaspoon ground cinnamon

DIRECTIONS

1. In your food processor, pulse all ingredients until it forms a sticky and uniform mixture.
2. Shape the batter into equal balls.
3. Place in your refrigerator until ready to serve.

NUTRITION: Calories: 495 Fat: 21.1g Carbs: 58.4g Protein: 22.1g

320. CRUNCHY SWEET POTATO BITES

COOKING: 10'   **PREPARATION: 15'**   **SERVES: 4**

INGREDIENTS

- 4 sweet potatoes, peeled and grated
- 2 chia eggs
- 1/4 cup nutritional yeast
- 2 tablespoons tahini
- 2 tablespoons chickpea flour
- 1 teaspoon shallot powder
- 1 teaspoon garlic powder
- 1 teaspoon paprika
- Sea salt and ground black pepper, to taste

DIRECTIONS

1. Start by preheating your oven to 395°F. Line a baking pan with parchment paper or Silpat mat.
2. Thoroughly combine all the ingredients until everything is well incorporated.
3. Roll the batter into equal balls and place them in your refrigerator for about 1 hour.
4. Bake these balls for approximately 25 minutes, turning them over halfway through the cooking time.

NUTRITION: Calories: 215, Fat: 4.5g, Carbs: 35g, Protein: 8.7g

THE PLANT BASED DIET COOKBOOK

321. ROASTED GLAZED BABY CARROTS

COOKING: 0'   **PREPARATION: 15'**   **SERVES: 4**

INGREDIENTS

- 2 lb.' baby carrots
- 1/4 cup olive oil
- 1/4 cup apple cider vinegar
- 1/2 teaspoon red pepper flakes
- Sea salt and freshly ground black pepper, to taste
- 1 tablespoon agave syrup
- 2 tablespoons soy sauce
- 1 tablespoon fresh cilantro, minced

DIRECTIONS

1. Start by preheating your oven 395°F.
2. Then, toss the carrots with the olive oil, vinegar, red pepper, salt, black pepper, agave syrup and soy sauce.
3. Roast the carrots for about 30 minutes, rotating the pan once or twice. Garnish with fresh cilantro and serve.

NUTRITION: Calories: 165, Fat: 10.1g, Carbs: 16.5g, Protein: 1.4g

322. OVEN-BAKED KALE CHIPS

COOKING: 10'   **PREPARATION: 10'**   **SERVES: 8**

INGREDIENTS

- 2 bunches kale, leaves separated
- 2 tablespoons olive oil
- 1/2 teaspoon mustard seeds
- 1/2 teaspoon celery seeds
- 1/2 teaspoon dried oregano
- 1/4 teaspoon ground cumin
- 1 teaspoon garlic powder
- Coarse sea salt and ground black pepper, to taste

DIRECTIONS

1. Start by preheating your oven to 340°F. Line a baking sheet with parchment paper or Silpat mar.
2. Toss the kale leaves with the remaining ingredients until well coated.
3. Bake in the preheated oven for about 13 minutes, rotating the pan once or twice.

NUTRITION: Calories: 65, Fat: 3.9g, Carbs: 5.3g, Protein: 2.4g

323. CHEESY CASHEW DIP

COOKING: 10'   **PREPARATION: 10'**   **SERVES: 8**

INGREDIENTS

- 1 cup raw cashews
- 1 lemon, freshly squeezed
- 2 tablespoons tahini
- 2 tablespoons nutritional yeast
- 1/2 teaspoon turmeric powder
- 1/2 teaspoon red pepper flakes, crushed
- Sea salt and ground black pepper, to taste

DIRECTIONS

1. Place all the ingredients in the bowl of your food processor. Blend until uniform, creamy and smooth. You can add a splash of water to thin it out, as needed.
2. Spoon your dip into a serving bowl; serve with veggie sticks, chips, or crackers.

NUTRITION: Calories: 115, Fat: 8.6g, Carbs: 6.6g, Protein: 4.4g

324. PEPPERY HUMMUS DIP

COOKING: 10' **PREPARATION: 10'** **SERVES: 8**

INGREDIENTS

- 20 oz. canned or boiled chickpeas, drained
- 1/4 cup tahini
- 2 garlic cloves, minced
- 2 tablespoons lemon juice, freshly squeezed
- 1/2 cup chickpea liquid
- 2 red roasted peppers, seeded and sliced
- 1/2 teaspoon paprika
- 1 teaspoon dried basil
- Sea salt and ground black pepper, to taste
- 2 tablespoons olive oil

DIRECTIONS

1. Blitz all the ingredients, except for the oil, in your blender or food processor until your desired consistency is reached.
2. Place in your refrigerator until ready to serve.
3. Serve with toasted pita wedges or chips, if desired.

NUTRITION: Calories: 155, Fat: 7.9g, Carbs: 17.4g, Protein: 5.9g

325. TRADITIONAL LEBANESE MUTABAL

COOKING: 10' **PREPARATION: 10'** **SERVES: 6**

INGREDIENTS

- 1-pound eggplant
- 1 onion, chopped
- 1 tablespoon garlic paste
- 4 tablespoons tahini
- 1 tablespoon coconut oil
- 2 tablespoons lemon juice
- 1/2 teaspoon ground coriander
- 1/4 cup ground cloves
- 1 teaspoon red pepper flakes
- 1 teaspoon smoked peppers
- Sea salt and ground black pepper, to taste

DIRECTIONS

1. Roast the eggplant until the skin turns black; peel the eggplant and transfer it to your food processor bowl.
2. Add in the remaining ingredients. Blend until everything is well incorporated.
3. Serve with crostini or pita bread, if desired.

NUTRITION: Calories: 115, Fat: 7.8g, Carbs: 9.8g, Protein: 2.9g

326. INDIAN-STYLE ROASTED CHICKPEAS

COOKING: 10' **PREPARATION: 10'** **SERVES: 6**

INGREDIENTS

- 2 cups canned chickpeas, drained
- 2 tablespoons olive oil
- 1/2 teaspoon garlic powder
- 1/2 teaspoon paprika
- 1 teaspoon curry powder
- 1 teaspoon garam masala
- Sea salt and red pepper, to taste

DIRECTIONS

1. Pat the chickpeas dry using paper towels. Drizzle olive oil over the chickpeas.
2. Roast the chickpeas in the preheated oven at 400°F for about 25 minutes, tossing them once or twice.
3. Toss your chickpeas with the spices and enjoy!

NUTRITION: Calories: 313 Fat: 22.1g Carbs: 15.4g Protein: 7g

THE PLANT BASED DIET COOKBOOK

327. AVOCADO WITH TAHINI SAUCE

COOKING: 10'   **PREPARATION: 10'**   **SERVES: 4**

INGREDIENTS

- 2 large-sized avocados, pitted and halved
- 4 tablespoons tahini
- 4 tablespoons soy sauce
- 1 tablespoon lemon juice
- 1/2 teaspoon red pepper flakes
- Sea salt and ground black pepper, to taste
- 1 teaspoon garlic powder

DIRECTIONS

1. Place the avocado halves on a serving platter.
2. Mix the tahini, soy sauce, lemon juice, red pepper, salt, black pepper and garlic powder in a small bowl. Divide the sauce between the avocado halves.

NUTRITION: Calories: 304 Fat: 25.7g Carbs: 17.6g Protein: 6g

328. SWEET POTATO TATER TOTS

COOKING: 10'   **PREPARATION: 15'**   **SERVES: 4**

INGREDIENTS

- 1 ½ lb. sweet potatoes, grated
- 2 chia eggs
- 1/2 cup plain flour
- 1/2 cup breadcrumbs
- 3 tablespoons hummus
- Sea salt and black pepper, to taste
- 1 tablespoon olive oil
- 1/2 cup salsa sauce

DIRECTIONS

1. Start by preheating your oven to 395°F. Line a baking pan with parchment paper or Silpat mat.
2. Thoroughly combine all the ingredients, except for the salsa, until everything is well incorporated.
3. Roll the batter into equal balls and place them in your refrigerator for about 1 hour.
4. Bake these balls for approximately 25 minutes, turning them over halfway through the cooking time.

NUTRITION: Calories: 232, Fat: 7.1g, Carbs: 37g, Protein: 8.4g

CHAPTER 15: WRAPS AND SANDWICHES

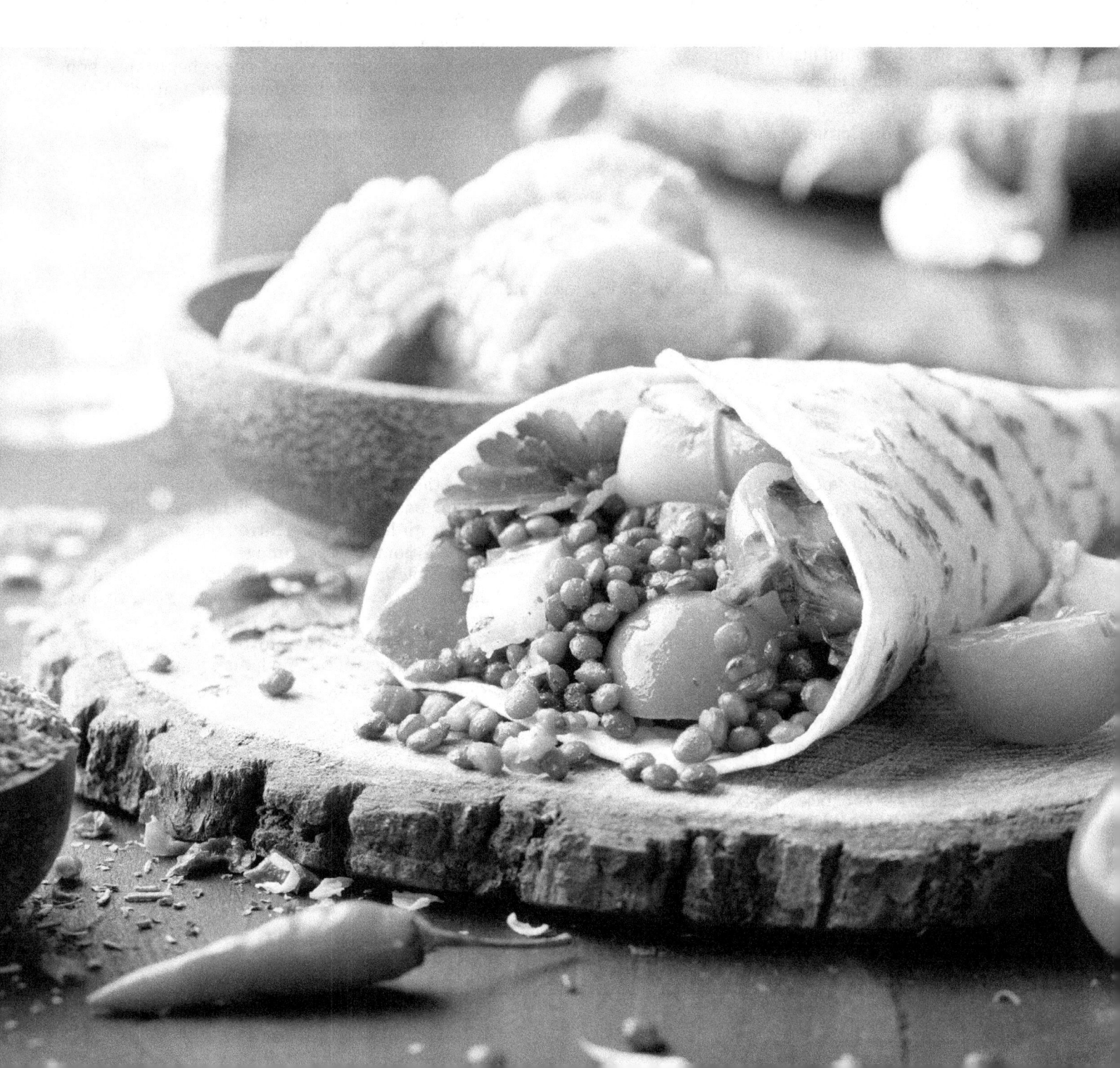

329. TOFU SALAD SANDWICHES

COOKING: 0'   **PREPARATION: 15'**   **SERVES: 6**

INGREDIENTS

- 1 (14-oz.) package extra-firm tofu, drained and pressed (see here)
- 2 celery stalks, finely chopped
- 1 scallion, finely chopped
- 1/3 cup Cashew Mayonnaise, or store-bought nondairy mayonnaise
- 1 teaspoon yellow mustard
- 1 teaspoon freshly squeezed lemon juice
- 1 teaspoon ground turmeric
- Salt. Freshly ground black pepper
- 12 slices bread of choice
- 1 large tomato, sliced
- 6 large romaine lettuce leaves

DIRECTIONS

1. Crumble the tofu into a medium bowl. Using a fork, gently mash it into small pieces.
2. Stir in the celery and scallion. Gently fold in the mayonnaise, mustard, lemon juice, and turmeric. Taste and season with salt and pepper.
3. Spoon the tofu mixture onto 6 slices of bread. Add the tomato slices and lettuce leaves and top with the remaining bread slices.
4. First-Timer tip: You can mix up your tofu salad by freezing the tofu beforehand, making it firmer and chewier. It also makes it a little spongy, which helps absorb dressings and sauces better. Just pop the package of tofu into the freezer. Once it's fully frozen, defrost it totally, then drain and press out the water as you normally would.

NUTRITION: Calories: 247 Fat: 9g Carbs: 30g Protein: 13g

330. CHICKPEA SALAD SANDWICHES

COOKING: 0'   **PREPARATION: 15'**   **SERVES: 4**

INGREDIENTS

- 1 (15-oz.) can chickpeas, drained and rinsed, or 1½ cups cooked chickpeas (see here)
- 2 celery stalks, chopped
- 1 small carrot, grated or shredded
- 1/4 cup finely chopped red onion
- 1/4 cup finely chopped dill pickle, or pickle relish
- 1/4 cup Cashew Mayonnaise, or store-bought nondairy mayonnaise
- 1 teaspoon dried dill
- ½ teaspoon garlic powder
- ½ teaspoon onion powder
- Salt. Freshly ground black pepper
- 8 slices bread of choice
- 1 large tomato, sliced
- 4 large romaine lettuce leaves

DIRECTIONS

1. Place the chickpeas in a large bowl and, using a potato masher or large fork, lightly mash them.
2. Gently stir in the celery, carrot, red onion, and dill pickle to combine everything.
3. Gently fold in the mayonnaise, dill, garlic powder, and onion powder. Taste and season with salt and pepper.
4. Spoon the chickpea mixture onto 4 slices of bread. Add the tomato slices and lettuce leaves and top with the remaining bread slices.

Variation tip: This recipe is reminiscent of chicken salad, but you can easily turn it into a vegan "tuna" salad by omitting the dill, garlic powder, and onion powder, and using 2 teaspoons seaweed flakes instead. You can usually find seaweed flakes in the Asian food aisle of the grocery store.

NUTRITION: Calories: 320 Fat: 9g Carbs: 49g Protein: 14g;

331. SEITAN SHAWARMA

COOKING: 15' **PREPARATION: 20'** **SERVES: 4**

INGREDIENTS

- 1/4 cup tahini
- 1/4 cup water
- 2 tablespoons freshly squeezed lemon juice
- 1 teaspoon garlic powder
- 2 teaspoons vegetable oil
- 1 small red onion, thinly sliced
- 1-pound Seitan, or store-bought seitan, thinly sliced
- 1/2 teaspoon ground cumin
- 1/2 teaspoon ground turmeric
- 1/2 teaspoon paprika
- 1/4 teaspoon salt
- ¼ teaspoon freshly ground black pepper
- 4 pitas, or flatbreads of choice
- 1 large tomato, sliced
- 1 cup sliced cucumber
- 2 cups sliced romaine lettuce

DIRECTIONS

1. In a small bowl, whisk the tahini, water, lemon juice, and garlic powder to blend. Set aside.
2. In a large pan over medium-high heat, heat the vegetable oil. Add the red onion and cook for about 5 minutes, stirring frequently, until it begins to soften and brown.
3. Add the seitan, cumin, turmeric, paprika, salt, and pepper. Cook, stirring frequently, for about 10 minutes until the seitan browns and some of the edges get crispy.
4. To assemble the sandwiches, stuff each pita with some of the seitan mixture. Add tomato and cucumber slices and romaine lettuce. Drizzle each with the tahini dressing.
5. Substitution tip: Swap store-bought vegan beef for the seitan, if you prefer. You can also use sliced portobello mushrooms to keep your shawarma veggie-centric.

NUTRITION: Calories: 354 Fat: 12g Carbs: 41g Protein: 20g

332. CHIPOTLE SEITAN TAQUITOS

COOKING: 15' **PREPARATION: 15'** **SERVES: 2**

INGREDIENTS

- ½ cup Cashew Cream Cheese, or store-bought nondairy cream cheese
- 2 canned chipotle peppers in adobo sauce, minced, sauce reserved
- 12 (6-inch) corn tortillas
- 1-pound Seitan, or store-bought seitan, cut into slices

DIRECTIONS

1. Preheat the oven to 400°F. Have a large baking dish or sheet nearby.
2. In a small bowl, stir together the cashew cream cheese, chipotle peppers, and 2 tablespoons of the reserved adobo sauce.
3. Place a tortilla on a clean surface and spread a line (about 2 teaspoons) of the chipotle cream cheese mixture down the middle. Top with a few slices of seitan. Roll up the tortilla as tightly as possible and place it, seam-side down, in the baking dish. Repeat with the remaining tortillas.
4. Bake for 15 minutes, or until the tortillas are crisp.

Fun fact: Chipotles are not their type of pepper. They're dried, smoked jalapeños. When buying them for this recipe, look for chipotles in adobo sauce, which come in small cans found in the grocery store's Mexican food section. You'll need both the peppers and the sauce.

NUTRITION: Calories: 193 Fat: 7g Carbs: 25g Protein: 8g;

333. MEDITERRANEAN CHICKPEA WRAPS

COOKING: 0'   **PREPARATION: 15'**   **SERVES: 4**

INGREDIENTS

- 1/4 cup extra-virgin olive oil
- 2 tablespoons freshly squeezed lemon juice
- 1 teaspoon dried dill
- 1 teaspoon dried oregano
- 1/4 teaspoon salt
- 1 (15-oz.) can chickpeas, drained and rinsed, or 1½ cups cooked chickpeas (see here)
- ½ cup Tofu Feta, or store-bought nondairy feta
- 1 cup chopped cucumber
- 1 large tomato, diced
- ¼ cup diced red onion
- 2 cups fresh baby spinach
- 4 (12-inch) tortillas, or flatbreads of choice

DIRECTIONS

1. In a small bowl, whisk the olive oil, lemon juice, dill, oregano, and salt to combine.
2. In a large bowl, gently toss together the chickpeas, feta, cucumber, tomato, and red onion. Add the dressing and toss to combine.
3. Assemble the wraps by placing ½ cup of spinach on each tortilla and topping it with ¼ of the chickpea mixture. Roll up the wrap, tucking in the sides as you go.

Substitution tip: If you'd like to keep your wraps gluten-free and you can't find gluten-free flatbread, use collard greens. You'll need 4 large collard leaves. Cut off the stem from each and shave off the thick part of the stem that's left in the center with a sharp knife. Assemble the wrap the way you would a tortilla, by filling it with the spinach and chickpea mixture and rolling the leaf, tucking in the sides as you go.

NUTRITION: Calories: 623 Fat: 25g Carbs: 80g Protein: 20g;

334. BARBECUE CHICKPEA BURGERS WITH SLAW

COOKING: 25'   **PREPARATION: 15'**   **SERVES: 4**

INGREDIENTS

- 1 cup rolled oats
- 1 (15-oz.) can chickpeas, drained and rinsed, or 1½ cup cooked chickpeas (see here)
- ½ cup Barbecue Sauce, or store-bought vegan barbecue sauce, divided
- 1 garlic clove, minced
- ½ teaspoon salt
- ½ teaspoon freshly ground black pepper
- 2 cups shredded cabbage
- 2 carrots, grated or shredded
- ¼ cup Cashew Mayonnaise, or store-bought nondairy mayonnaise
- 4 burger buns of choice

DIRECTIONS

1. Preheat the oven to 400°F. Line a large baking sheet with parchment paper.
2. In a food processor, pulse the rolled oats until they resemble a coarse meal. Add the chickpeas, ¼ cup of barbecue sauce, the garlic, salt, and pepper.
3. Pulse until the chickpeas are mashed and everything is well combined. It's okay if there are a few whole chickpeas. Form the mixture into 4 patties and place them on the prepared baking sheet.
4. Bake the burgers for 20 to 25 minutes, flipping them at the halfway point. They should be golden brown and firm.
5. While the burgers bake, make the slaw. In a large bowl, stir together the cabbage, carrots, and mayonnaise.
6. Serve each burger on a bun topped with 1 tablespoon of the remaining barbecue sauce and ¼ cup of slaw.

First-Timer tip: If you don't have a food processor, mash your chickpeas well using a potato masher or large fork. Rolled oats won't mash well by hand, so use oat flour or all-purpose flour instead. Combine the mashed chickpeas, flour, barbecue sauce, garlic, salt, and pepper in a large bowl before shaping into patties.

NUTRITION: Calories: 433 Fat: 10g Carbs: 73g Protein: 13g

335. BASIC HUMMUS AND VEGETABLE SANDWICH

COOKING: 0'   **PREPARATION: 15'**   **SERVES: 1**

INGREDIENTS

- Salad Greens (½ cup)
- Avocado (1/4, Mashed)
- Bell Pepper (1/4, Sliced)
- Hummus (3 tablespoons)
- Whole-grain Bread (2 Slices)
- Carrots (1/4 cup, Sliced)
- Cucumber (1/4 cup, Sliced)

DIRECTIONS

1. For a quick and easy lunch, you will first want to lay the bread out and spread hummus on one side and avocado on the other.
2. Once the spread is placed, put the vegetables in between, and your sandwich is ready to go!

NUTRITION: Calories: 350 Carbs: 45g Fat: 15g Proteins: 15g

336. GREEN PESTO SANDWICH

COOKING: 5'   **PREPARATION: 5'**   **SERVES: 1**

INGREDIENTS

- Whole Wheat Bread (2 Sliced)
- Vegan Pesto (1 tablespoon)
- Artichoke Hearts
- Cannellini Beans (½ cup)
- Avocado (1/2, Sliced)
- Arugula (½ cup)
- Olive Oil (2 tablespoons)
- Pepper (to Taste)

DIRECTIONS

1. The first step of making this sandwich will be placing the cannellini beans into a bowl and mashing them with a fork.
2. Once this is done, you can mix in your pesto and spread the mixture on both slices of bread.
3. Next, you will place the spinach, avocado, and artichoke hearts in the center and then close your sandwich.
4. With the sandwich set, take a skillet and place it over medium heat. Once warm, toss in some olive oil and grill your sandwich until browned on both sides.
5. Typically, this will only take you about five minutes, and then you can slice and enjoy your sandwich.

NUTRITION: Calories: 350 Carbs: 50g Fat: 20g Proteins: 10g

337. CHICKPEA SALAD SANDWICH

COOKING: 0'   **PREPARATION: 10'**   **SERVES: 4**

INGREDIENTS

- Chickpeas (1 Can)
- Sweet Pickle Relish (2 tablespoons)
- Red Bell Pepper (1/4 cup)
- Celery (1, Chopped)
- Vegan Mayo (1/4 cup)
- Lettuce Leaves
- Bread (4 Slices)
- Salt (to taste)
- Dill (1/4 teaspoon)
- Onion (2 tablespoons, Chopped)

DIRECTIONS

1. This sandwich is the vegan version of a tuna sandwich! You can begin the recipe by taking out a mixing bowl and adding in the chickpeas.
2. At this point, mash the chickpeas down and then add in the mayo, dill, relish, celery, onion, and bell pepper.
3. Once you stir everything together, season with salt and pepper to your desired flavoring.
4. Now, lay out your bread and spread one side with the mayo before placing the lettuce and chickpea mixture. Close the sandwich, slice in half, and lunch is served!

NUTRITION: Calories: 200 Carbs: 40g Fat: 5g Proteins: 8g

338. AVOCADO AND WHITE BEAN SANDWICH

COOKING: 0'   **PREPARATION: 10'**   **SERVES: 4**

INGREDIENTS

- Whole-grain Bread (8 Sliced)
- Lettuce (3 Leaves)
- Alfalfa Sprouts (1 cup)
- Avocado (1, Sliced)
- Lemon
- White Beans (1 Can)
- Pepper (to Taste)

DIRECTIONS

1. Start this sandwich by first taking your beans and place them into a food processor or blender. You will want to puree the beans until the mixture is smooth.
2. At this point, you can season with pepper, salt, and squeeze the lemon juice in.
3. Now that your bean mix is made go ahead and spread it in between the bread slices. With that in place, build your sandwich with avocado slices, lettuce, and some alfalfa sprouts.
4. Slice the sandwich, and then you can enjoy it!

NUTRITION: Calories: 300 Carbs: 50g Fat: 10g Proteins: 10g

339. SWEET POTATO AND KALE SANDWICH SANDWICH

COOKING: 30'   **PREPARATION: 10'**   **SERVES: 4**

INGREDIENTS

- Hummus (½ cup)
- Kale (2 cups)
- Salt (to Taste)
- Whole-grain Roll
- Olive Oil (2 tablespoons)
- Sweet Potato (1, Sliced)

DIRECTIONS

1. While this sandwich seems simple, the sweet potato adds nice flavor and texture to switch up your typical sandwich choices. You will want to begin by Preparing the oven to 400.
2. As the oven warms, take out a small mixing bowl and toss your sweet potato pieces in the olive oil, pepper, and salt.
3. When the potato is well coated, lay the pieces across a roasting sheet and pop into the cooker for thirty minutes.
4. At the end of thirty minutes, take out the rolls, and spread hummus on either side. Finally, layer your kale, and sweet potato in between the bread and the sandwich will be all set.

NUTRITION: Calories: 100 Carbs: 10g Fat: 5g Proteins: 3g

340. HUMMUS AND QUINOA WRAP

COOKING: 10'   **PREPARATION: 10'**   **SERVES: 4**

INGREDIENTS

- Lettuce Leaves
- Cooked Quinoa (1 cup)
- Cabbage (½ cup)
- Sprouts (½ cup)
- Avocado (1 cup, Sliced)
- Hummus (1 cup)

DIRECTIONS

1. For this recipe, the lettuce leaves are going to act as your wrap! When you are all set, spread the wrap out and place the hummus and avocado into each leaf.
2. Once this is set, layer your quinoa and cabbage on top before wrapping the leaf up and eating!

NUTRITION: Calories: 280 Carbs: 40g Fat: 10g Proteins: 10g

341. MEDITERRANEAN VEGGIE WRAP

COOKING: 0'   **PREPARATION: 15'**   **SERVES: 4**

INGREDIENTS

- Whole-grain Tortillas
- Chickpeas (3 cups)
- Onion (1/4 cup, Diced)
- Tomato (1, Diced)
- Salt (to Taste)
- Kalamata Olives (4 tablespoons)
- Garlic Clove (1, Minced)
- Lettuce (2 cups)
- Lemon Juice (2 tablespoons)
- Cucumber (1, Grated)
- Fresh Dill (2 tablespoons)
- Plant-based Yogurt (7 Oz.)
- Green Pepper (1/4 cup, Diced)
- Pepper (to Taste)

DIRECTIONS

1. Before you begin preparing this wrap, you will want to take half of your cucumber and grate it into a mixing bowl.
2. After this step is complete, lightly sprinkle the cucumber with salt to help get some of the excess water out.
3. As this process happens, you can now take your chickpeas and mash them down well with a fork.
4. With that, all set, take out a dish, and combine the cucumber, yogurt, citrus juice, garlic, and dill altogether. Once this is done, season with pepper and salt to your liking.
5. When you are ready, lay out your wraps and layer your smashed chickpeas, lettuce, and the mixed vegetables. For some extra flavor, try adding some tzatziki sauce over the top before rolling up.

NUTRITION: Calories: 400 Carbs: 30g Fat: 5g Proteins: 15g

342. QUICK LENTIL WRAP

COOKING: 30'   **PREPARATION: 10'**   **SERVES: 4**

INGREDIENTS

- Whole-grain Wraps
- Garlic Clove (1, Minced)
- Olive Oil (2 tablespoons)
- Onion (1, Diced)
- Cilantro (1/3 cup, Cilantro)
- Lentils (2 cups)
- Tomato Paste (1/3 cup)

DIRECTIONS

1. Begin this recipe by taking out a skillet and place two cups of water and lentils in.
2. You will want to get everything to a boil before turning the temperature down and simmer for ten minutes or until the lentils are soft.
3. Once the lentils are cooked through, add in the tomato paste, garlic, and onion. Go ahead and cook all of these ingredients together for another five minutes before turning off heat and seasoning to your liking.
4. Finally, lay out your wraps, spread the mixture in the center, and then roll the wrap up for lunch.

NUTRITION: Calories: 400 Carbs: 50g Fat: 5g Proteins: 20g

343. THAI VEGETABLE AND TOFU WRAP SANDWICH

COOKING: 30' **PREPARATION: 5'** **SERVES: 1**

INGREDIENTS

- Extra-firm Tofu (1 cup, Diced)
- Peanut Sauce (1/4 cup)
- Olive Oil (1 teaspoon)
- Cucumber (1/3 cup, Diced)
- Carrot (1/3 cup, Shredded)
- Cilantro (1/4 cup)
- Garlic Cloves (1, Minced)
- Whole-wheat Wrap

DIRECTIONS

1. Tofu is an excellent Protein: to have on hand because it is so versatile! To begin this recipe, you will want to take a skillet and place it over medium heat.
2. As it warms, add in your olive oil and begin cooking the tofu for around five minutes.
3. After five minutes, combine in the garlic and cook for an additional minute. At this point, all of the liquid from the tofu should be gone.
4. Next, eliminate the skillet from the cooker and add in the peanut sauce. Be sure to stir very well to help coat the tofu pieces evenly!
5. When you are set to make your wraps, spread the tofu into your wrap, top with the diced and shredded vegetables, and roll everything up together nice and tight before serving.
6. For extra flavor, feel free to add some fresh cilantro to your wrap!

NUTRITION: Calories: 270 Carbs: 12g Fat: 15g Proteins: 20g

344. PLANT-BASED BUFFALO WRAP

COOKING: 15' **PREPARATION: 5'** **SERVES: 4**

INGREDIENTS

- Olive Oil (1 teaspoon)
- Kale (2 cups, Chopped)
- Buffalo Sauce (½ cup)
- Seitan (1 cup, Chopped)
- Whole Wheat Wraps (
- Tomatoes (1 cup, Diced)
- Cashews (1 cup)
- Salt (to taste)
- Dried Dill (1/2 teaspoon)
- Pepper (to Taste)
- Dried Parsley (1/2 teaspoon)
- Almond Milk (8 tablespoons)
- Apple Cider Vinegar (1 ½ tablespoons)

DIRECTIONS

1. This recipe is the perfect way to get a buffalo chicken wrap, without the chicken! You will want to start by making your ranch dressing.
2. You can accomplish this by taking out your blender and mixing the almond milk, apple cider vinegar, cashews, pepper, salt, parsley, and dill.
3. Once this is done, set your sauce to the side.
4. Next, you will need to get out a saucepan and place it over medium heat. Once warm, add in some olive oil and begin cooking your seitan pieces. Normally, this will take you eight minutes.
5. When the seitan is cooked through, add in the buffalo sauce and cook for another minute.
6. With these steps done, you will want to now take a moment to take the kale and mix it in a bowl with olive oil and seasoning.
7. Finally, it is time to assemble your wrap! You can do this by taking out your wrap and spreading your ranch dressing across the surface.
8. Once this is in place, begin building your wrap by layering the kale, tomato, and seitan pieces. For a final touch, add some more buffalo sauce over the top and then wrap it up!

NUTRITION: Calories: 250 Carbs: 25g Fat: 15g Proteins: 20g

THE PLANT BASED DIET COOKBOOK

345. COLORFUL VEGGIE WRAP

COOKING: 0'   **PREPARATION: 10'**   **SERVES: 4**

INGREDIENTS

- Large Lettuce Leaves
- Soy Sauce (1 tablespoon)
- Olive Oil (1 tablespoon)
- Seed Butter (½ cup)
- Garlic Powder (1 tablespoon)
- Lime Juice (2 tablespoons)
- Red Cabbage (1 cup, Shredded)
- Cucumber (1 cup, Chopped)
- Red Pepper (1 cup, Chopped)
- Carrot (1 cup, Chopped)
- Ground Ginger (1/4 teaspoon)

DIRECTIONS

1. This wrap looks pretty at and full of flavor! You can start this recipe off by making the sauce.
2. For the sauce, take out a petite bowl and combine the oil, garlic, soy sauce, juice of the lime, ground ginger, pepper flakes, and the seed butter.
3. Once everything is mixed together well, place it to the side.
4. Next, it is time to build your wrap! Go ahead and lay the lettuce leaves out flat before spreading sauce across the surface.
5. Once this is in place, you will want to layer the other vegetables before rolling the leaf up and enjoying your veggie-packed wrap!

NUTRITION: Calories: 250 Carbs: 15g Fat: 20g Proteins: 10g

346. BBQ CHICKPEA WRAP

COOKING: 0'   **PREPARATION: 10'**   **SERVES: 4**

INGREDIENTS

- Whole-wheat Tortillas
- Coleslaw (2 cups)
- BBQ Sauce (½ cup)
- Chickpeas (2 cups)

DIRECTIONS

1. Are you in a rush for lunch? You can slap this wrap together in a snap! Start by taking out a blending bowl and combine the BBQ with the chickpeas.
2. Next, you will want to lay out your tortillas and place the coleslaw and chickpeas in the center.
3. For a nice touch, wrap your tortilla up and pop into the microwave for a few seconds to heat it before enjoying it!

NUTRITION: Calories: 450 Carbs: 50g Fat: 5g Proteins: 10g

347. CHICKPEA AND MANGO WRAPS

COOKING: 0'   **PREPARATION: 15'**   **SERVES: 3**

INGREDIENTS

- 3 tablespoons tahini
- 1 tablespoon curry powder
- ¼ teaspoon sea salt (optional)
- Zest and juice of 1 lime
- 3 to 4 tablespoons water
- 1½ cups cooked chickpeas
- 1 cup diced mango
- ½ cup fresh cilantro, chopped
- 1 red bell pepper, deseeded and diced
- 3 large whole-wheat wraps
- 1½ cups shredded lettuce

DIRECTIONS

1. Tofu is an excellent Protein: to have on hand because it is so versatile! To begin this recipe, you will want to take a skillet and place it over medium heat.
2. As it warms, add in your olive oil and begin cooking the tofu for around five minutes.
3. After five minutes, combine in the garlic and cook for an additional minute. At this point, all of the liquid from the tofu should be gone.
4. Next, eliminate the skillet from the cooker and add in the peanut sauce. Be sure to stir very well to help coat the tofu pieces evenly!
5. When you are set to make your wraps, spread the tofu into your wrap, top with the diced and shredded vegetables, and roll everything up together nice and tight before serving.
6. For extra flavor, feel free to add some fresh cilantro to your wrap!

NUTRITION: Calories: 270 Carbs: 12g Fat: 15g   Proteins: 20g

344. PLANT-BASED BUFFALO WRAP

COOKING: 15'   **PREPARATION: 5'**   **SERVES: 4**

INGREDIENTS

- Olive Oil (1 teaspoon)
- Kale (2 cups, Chopped)
- Buffalo Sauce (½ cup)
- Seitan (1 cup, Chopped)
- Whole Wheat Wraps (
- Tomatoes (1 cup, Diced)
- Cashews (1 cup)
- Salt (to taste)
- Dried Dill (1/2 teaspoon)
- Pepper (to Taste)
- Dried Parsley (1/2 teaspoon)
- Almond Milk (8 tablespoons)
- Apple Cider Vinegar (1 ½ tablespoons)

DIRECTIONS

1. In a large bowl, stir together the tahini, curry powder, lime zest, lime juice and sea salt (if desired) until smooth and creamy. Whisk in 3 to 4 tablespoons water to help thin the mixture.
2. Add the cooked chickpeas, mango, cilantro and bell pepper to the bowl. Toss until well coated.
3. On a clean work surface, lay the wraps. Divide the chickpea and mango mixture among the wraps. Spread the shredded lettuce on top and roll up tightly.
4. Serve immediately.

NUTRITION: Calories: 436 Fat: 17.9g Carbs: 8.9g Protein: 15.2g

THE PLANT BASED DIET COOKBOOK

348. TOFU AND PINEAPPLE IN LETTUCE

COOKING: 15' **PREPARATION: 2H** **SERVES: 4**

INGREDIENTS

- ¼ cup low-sodium soy sauce
- 1 garlic clove, minced
- 2 tablespoons sesame oil (optional)
- 1 tablespoons coconut sugar (optional)
- 1 (14-oz. / 397-g) package extra firm tofu, drained, cut into ½-inch cubes
- 1 small white onion, diced
- ½ pineapple, peeled, cored, cut into cubes
- Salt and ground black pepper, to taste (optional)
- 4 large lettuce leaves
- 1 tablespoon roasted sesame seeds

DIRECTIONS

1. Combine the soy sauce, garlic, sesame oil (if desired), and coconut sugar in a bowl. Stir to mix well.
2. Add the tofu cubes to the bowl of soy sauce mixture, then press to coat well. Wrap the bowl in plastic and refrigerate to marinate for at least 2 hours.
3. Pour the marinated tofu and marinade in a skillet and heat over medium heat. Add the onion and pineapple cubes to the skillet and stir to mix well.
4. Sprinkle with salt (if desired) and pepper and sauté for 15 minutes or until the onions are lightly browned and the pineapple cubes are tender.
5. Divide the lettuce leaves among 4 plates, then top the leaves with the tofu and pineapple mixture. Sprinkle with sesame seeds and serve immediately.

NUTRITION: Calories: 259 Fat: 15.4g Carbs: 20.5g Protein: 12.1g

349. QUINOA AND BLACK BEAN LETTUCE WRAPS

COOKING: 15' **PREPARATION: 30'** **SERVES: 6**

INGREDIENTS

- 2 tablespoons avocado oil (optional)
- ¼ cup deseeded and chopped bell pepper
- ½ onion, chopped
- 2 tablespoons minced garlic
- 1 teaspoon salt (optional)
- 1 teaspoon pepper (optional)
- ½ cup cooked quinoa
- 1 cup cooked black beans
- ½ cup almond flour
- ½ teaspoon paprika
- ½ teaspoon red pepper flakes
- 6 large lettuce leaves

DIRECTIONS

1. Heat 1 tablespoon of the avocado oil (if desired) in a skillet over medium-high heat.
2. Add the bell peppers, onions, garlic, salt (if desired), and pepper. Sauté for 5 minutes or until the bell peppers are tender.
3. Turn off the heat and cool for 10 minutes, then pour the vegetables in a food processor. Add the quinoa, beans, flour.
4. Sprinkle with paprika and red pepper flakes. Pulse until thick and well combined.
5. Line a baking pan with parchment paper, then shape the mixture into 6 patties with your hands and place on the baking pan.
6. Put the pan in the freezer for 5 minutes to make the patties firm.
7. Heat the remaining avocado oil (if desired) in the skillet over high heat.
8. Add the patties and cook for 6 minutes or until well browned on both sides. Flip the patties halfway through.
9. Arrange the patties in the lettuce leaves and serve immediately.

NUTRITION: Calories: 200 Fat: 10.6g Carbs: 40.5g Protein: 9.5g

CHAPTER 16: SAUCES, DRESSINGS, AND DIPS

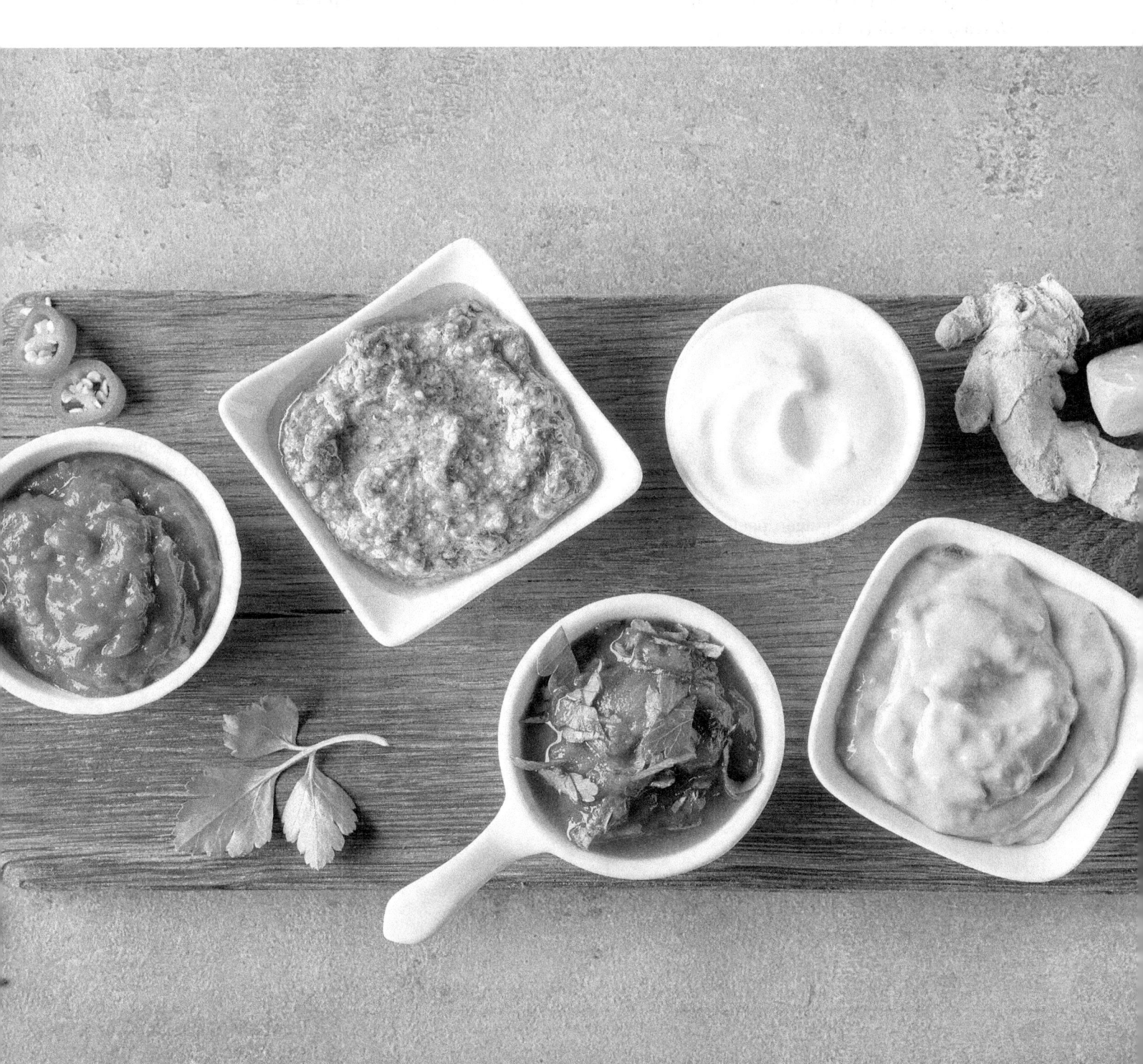

350. SATAY SAUCE

COOKING: 8'   **PREPARATION: 5'**   **SERVES: 2**

INGREDIENTS

- ½ yellow onion, diced
- 3 garlic cloves, minced
- 1 fresh red chile, thinly sliced (optional)
- 1-inch piece fresh ginger, peeled and minced
- ¼ cup smooth peanut butter
- 2 tablespoons coconut aminos
- 1 (13.5-oz.) can unsweetened coconut milk
- ¼ teaspoon freshly ground black pepper
- ¼ teaspoon salt (optional)

DIRECTIONS

1. ½ yellow onion, diced
2. 3 garlic cloves, minced
3. 1 fresh red chile, thinly sliced (optional)
4. 1-inch piece fresh ginger, peeled and minced
5. ¼ cup smooth peanut butter
6. 2 tablespoons coconut aminos
7. 1 (13.5-oz.) can unsweetened coconut milk
8. ¼ teaspoon freshly ground black pepper
9. ¼ teaspoon salt (optional)

NUTRITION: Calories: 322 Fat: 28.8g Carbs: 9.4g Protein: 6.3g

351. TAHINI BBQ SAUCE

COOKING: 0'   **PREPARATION: 10'**   **SERVES: 4**

INGREDIENTS

- ½ cup water
- ¼ cup red miso
- 3 cloves garlic, minced
- 1-inch (2.5 cm) piece ginger, peeled and minced
- 2 tablespoons rice vinegar
- 2 tablespoons tahini
- 2 tablespoons chili paste or chili sauce
- 1 tablespoon date sugar
- ½ teaspoon crushed red pepper (optional)

DIRECTIONS

1. Place all the ingredients in a food processor, and purée until thoroughly mixed and smooth. You can thin the sauce out by stirring in ½ cup of water, or keep it thick.
2. Transfer to the refrigerator to chill until ready to serve.

NUTRITION: Calories: 206 Fat: 10.2g Carbs: 21.3g Protein: 7.2g

352. TAMARI VINEGAR SAUCE

COOKING: 0'   **PREPARATION:** 10'   **SERVES:** 1

INGREDIENTS

- ¼ cup tamari
- ½ cup nutritional yeast
- 2 tablespoons balsamic vinegar
- 2 tablespoons apple cider vinegar
- 2 tablespoons Worcestershire sauce
- 2 teaspoons Dijon mustard
- 1 tablespoon plus 1 teaspoon maple syrup
- ½ teaspoon ground turmeric
- ¼ teaspoon black pepper

DIRECTIONS

1. Place all the ingredients in an airtight container, and whisk until everything is well incorporated. Store in the refrigerator for up to 3 weeks.

NUTRITION: Calories: 216 Fat: 9.9g Carbs: 18.0g Protein: 13.7g

353. SWEET AND TANGY KETCHUP

COOKING: 15'   **PREPARATION:** 5'   **SERVES:** 2

INGREDIENTS

- 1 cup water
- ¼ cup maple syrup
- 1 cup tomato paste
- 3 tablespoons apple cider vinegar
- 1 teaspoon onion powder
- 1 teaspoon garlic powder

DIRECTIONS

1. Add the water to a medium saucepan and bring to a rolling boil over high heat.
2. Reduce the heat to low, stir in the maple syrup, tomato paste, vinegar, onion powder, and garlic powder. Cover and bring to a gently simmer for about 10 minutes, stirring frequently, or until the sauce begins to thicken and bubble.
3. Let the sauce rest for 30 minutes until cooled completely. Transfer to an airtight container and refrigerate for up to 1 month.

NUTRITION: Calories: 46 Fat: 5.2g Carbs: 1.0g Protein: 1.1g

354. HOMEMADE TZATZIKI SAUCE

COOKING: 0' **PREPARATION: 20'** **SERVES: 1**

INGREDIENTS

- 2 oz. raw, unsalted cashews (about ½ cup)
- 2 tablespoons lemon juice
- 1/3 cup water
- 1 small clove garlic
- 1 cup chopped cucumber, peeled
- 2 tablespoons fresh dill

DIRECTIONS

1. In a blender, add the cashews, lemon juice, water, and garlic. Keep it aside for at least 15 minutes to soften the cashews.
2. Blend the ingredients until smooth. Stir in the chopped cucumber and dill, and continue to blend until it reaches your desired consistency. It doesn't need to be smooth. Feel free to add more water if you like a thinner consistency.
3. Transfer to an airtight container and chill for at least 30 minutes for best flavors.
4. Bring the sauce to room temperature and shake well before serving.

NUTRITION: Calories: 208 Fat: 13.5g carbs:15.0 g Protein: 6.7g

355. TANGY CASHEW MUSTARD DRESSING

COOKING: 0' **PREPARATION: 20'** **SERVES: 1**

INGREDIENTS

- 2 oz. raw, unsalted cashews (about ½ cup)
- ½ cup water
- 3 tablespoons lemon juice
- 2 teaspoons apple cider vinegar
- 2 tablespoons Dijon mustard
- 1 medium clove garlic

DIRECTIONS

1. Put all the ingredients in a food processor and keep it aside for at least 15 minutes.
2. Purée until the ingredients are combined to a smooth and creamy mixture. Thin the dressing with a little extra water as needed to achieve your preferred consistency.
3. Store in an airtight container in the refrigerator for up to 5 days.

NUTRITION: Calories: 187 Fat: 13.0g Carbs: 11.5g Protein: 5.9g

356. AVOCADO-DILL DRESSING

COOKING: 0'   **PREPARATION: 20'**   **SERVES: 1**

INGREDIENTS

- 2 oz. raw, unsalted cashews (about ½ cup)
- ½ cup water
- 3 tablespoons lemon juice
- ½ medium, ripe avocado, chopped
- 1 medium clove garlic
- 2 tablespoons chopped fresh dill
- 2 green onions, white and green parts, chopped

DIRECTIONS

1. Put the cashews, water, lemon juice, avocado, and garlic into a blender. Keep it aside for at least 15 minutes to soften the cashews.
2. Blend until everything is fully mixed. Fold in the dill and green onions, and blend briefly to retain some texture.
3. Store in an airtight container in the fridge for up to 3 days and stir well before serving.

NUTRITION: Calories: 312 Fat: 21.1g Carbs: 22.6g Protein: 8.0g

357. EASY LEMON TAHINI DRESSING

COOKING: 0'   **PREPARATION: 5'**   **SERVES: 1**

INGREDIENTS

- 1½ cup tahini
- ¼ cup fresh lemon juice (about 2 lemons)
- 1 teaspoon maple syrup
- 1 small garlic clove, chopped
- 1/8 teaspoon black pepper
- ¼ teaspoon salt (optional)
- ¼ to ½ cup water

DIRECTIONS

1. Process the tahini, lemon juice, maple syrup, garlic, black pepper, and salt (if desired) in a blender (high-speed blenders work best for this). Gradually add the water until the mixture is completely smooth.
2. Store in an airtight container in the fridge for up to 5 days.

NUTRITION: Calories: 128 Fat: 9.6g Carbs: 6.8g Protein: 3.6g

358. SWEET MANGO AND ORANGE DRESSING

COOKING: 0' **PREPARATION: 0'** **SERVES: 1**

INGREDIENTS

- 1 cup diced mango, thawed if frozen
- ½ cup orange juice
- 2 tablespoons rice vinegar
- 2 tablespoons fresh lime juice
- ¼ teaspoon salt (optional)
- 1 teaspoon date sugar (optional)
- 2 tablespoons chopped cilantro

DIRECTIONS

1. Pulse all the ingredients except for the cilantro in a food processor until it reaches the consistency you like. Add the cilantro and whisk well.
2. Store in an airtight container in the fridge for up to 2 days.

NUTRITION: Calories: 32 Fat: 0.1g Carbs: 7.4g Protein: 0.3g

359. CREAMY AVOCADO CILANTRO LIME DRESSING

COOKING: 0' **PREPARATION: 5'** **SERVES: 1**

INGREDIENTS

- 1 avocado, diced
- ½ cup water
- ¼ cup cilantro leaves
- ¼ cup fresh lime or lemon juice (about 2 limes or lemons)
- ½ teaspoon ground cumin
- ¼ teaspoon salt (optional)

DIRECTIONS

1. Put all the ingredients in a blender (high-speed blenders work best for this), and pulse until well combined. Taste and adjust the seasoning as needed. It is best served within 1 day.

NUTRITION: Calories: 94 Fat: 7.4g Carbs: 5.7g Protein: 1.1g

360. MAPLE DIJON DRESSING

COOKING: 0' **PREPARATION: 5'** **SERVES: 1**

INGREDIENTS

- ¼ cup apple cider vinegar
- 2 teaspoons Dijon mustard
- 2 tablespoons maple syrup
- 2 tablespoons low-sodium vegetable broth
- ¼ teaspoon black pepper
- Salt, to taste (optional)

DIRECTIONS

1. Mix the apple cider vinegar, Dijon mustard, maple syrup, vegetable broth, and black pepper in a resealable container until well incorporated. Season with salt to taste, if desired.
2. The dressing can be refrigerated for up to 5 days.

NUTRITION: Calories: 82 Fat: 0.3g Carbs: 19.3g Protein: 0.6g

361. AVOCADO HUMMUS

COOKING: 0' | **PREPARATION: 10'** | **SERVES: 4**

INGREDIENTS

- 2 Ripe Avocados
- ½ Cup Coconut Cream
- ¼ Cup Sesame Paste
- ½ Lemon Juice
- 1 Tsp. Clove, Pressed
- ½ Tsp Ground Cumin
- ½ Tsp Salt
- ¼ Tsp Ground Black Pepper

DIRECTIONS

1. Cut the avocado lengthways and remove seed from the fruit.
2. Put all ingredients in a blender or food processor and mix until thoroughly smooth.
3. Add more cream, lemon juice or water if you want to have a looser texture.
4. Adjust seasonings as needed.
5. Serve with naan and enjoy.

NUTRITION: Calories 289, Fat: 9g, Carbs: 6g, Sugar: 6g, Protein: 21g

---

362. AVOCADO-CHICKPEA DIP

COOKING: 0' | **PREPARATION: 15'** | **SERVES: 2**

INGREDIENTS

- 1 (15-oz. / 425-g) can cooked chickpeas, drained and rinsed
- 2 large, ripe avocados, chopped
- ¼ cup red onion, finely chopped
- 1 tablespoon Dijon mustard
- 1 to 2 tablespoons lemon juice
- 2 teaspoons chopped fresh oregano
- 1/2 teaspoon garlic clove, finely chopped

DIRECTIONS

1. In a medium bowl, mash the cooked chickpeas with a potato masher or the back of a fork, or until the chickpeas pop open (a food processor works best for this).
2. Stir in the remaining ingredients and continue to mash until completely smooth.
3. Place in the refrigerator to chill until ready to serve.

NUTRITION: Calories: 101 Fat: 1.9g Carbs: 16.2g Protein: 4.7g

---

363. BEER "CHEESE" DIP

COOKING: 7' | **PREPARATION: 10'** | **SERVES: 3**

INGREDIENTS

- ¾ cup water
- ¾ cup brown ale
- ½ cup raw walnuts, soaked in hot water for at least 15 minutes, then drained
- ½ cup raw cashews, soaked in hot water for at least 15 minutes, then drained
- 2 tablespoons tomato paste
- 2 tablespoons fresh lemon juice
- 1 tablespoon apple cider vinegar
- ½ cup nutritional yeast
- ½ teaspoon sweet or smoked paprika
- 1 tablespoon arrowroot powder
- 1 tablespoon red miso

DIRECTIONS

1. Place the water, brown ale, walnuts, cashews, tomato paste, lemon juice, apple cider vinegar into a high-speed blender, and purée until thoroughly mixed and smooth.
2. Transfer the mixture to a saucepan over medium heat. Add the nutritional yeast, paprika, and arrowroot powder, and whisk well. Bring to a simmer for about 7 minutes, stirring frequently, or until the mixture begins to thicken and bubble.
3. Remove from the heat and whisk in the red miso. Let the dip cool for 10 minutes and refrigerate in an airtight container for up to 5 days.

NUTRITION: Calories: 113 Fat: 5.1g Carbs: 10.4g Protein: 6.3g

---

THE PLANT BASED DIET COOKBOOK

364. CREAMY BLACK BEAN DIP

COOKING: 0'   PREPARATION: 10'   SERVES: 3

INGREDIENTS

- 4 cups cooked black beans, rinsed and drained
- 2 tablespoons Italian seasoning
- 2 tablespoons minced garlic
- 2 tablespoon low-sodium vegetable broth
- 2 tablespoons onion powder
- 1 tablespoon lemon juice, or more to taste
- ¼ teaspoon salt (optional)

DIRECTIONS

1. In a large bowl, mash the black beans with a potato masher or the back of a fork until mostly smooth.
2. Add the remaining ingredients to the bowl and whisk to combine.
3. Taste and add more lemon juice or salt, if needed. Serve immediately, or refrigerate for at least 30 minutes to better incorporate the flavors.

NUTRITION: Calories: 387 Fat: 6.5g Carbs: 63.0g Protein: 21.2g

365. SPICY AND TANGY BLACK BEAN SALSA

COOKING: 0'   PREPARATION: 15'   SERVES: 3

INGREDIENTS

- 1 (15-oz. / 425-g) can cooked black beans, drained and rinsed
- 1 cup chopped tomatoes
- 1 cup corn kernels, thaw if frozen
- ½ cup cilantro or parsley, chopped
- ¼ cup finely chopped red onion
- 1 tablespoon lemon juice
- 1 tablespoon lime juice
- 1 teaspoon chili powder
- ½ teaspoon ground cumin
- ½ teaspoon regular or smoked paprika
- 1 medium clove garlic, finely chopped

DIRECTIONS

1. Put all the ingredients in a large bowl and stir with a fork until well incorporated.
2. Serve immediately, or chill for 2 hours in the refrigerator to let the flavors blend.

NUTRITION: Calories: 83 Fat: 0.5g Carbs: 15.4g Protein: 4.3g

366. HOMEMADE CHIMICHURRI

COOKING: 0'   PREPARATION: 5'   SERVES: 1

INGREDIENTS

- 1 cup finely chopped flat-leaf parsley leaves
- Zest and juice of 2 lemons
- ¼ cup low-sodium vegetable broth
- 4 garlic cloves
- 1 teaspoon dried oregano

DIRECTIONS

1. Place all the ingredients into a food processor, and pulse until it reaches the consistency you like.
2. Refrigerate the chimichurri in an airtight container for up to 5 days. It's best served within 1 day.

NUTRITION: Calories: 19 Fat: 0.2g Carbs: 3.7g Protein: 0.7g

367. CILANTRO COCONUT PESTO

COOKING: 0'   **PREPARATION: 5'**   **SERVES: 2**

INGREDIENTS

- 1 (13.5-oz.) can unsweetened coconut milk
- 2 jalapeños, seeds and ribs removed
- 1 bunch cilantro, leaves only
- 1 tablespoon white miso
- 1-inch piece ginger, peeled and minced
- Water, as needed

DIRECTIONS

1. Pulse all the ingredients in a blender until creamy and smooth.
2. Thin with a little extra water as needed to reach your preferred consistency.
3. Store in an airtight container in the fridge for up to 2 days or in the freezer for up to 6 months.

NUTRITION: Calories: 141 Fat: 13.7g Carbs: 2.8g Protein: 1.6g

368. FRESH MANGO SALSA

COOKING: 0'   **PREPARATION: 10'**   **SERVES: 6**

INGREDIENTS

- 2 small mangoes, diced
- 1 red bell pepper, finely diced
- ½ red onion, finely diced
- Juice of ½ lime, or more to taste
- 2 tablespoon low-sodium vegetable broth
- Handful cilantro, chopped
- Freshly ground black pepper, to taste
- Salt, to taste (optional)

DIRECTIONS

1. Stir together all the ingredients in a large bowl until well incorporated.
2. Taste and add more lime juice or salt, if needed.
3. Store in an airtight container in the fridge for up to 5 days.

NUTRITION: Calories: 86 Fat: 1.9g Carbs: 13.3g Protein: 1.2g

369. PINEAPPLE MINT SALSA

COOKING: 0'   **PREPARATION: 10'**   **SERVES: 3**

INGREDIENTS

- 1 pound fresh pineapple, finely diced and juices reserved
- 1 bunch mint, leaves only, chopped
- 1 minced jalapeño, (optional)
- 1 white or red onion, finely diced
- Salt, to taste (optional)

DIRECTIONS

1. In a medium bowl, mix the pineapple with its juice, mint, jalapeño (if desired), and onion, and whisk well. Season with salt to taste, if desired.
2. Refrigerate in an airtight container for at least 2 hours to better incorporate the flavors.

NUTRITION: Calories: 58 Fat: 0.1g Carbs: 13.7g Protein: 0.5g

370. ASPARAGUS SPANAKOPITA

COOKING: 25' **PREPARATION: 25'** **SERVES: 12**

INGREDIENTS

- 2 cups cut fresh asparagus (1-inch pieces)
- 20 sheets phyllo dough, (14 inches' x 9 inches)
- Nonstick cooking spray
- Refrigerated butter-flavored spray
- 2 cups torn fresh spinach
- 3 oz. crumbled feta cheese
- 2 tablespoon butter
- 1/4 cup all-purpose flour
- 1-1/2 cups fat-free milk
- 3 tablespoon lemon juice
- 1 teaspoon dill weed
- 1 teaspoon dried thyme
- 1/4 teaspoon salt

DIRECTIONS

1. Put the asparagus in a steamer basket and place it on top of a saucepan with 1-inch of water, then boil. Put the cover and let it steam for 5 minutes or until it becomes crisp-tender.
2. Put 1 sheet of phyllo dough in a cooking spray-coated 13x9-inch baking dish, then cut if needed. Use the butter-flavored spray to spritz the dough. Redo the layers 9 times. Lay the asparagus, feta cheese, and spinach on top. Cover it using a sheet of phyllo dough, then spritz it using the butter-flavored spray. Redo the process using the leftover phyllo. Slice it into 12 pieces. Let it bake for 15 minutes at 350°F without cover, or until it turns golden brown.
3. To make the sauce, in a small saucepan, melt the butter. Mix in the flour until it becomes smooth, then slowly add the milk. Stir in salt, thyme, dill, and lemon juice, then boil. Let it cook and stir for 5 minutes until it becomes thick. Serve the spanakopita with the sauce.

NUTRITION: Calories: 112 Fat: 4g Carbs: 14g Protein: 5g

371. BLACK BEAN AND CORN SALSA FROM RED GOLD

COOKING: 15' **PREPARATION: 15'** **SERVES: 25**

INGREDIENTS

- 2 cans black beans, drained and rinsed
- 1 can whole kernel corn, drained
- 2 cans Petite Diced Tomatoes & Green Chilies
- 1 can Diced Tomatoes, drained
- 1/2 cup chopped green onions
- 2 tablespoon chopped fresh cilantro
- Salt and black pepper to taste

DIRECTIONS

1. Mix all ingredients to combine in a big bowl. Refrigerate to blend flavors for a few hours to overnight. Serve with chips or crackers.

NUTRITION: Calories: 65 Fat: 3g Carbs: 8g Protein: 9g

372. AVOCADO BEAN DIP

COOKING: 15' **PREPARATION: 15'** **SERVES: 2**

INGREDIENTS

- 1 medium ripe avocado, peeled and cubed
- 1/2 cup fresh cilantro leaves
- 3 tablespoon lime juice
- 1/2 teaspoon onion powder
- 1/2 teaspoon garlic powder
- 1/2 teaspoon chipotle hot pepper sauce
- 1/4 teaspoon salt
- 1/4 teaspoon ground cumin
- Baked tortilla chips

DIRECTIONS

1. Mix the first 9 ingredients in a food processor, then cover and blend until smooth. Serve along with chips.

NUTRITION: Calories: 85 Fat: 4g Carbs: 13g Protein: 6g

373. CRUNCHY PEANUT BUTTER APPLE DIP

COOKING: 10'   **PREPARATION: 10'**   **SERVES: 2**

INGREDIENTS

- 1 carton (8 oz.) reduced-Fat: spreadable cream cheese
- 1 cup creamy peanut butter
- 1/4 cup fat-free milk
- 1 tablespoon brown sugar
- 1 teaspoon vanilla extract
- 1/2 cup chopped unsalted peanuts
- Apple slices

DIRECTIONS

1. Beat the initial 5 ingredients in a small bowl until combined. Mix in peanuts. Serve with slices of apple, then put the leftovers in the fridge.

NUTRITION: Calories: 125 Fat: 5g Carbs: 23g Protein: 9g

---

374. HERB POCKETS

COOKING: 25'   **PREPARATION: 25'**   **SERVES: 3**

INGREDIENTS

- 2/3 cup reduced-Fat: garlic-herb spreadable cheese
- 4 oz. reduced-Fat: cream cheese
- 2 tablespoons half-and-half cream
- 1 garlic clove, minced
- 1 tablespoon dried basil
- 1 teaspoon dried thyme
- 1/2 teaspoon celery salt
- 1/4 teaspoon dill weed
- 1/4 teaspoon salt
- 1/4 teaspoon pepper
- 3 to 4 drops hot pepper sauce
- 1/2 cup chopped canned water-packed artichoke hearts, rinsed and drained
- 1/4 cup chopped roasted red peppers
- 2 tubes (8 oz. each) refrigerated reduced-fat: crescent rolls

DIRECTIONS

1. Beat garlic, cream, cream cheese, and spreadable cheese until blended in a small bowl. Beat in hot pepper sauce, pepper, salt, and herbs. Fold in red peppers and artichokes. Refrigerate, covered, for at least an hour.
2. Unroll both crescent roll dough tubes. Form every dough tube to a long rectangle on a lightly floured surface. Seal perforations and seams. Roll each to a 16x12-in. rectangle. Cut to 4 strips, lengthwise and 3 strips, width wise. Separate squares.
3. In the middle of each square, put 1 rounded tablespoon filling. Fold into half, making triangles. Seal by crimping edges. Trim if needed. Put onto ungreased baking sheets. Bake for 10-15 minutes or until golden brown at 375°F. Serve warm.

NUTRITION: Calories: 245 Fat: 5g Carbs: 10g Protein: 7g

---

375. CREAMY CUCUMBER YOGURT DIP

COOKING: 15'   **PREPARATION: 15'**   **SERVES: 4**

INGREDIENTS

- 1 cup (8 oz.) reduced-Fat: plain yogurt
- 4 oz. reduced-Fat: cream cheese
- 1/2 cup chopped seeded peeled cucumber
- 1-1/2 teaspoon. finely chopped onion
- 1-1/2 teaspoon. snipped fresh dill or 1/2 teaspoon dill weed
- 1 teaspoon lemon juice
- 1 teaspoon grated lemon peel
- 1 garlic clove, minced
- 1/4 teaspoon salt
- 1/4 teaspoon pepper
- Assorted fresh vegetables

DIRECTIONS

1. Mix the cream cheese and yogurt in a small bowl. Stir in pepper, salt, garlic, peel, lemon juice, dill, onion, and cucumber. Put on the cover and let it chill in the fridge. Serve it with the veggies.

NUTRITION: Calories: 55 Fat: 4g Carbs: 12g Protein: 6g

THE PLANT BASED DIET COOKBOOK

376. CHUNKY CUCUMBER SALSA

COOKING: 20' | **PREPARATION: 20'** | **SERVES: 4**

INGREDIENTS

- 3 medium cucumbers, peeled and coarsely chopped
- 1 medium mango, coarsely chopped
- 1 cup frozen corn, thawed
- 1 medium sweet red pepper, coarsely chopped
- 1 small red onion, coarsely chopped
- 1 jalapeno pepper, finely chopped
- 3 garlic cloves, minced
- 2 tablespoons white wine vinegar
- 1 tablespoon minced fresh cilantro
- 1 teaspoon salt
- 1/2 teaspoon sugar
- 1/4 to 1/2 teaspoon cayenne pepper

DIRECTIONS

1. Mix all ingredients in a big bowl, then chill, covered, about 2 to 3 hours before serving.

NUTRITION: Calories: 215 Fat: 5g Carbs: 23g Protein: 10g

377. HEALTHIER GUACAMOLE

COOKING: 10' | **PREPARATION: 10'** | **SERVES: 4**

INGREDIENTS

- 3/4 cup crumbled tofu
- 2 avocados - peeled and pitted, divided
- 1 teaspoon salt
- 1 teaspoon minced garlic
- 1 pinch cayenne pepper (optional)

DIRECTIONS

1. Prepare a food processor then put one avocado and tofu in it then blend well until it becomes smooth. Combine salt, lime juice, and the left avocado in a bowl.
2. Add in the garlic, tomatoes, cilantro, onion, and tofu-avocado mixture. Put in cayenne pepper.
3. Let it chill in the refrigerator for 1 hour to enhance the flavor or you can serve it right away.

NUTRITION: Calories: 534 Fat: 5g Carbs: 23g Protein: 11g

378. GARLIC WHITE BEAN DIP

COOKING: 15' | **PREPARATION: 15'** | **SERVES: 2**

INGREDIENTS

- 1/4 cup soft bread crumbs
- 2 tablespoon dry white wine or water
- 2 tablespoons olive oil
- 2 tablespoon lemon juice
- 4-1/2 teaspoon. minced fresh parsley
- 3 garlic cloves, peeled and halved
- 1/2 teaspoon salt
- 1/2 teaspoon snipped fresh dill or 1/4 teaspoon dill weed
- 1/8 teaspoon cayenne pepper
- Assorted fresh vegetables

DIRECTIONS

1. Mix wine and bread crumbs in a small bowl. Mix cayenne, dill, salt, garlic, parsley, beans, lemon juice, and oil in a food processor, then cover and blend until smooth.
2. Put in bread crumb mixture and process until well combined. Serve together with vegetables.

NUTRITION: Calories: 105 Fat: 5g Carbs: 12g Protein: 6g

379. FRUIT SKEWERS

COOKING: 20'   **PREPARATION: 20'**   **SERVES: 2**

INGREDIENTS

- cream cheese
- Fat sour cream
- lime juice
- honey
- 1/2 teaspoon ground ginger
- 2 cups green grapes
- 2 cups fresh or canned unsweetened pineapple chunks
- 2 large red apples, cut into 1-inch pieces

DIRECTIONS

1. To make the dip, beat the sour cream and cream cheese in a small bowl until it becomes smooth. Beat in the ginger, honey, and lime juice until it becomes smooth.
2. Put the cover and let it chill in the fridge for a minimum of 1 hour.
3. Alternately thread the apples, pineapple, and grapes on 8 12-inch skewers. Serve it right away with the dip.

NUTRITION: Calories: 180 Fat: 5g Carbs: 28g Protein: 4g

---

380. LOW-FAT: STUFFED MUSHROOMS

COOKING: 25'   **PREPARATION: 20'**   **SERVES: 6**

INGREDIENTS

- 1 lb. large fresh mushrooms
- 3 tablespoons seasoned bread crumbs
- 3 tablespoons fat-free sour cream
- 2 tablespoons grated Parmesan cheese
- 2 tablespoons minced chives
- 2 tablespoons reduced-Fat: mayonnaise
- 2 teaspoons balsamic vinegar
- 2 to 3 drops hot pepper sauce, optional

DIRECTIONS

1. Take out the stems from the mushrooms, then put the cups aside. Chop the stems and set aside 1/3 cup (eliminate the leftover stems or reserve for later use).
2. Mix the reserved mushroom stems, hot pepper sauce if preferred, vinegar, mayonnaise, chives, Parmesan cheese, sour cream, and breadcrumbs in a bowl, then stir well.
3. Put the mushroom caps on a cooking spray-coated baking tray and stuff it with the crumb mixture.
4. Let it boil for 5 to 7 minutes, placed 4-6 inches from the heat source, or until it turns light brown.

NUTRITION: Calories: 435 Fat: 4g Carbs: 23g Protein: 9g

---

381. MARINATED MUSHROOMS

COOKING: 25'   **PREPARATION: 15'**   **SERVES: 8**

INGREDIENTS

- 1 cup red wine
- 1/2 cup red wine vinegar
- 1/3 cup olive oil
- 2 tablespoon brown sugar
- 2 cloves garlic, minced
- 1 teaspoon crushed red pepper flakes
- 1/4 cup red bell pepper, diced
- 1 lb. small fresh mushrooms, washed and trimmed
- 1/4 cup chopped green onions
- 1/4 teaspoon dried oregano
- 1/2 teaspoon salt
- 1/4 teaspoon ground black pepper

DIRECTIONS

1. Mix the mushrooms, red pepper flakes, bell pepper, garlic, sugar, oil, vinegar, and wine in a saucepan on medium heat, then boil.
2. Put the cover and put it aside to let it cool.
3. Mix in pepper, salt, oregano, and green onions once cooled. Serve it at room temperature or chilled.

NUTRITION: Calories: 135 Fat: 5g Carbs: 13g Protein: 8g

382. PUMPKIN SPICE SPREAD

COOKING: 10' — **PREPARATION: 10'** — **SERVES: 4**

INGREDIENTS

- 1 package (8 oz.) fat-free cream cheese
- 1/2 cup canned pumpkin
- Sugar substitute equivalent to 1/2 cup sugar
- 1 teaspoon ground cinnamon
- 1 teaspoon vanilla extract
- 1 teaspoon maple flavoring
- 1/2 teaspoon pumpkin pie spice
- 1/2 teaspoon ground nutmeg
- 1 carton (8 oz.) frozen reduced-Fat: whipped topping, thawed

DIRECTIONS

1. Mix well together sugar substitute, pumpkin, and cream cheese in a big bowl. Beat in nutmeg, pumpkin pie spice, maple flavoring, vanilla, and cinnamon.
2. Fold in whipped topping and chill until serving.

NUTRITION: Calories: 177 Fat: 6g Carbs: 21g Protein: 11g

---

383. MAPLE BAGEL SPREAD

COOKING: 10' — **PREPARATION: 10'** — **SERVES: 1**

INGREDIENTS

- cream cheese
- maple syrup
- cinnamon
- walnuts

DIRECTIONS

1. Beat the cinnamon, syrup, and cream cheese in a big bowl until it becomes smooth, then mix in walnuts.
2. Let it chill until ready to serve. Serve it with bagels.

NUTRITION: Calories: 586 Fat: 7g Carbs: 23g Protein: 4g

---

384. ITALIAN STUFFED ARTICHOKES

COOKING: 25' — **PREPARATION: 20'** — **SERVES: 4**

INGREDIENTS

- 4 large artichokes
- 2 teaspoon lemon juice
- 2 cups soft Italian bread crumbs, toasted
- 1/2 cup grated Parmigiano-Reggiano cheese
- 1/2 cup minced fresh parsley
- 2 teaspoon Italian seasoning
- 1 teaspoon grated lemon peel
- 1/2 teaspoon pepper
- 1/4 teaspoon salt
- 1 tablespoon olive oil

DIRECTIONS

1. Level the bottom of each artichoke using a sharp knife and trim off 1-inch from the tops. Snip off tips of outer leaves using kitchen scissors, then brush lemon juice on cut edges. In a Dutch oven, stand the artichokes and pour 1-inch of water, then boil. Lower the heat, put the cover, and let it simmer for 5 minutes or until the leaves near the middle pull out effortlessly.
2. Turn the artichokes upside down to drain. Allow it to stand for 10 minutes. Carefully scrape out the fuzzy middle part of the artichokes using a spoon and get rid of it.
3. Mix the salt, pepper, lemon peel, Italian seasoning, garlic, parsley, cheese, and breadcrumbs in a small bowl, then add olive oil and stir well. Gently spread the artichoke leaves apart, then fill it with breadcrumb mixture.
4. Put it in a cooking spray-coated 11x7-inch baking dish. Let it bake for 10 minutes at 350°F without cover, or until the filling turns light brown.

NUTRITION: Calories: 543 Fat: 5g Carbs: 44g Protein: 6g

385. ENCHILADA SAUCE

COOKING: 10' **PREPARATION: 10'** **SERVES: 3**

INGREDIENTS

- 1½ tablespoon MCT oil
- ½ tablespoon chili powder
- ½ tablespoon whole wheat flour
- ½ teaspoon ground cumin
- ¼ teaspoon oregano (dried or fresh)
- ¼ teaspoon salt (or to taste)
- 1 garlic clove (minced)
- 1 tablespoon tomato paste
- 1 cup vegetable broth
- ½ teaspoon apple vinegar
- ½ teaspoon ground black pepper

DIRECTIONS

1. Heat a small saucepan over medium heat.
2. Add the MCT oil and minced garlic to the pan and sauté for about 1 minute.
3. Mix the dry spices and flour in a medium bowl and pour the dry mixture into the saucepan.
4. Stir in the tomato paste immediately, slowly pour in the vegetable broth, and make sure that everything combines well.
5. When everything is mixed thoroughly, bring up the heat to medium-high until it gets to a simmer and cook for about 3 minutes or until the sauce becomes a bit thicker.
6. Remove the pan from the heat and add the vinegar with the black pepper, adding more salt and pepper to taste.

NUTRITION: Calories: 225 Fat: 4 Carbs: 33g Protein: 5g

386. KETO SALSA VERDE

COOKING: 5' **PREPARATION: 10'** **SERVES: 5**

INGREDIENTS

- 4 tablespoons fresh cilantro, finely chopped
- 1/4 cup fresh parsley, finely chopped
- 2 garlic cloves, grated
- 2 teaspoon lemon juice
- 3/4 cup of olive oil
- 2 tablespoon small capers
- 1 teaspoon of salt
- 1/2 teaspoon black pepper

DIRECTIONS

1. Add all ingredients to a large mixing bowl. Can be mixed with by hand or with an immersion blender. Mix until desired consistency is achieved.
2. Can be served over burgers, sandwiches, salads and more. Can be stored in the refrigerator for up to 5 days or for longer in the freezer.

NUTRITION: Calories: 110 Fat: 25.3g Carbs: 2g Protein: 0.2g

387. CHIMICHURRI

COOKING: 5' **PREPARATION: 10'** **SERVES: 8**

INGREDIENTS

- 1/2 yellow bell pepper, deseeded and finely chopped
- 1 green chili pepper, deseeded and finely chopped
- Juice and zest of 1 lemon
- 1 cup olive oil
- 1/2 cup parsley, chopped
- 2 garlic cloves, grated
- Salt and pepper to taste

DIRECTIONS

1. Add all ingredients to a large mixing bowl. Can be mixed with by hand or with an immersion blender. Mix until desired consistency is achieved.
2. Can be served over burgers, sandwiches, salads and more. Can be stored in the refrigerator for up to 5 days or for longer in the freezer.

NUTRITION: Calories: 278 Fat: 15.5g Carbs: 6.31g Protein: 4.2g

THE PLANT BASED DIET COOKBOOK

388. KETO VEGAN RAW CASHEW CHEESE SAUCE

COOKING: 5' **PREPARATION:** 5' **SERVES:** 6

INGREDIENTS

- 1 cup raw cashews, soaked in water for at least 3 hours before making recipe
- 2 tablespoons olive oil
- 2 tablespoon nutritional yeast
- 1/4 teaspoon garlic powder
- 2 tablespoons fresh lemon juice
- 1/2 cup water
- Salt to taste

DIRECTIONS

1. To prepare cashews before making the sauce, boil 2 cups of water turn off heat and add cashews. This can be allowed to soak overnight. Rinse and strained cashews. Discard water.
2. Add all ingredients to a food processor and blend until a smooth consistency is achieved. Can be used to make pizzas, over roasted veggies, in lasagna, as a dip and more.

NUTRITION: Calories: 312 Fat: 15.5g Carbs: 9.23g Protein: 5.1g

389. SPICY AVOCADO MAYONNAISE

COOKING: 10' **PREPARATION:** 10' **SERVES:** 8

INGREDIENTS

- 2 ripe avocados, pitted and peeled
- 1/4 jalapeno pepper, minced
- 2 tablespoon lemon juice
- 1/2 teaspoon onion powder
- 2 tablespoons fresh cilantro, chopped
- Salt to taste

DIRECTIONS

1. Add all ingredients to a food processor and blender until a smooth creamy consistency is achieved.
2. The jalapeno peppers can be foregone if you prefer a cooler mayo. Can be enjoyed in sandwiches, on toast, as a topping, in veggie wraps and salads

NUTRITION: Calories: 456 Fat: 9.8g Carbs: 4.6g Protein: 1g

390. GREEN COCONUT BUTTER

COOKING: 10' **PREPARATION:** 10' **SERVES:** 8

INGREDIENTS

- 2 cups unsweetened shredded coconut
- 2 teaspoon matcha powder
- 1 tablespoon coconut oil

DIRECTIONS

1. Add shredded coconut to a food processor and blend for 5 minutes or until a smooth but runny consistency is achieved.
2. Add matcha powder and olive oil. Blend for 1 more minute.
3. Can be stored in an airtight container at room temperature for up to 2 weeks. Makes a delicious fruit dip and can be added to smoothies, on pancakes and toast.

NUTRITION: Calories: 221 Fat: 5.2g Carbs: 1.7g Protein: 0.7g

391. SPICED ALMOND BUTTER SAUCE

COOKING: 5' **PREPARATION: 10'** **SERVES: 10**

INGREDIENTS

- 2 cups raw almond
- 1/8 teaspoon allspice
- 1/8 teaspoon cinnamon
- 1/8 teaspoon cardamom
- 1/8 teaspoon ground ginger
- 1/8 teaspoon ground cloves
- 1/2 teaspoon salt

DIRECTIONS

1. Place all ingredients in a food processor and blend until a smooth consistency is achieved. Makes a delicious fruit and veggie dip and can be added to smoothies, on toast, on pancakes and waffles.

NUTRITION: Calories: 312 Fat: 9.5g Carbs: 4.1g Protein: 4g

392. KETO STRAWBERRY JAM

COOKING: 5' **PREPARATION: 25'** **SERVES: 18**

INGREDIENTS

- 1 cup fresh strawberries, chopped
- 1 tablespoon lemon juice
- 4 teaspoon xylitol
- 1 tablespoon water

DIRECTIONS

1. Add all ingredients to a small saucepan and place over medium heat. Stir to combine and cook for about 15 minutes. Stir occasionally.
2. After 15 minutes are up, mash-up strawberries with a potato masher or fork.
3. Pour into a heat-safe container such as a mason jar.
4. Allow to cool then cover with a lid and refrigerate. Can be stored in the refrigerator for up to 3 days. Goes great with toast and sweet sandwiches.

NUTRITION: Calories: 219 Fat: 0g Carbs: 1g Protein: 0.1g

390. GREEN COCONUT BUTTER

COOKING: 10' **PREPARATION: 10'** **SERVES: 8**

INGREDIENTS

- 2 cups unsweetened shredded coconut
- 2 teaspoon matcha powder
- 1 tablespoon coconut oil

DIRECTIONS

1. Add shredded coconut to a food processor and blend for 5 minutes or until a smooth but runny consistency is achieved.
2. Add matcha powder and olive oil. Blend for 1 more minute.
3. Can be stored in an airtight container at room temperature for up to 2 weeks. Makes a delicious fruit dip and can be added to smoothies, on pancakes and toast.

NUTRITION: Calories: 221 Fat: 5.2g Carbs: 1.7g Protein: 0.7g

THE PLANT BASED DIET COOKBOOK

393. CHOCOLATE COCONUT BUTTER SAUCE

COOKING: 20' | **PREPARATION: 10'** | **SERVES: 20**

INGREDIENTS

- 1/2 lb. unsweetened shredded coconut
- 3 tablespoon cocoa butter
- 1/8 teaspoon salt

DIRECTIONS

1. Preheat your oven to 350°F.
2. Place shredded coconut on a greased baking sheet. Spread out into a thin, even layer.
3. Bake for up to 15 minutes or until the coconut flakes are golden brown. Stir the coconut shreds every 3 minutes and watch them closely because they burn very easily and quickly.
4. Allow the coconut flakes to cool for 15 minutes.
5. Add coconut flakes to a food processor and blend until smooth and creamy yet runny in consistency.
6. Adding cocoa butter and salt and blend to incorporate well.
7. Pour into an airtight jar and seal lid. The consistency will thicken up as the butter cools. The oil may separate and float to the top of the container as the butter cools.
8. Simply reheat a portion in the microwave just before using. Can be stored for up to a whole year at room temperature!

NUTRITION: Calories: 457 Fat: 17.4g Carbs: 0.9g Protein: 0.3g

394. ORANGE DILL BUTTER

COOKING: 15' | **PREPARATION: 10'** | **SERVES: 12**

INGREDIENTS

- 1/2 cup vegan butter
- 2 tablespoons fresh dill, finely chopped
- 2 tablespoons orange zest
- 1 teaspoon salt

DIRECTIONS

1. Add 4 cups of water to a small pot and bring to a boil over high heat. Reduce heat to low and allow water to simmer.
2. Add vegan butter to a glass Mason jar and screw on lid loosely.
3. Place Mason jar in the boiling water. Ensure that the jar does not get submerged or over turn.
4. Allow the butter to melt and add remaining ingredients
5. Remove the Mason jar from the pot and allow to cool until the mixture becomes partially solidified.
6. Can be used alongside your favorite veggies to infuse them with flavor and fat. Can be stored in the refrigerator for up to 2 weeks.

NUTRITION: Calories: 287 Fat: 1.5g Carbs: 1g Protein: 0.1g

395. KETO CARAMEL SAUCE

COOKING: 35' | **PREPARATION: 10'** | **SERVES: 8**

INGREDIENTS

- 1/2 cup raw cashews
- 1/2 cup coconut cream, melted
- 10 drops liquid stevia
- 2 tablespoon vegan butter
- 3 teaspoon vanilla extract
- A pinch of salt

DIRECTIONS

1. Preheat your oven to 325°F
2. Place nuts on a greased baking tray and toast for 20 minutes or until lightly golden and crunchy.
3. Allow the nuts to cool slightly then add to a food processor and blend to a slightly lumpy consistency.
4. Add remaining ingredients and blend until a smooth and creamy consistency is achieved. Do not over blend or the coconut cream will become separated from the rest of the ingredients
5. Can be stored in a glass, airtight container in the refrigerator if not being served immediately. To reheat the caramel to make it more flow able, add to a saucepan and gently warm on low heat. Can be served with your favorite keto vegan treats such as ice-cream.

NUTRITION: Calories: 398 Fat: 9.8g Carbs: 4.6g Protein: 7.2g

396. PECAN BUTTER

COOKING: 10'   **PREPARATION: 10'**   **SERVES: 8**

INGREDIENTS

- 3 cups pecans, soaked well at least 3 hours, rinsed, strained and dried

DIRECTIONS

1. Add the pecans to a food processor and blend until a smooth and creamy consistency is achieved. Scrape down the sides of the bowl when necessary.
2. Transfer to a Mason jar and store in the refrigerator. Can be stored in the refrigerator for several months. Makes a great spread on toast and sandwiches and a great fruit and veggie dip.

NUTRITION: Calories: 312 Fat: 25g Carbs: 5g Protein: 6.9g

397. KETO VEGAN RANCH DRESSING

COOKING: 10'   **PREPARATION: 5'**   **SERVES: 3**

INGREDIENTS

- 1 cup vegan mayo
- 1 1/2 cup coconut milk
- 2 scallions
- 2 garlic cloves, peeled
- 1 cup fresh dill
- 1 teaspoon garlic powder
- Salt and pepper to taste

DIRECTIONS

1. Add scallion, fresh dill and garlic cloves to a food processor and pulse until finely chopped.
2. Add the rest of the ingredients and blend until a smooth, creamy consistency is achieved. Makes a great creamy salad dressing. Store in the refrigerator.

NUTRITION: Calories: 311 Fat: 11.9g Carbs: 6.2g Protein: 4g

398. CAULIFLOWER HUMMUS

COOKING: 20'   **PREPARATION: 10'**   **SERVES: 7**

INGREDIENTS

- 1 large head cauliflower
- 1 tablespoon almond butter
- 1 garlic clove, finely chopped
- 1 tablespoon lemon juice
- 2 teaspoons olive oil
- 1/4 teaspoon cumin
- Salt and pepper to taste

DIRECTIONS

1. Cut cauliflower into florets and place in a large microwave-safe bowl. Microwave for 10 minutes on high heat or until completely cooked through.
2. Transfer cauliflower florets to a food processor. Add the rest of the ingredients
3. Blend until smooth, creamy consistency is reached. Can be stored in the refrigerator in an airtight container for up to 5 days. Makes a great dip for fruits and veggies.

NUTRITION: Calories: Fat: 2.7g Carbs: 2.7g Protein: 4.3g

THE PLANT BASED DIET COOKBOOK

399. WHITE BEANS DIP

COOKING: 15'   **PREPARATION: 15'**   **SERVES: 6**

INGREDIENTS

- 1/2 cup olive oil
- 2 tablespoons garlic cloves, chopped
- 2 (15. 8-oz.) cans white beans, drained and rinsed
- 1/4 cup fresh lemon juice
- 4 tablespoons fresh parsley, chopped and divided
- 1 teaspoon ground cumin
- 1/4 tablespoon salt
- 1 teaspoon ground white pepper

DIRECTIONS

1. In a small saucepan, place the olive oil and garlic over medium-low heat and cook for about 2 minutes, stirring continuously.
2. Remove the pan of garlic oil from heat and let it cool slightly.
3. Strain the garlic oil, reserving both the oil and garlic in separate bowls.
4. In a food processor, place the beans, garlic, lemon juice, 2 tablespoons of parsley, cumin, and pulse until smooth.
5. While motor is running, add the reserved oil and pulse until light and smooth.
6. Transfer the dip into a bowl and stir in salt and white pepper.
7. Serve with the garnishing of remaining parsley.

NUTRITION: Calories: 263 Fat: 18.1g Carbs: 20.2 g Protein: 7g

---

400. EDAMAME HUMMUS

COOKING: 11'   **PREPARATION: 15'**   **SERVES: 5**

INGREDIENTS

- 10 oz. frozen edamame pods
- 1 ripe avocado, peeled, pitted, and chopped roughly
- 1/2 cup fresh cilantro, chopped
- 1/4 cup scallion, chopped
- 1 jalapeño pepper
- 1 garlic clove, peeled
- 2–3 tablespoons fresh lime juice
- Salt and ground black pepper, to taste
- 1/4 cup avocado oil
- 2 tablespoons fresh basil leaves

DIRECTIONS

1. In a small pot of boiling water, cook the edamame pods edamame pods for 6–8 minutes.
2. Drain the edamame pods and let them cool completely.
3. Remove soybeans from the pods.
4. In a food processor, add edamame and remaining ingredients (except for oil) and pulse until mostly pureed.
5. While motor is running, add the reserved oil and pulse until light and smooth.
6. Transfer the hummus into a bowl and serve with the garnishing of remaining basil leaves.

NUTRITION: Calories: 339 Fat: 33.8g Carbs: 6.3 g Protein: 5.1g

---

401. BEANS MAYONNAISE

COOKING: 2'   **PREPARATION: 10'**   **SERVES: 4**

INGREDIENTS

- 1 (15-oz.) can white beans, drained and rinsed
- 2 tablespoons apple cider vinegar
- 1 tablespoon fresh lemon juice
- 2 tablespoons yellow mustard
- 3/4 teaspoon salt
- 2 garlic cloves, peeled
- 2 tablespoons aquafaba (liquid from the can of beans)

DIRECTIONS

1. In a food processor, add all ingredients (except for oil) and pulse until mostly pureed.
2. While motor is running, add the reserved oil and pulse until light and smooth.
3. Transfer the mayonnaise into a container and refrigerate to chill before serving.

NUTRITION: Calories: 8 Fat: 1.1g Carbs: 14.3g Protein: 5.2g

402. CASHEW CREAM

COOKING: 0'   **PREPARATION: 10'**   **SERVES: 5**

INGREDIENTS

- 1 cup raw, unsalted cashews, soaked for 12 hours and drained
- 1/2 cup water
- 1 tablespoon nutritional yeast
- 1 teaspoon fresh lemon juice
- 1/8 teaspoon salt

DIRECTIONS

1. In a food processor, add all ingredients and pulse on high speed until creamy and smooth.
2. Serve immediately.

NUTRITION: Calories: 165 Fat: 12.8g Carbs: 9.9 g Protein: 5.1g

403. LEMON TAHINI

COOKING: 0'   **PREPARATION: 15'**   **SERVES: 4**

INGREDIENTS

- 1/4 cup fresh lemon juice
- 4 medium garlic cloves, pressed
- 1/2 cup tahini
- 1/2 teaspoon fine sea salt
- Pinch of ground cumin
- 6 tablespoons ice water

DIRECTIONS

1. In a medium bowl, combine the lemon juice and garlic and set aside for 10 minutes.
2. Through a fine-mesh sieve, strain the mixture into another medium bowl, pressing the garlic solids.
3. Discard the garlic solids.
4. In the lemon juice bowl, add the tahini, salt, and cumin, and whisk until well blended.
5. Slowly, add water, 2 tablespoons at a time, whisking well after each addition.

NUTRITION: Calories: 187 Fat: 16.3g Carbs: 7.7 g Protein: 5.4g

404. KETO-VEGAN KETCHUP

COOKING: 11'   **PREPARATION: 35'**   **SERVES: 10**

INGREDIENTS

- 1/8 t of the following:
- Mustard powder
- Cloves, ground
- 1/4 teaspoon paprika
- 1/2 teaspoon garlic powder
- 3/4 teaspoon onion powder
- 1 teaspoon sea salt
- 3 tablespoons. apple cider vinegar
- 1/4 cup powdered monk fruit
- 1 cup water
- 6 oz. tomato paste

DIRECTIONS

1. In a little saucepan, whisk together all the ingredients
2. Cover the pan and bring to low heat and simmer for 30 minutes, stirring occasionally.
3. Once reduced, add to the blender and puree until it's a smooth consistency.

NUTRITION: Calories: 13 Carbs: 2g Proteins: 0g Fat: 0g

405. GUACAMOLE

COOKING: 5' **PREPARATION: 5'** **SERVES: 6**

INGREDIENTS

- 3 tablespoons of the following:
- Tomato, diced
- Onion, diced
- 2 tablespoons of the following:
- Cilantro, chopped
- Jalapeno juice
- 1/4 teaspoon garlic powder
- 1/2 teaspoon salt
- 1/2 lime, squeezed
- 2 big avocados
- 1 jalapeno, diced

DIRECTIONS

1. Using a molcajete, crush the diced jalapenos until soft.
2. Add the avocados to the molcajete.
3. Squeeze the lime juice from ½ of the lime on top of the avocados.
4. Add the jalapeno juice, garlic, and salt and mix until smooth.
5. Once smooth, add in the onion, cilantro, and tomato and stir to incorporate.

NUTRITION: Calories: 127 Carbs: 9.3g Proteins: 2.4g Fat: 10.2g

406. KETO-VEGAN MAYO

COOKING: 5' **PREPARATION: 5'** **SERVES: 6**

INGREDIENTS

- ½ cup of the following:
- Extra virgin olive oil
- Almond milk, unsweetened
- 1/4 teaspoon xanthan gum
- Pinch of white pepper, ground
- Pinch of Himalayan salt
- 1 teaspoon Dijon mustard
- 2 teaspoons apple cider vinegar

DIRECTIONS

1. In a blender, place milk, pepper salt, mustard, and vinegar.
2. Turn the blender to high speed and slowly add xanthan then the olive oil.
3. Remove from the blender and allow cooling for 2 hours in the refrigerator.
4. During cooling, the mixture will thicken.

NUTRITION: Calories: 160.4 Carbs: 0.2g Proteins: 0g Fat: 18g

407. PEANUT SAUCE

COOKING: 10' **PREPARATION: 10'** **SERVES: 4**

INGREDIENTS

- 1/2 teaspoon Thai red curry paste
- 1 teaspoon of the following: Coconut oil, Soy Sauce, Chili garlic sauce
- 1 tablespoon sweetener of your choice
- 1/3 cup coconut milk
- 1/4 cup peanut butter, smooth

DIRECTIONS

1. Using a microwave-safe dish, add the peanut butter and heat for about 30 seconds.
2. Whisk into the peanut butter, the soy sauce, sweetener, and chili garlic then set to the side.
3. Warm a little saucepan over medium heat and add oil.
4. Cook the Thai red curry paste until fragrant then add to a microwave-safe bowl.
5. Continuously stir the peanut mixture as you add the coconut milk. Stir until well-combined.
6. Enjoy at room temperature or warmed.

NUTRITION: Calories: 151 Carbs: 4g Proteins: 4g Fat: 13g

408. PISTACHIO DIP

COOKING: 10' | **PREPARATION: 10'** | **SERVES: 8**

INGREDIENTS

- 2 tablespoon lemon juice
- 1 teaspoon extra virgin olive oil
- 2 tablespoons of the following:
- Tahini
- Parsley, chopped
- 2 cloves of garlic
- ½ cup pistachios shelled
- 15 oz. garbanzo beans, save the liquid from the can
- Salt and pepper to taste

DIRECTIONS

1. Using a food processor, add pistachios, pepper, sea salt, lemon juice, olive oil, tahini, parsley, garlic, and garbanzo beans. Pulse until mixed.
2. Using the liquid from the garbanzo beans, add to the dip while slowly blending until it reaches your desired consistency.
3. Enjoy at room temperature or warmed.

NUTRITION: Calories: 88 Carbs: 9g Proteins: 2.5g Fat: 3g

409. SMOKEY TOMATO JAM

COOKING: 45' | **PREPARATION: 45'** | **SERVES: 1 CUP**

INGREDIENTS

- 1/2 teaspoon of the following:
- White wine vinegar
- Salt
- 1/3 teaspoon smoked paprika
- Pinch Black pepper
- 1/4 cup coconut sugar
- 2 lb.' tomatoes

DIRECTIONS

1. Over medium-high heat, bring a big pot of water to a boil.
2. Fill a big bowl with ice and water.
3. Carefully place the tomatoes into the boiling water for 1 minute and then remove, and immediately put into the ice water.
4. While tomatoes are in the ice water, peel them by hand and then transfer to a clean cutting surface.
5. Empty the pot of water.
6. Chop the tomatoes and place back into the pot; add the coconut sugar and stir to combine.
7. Bring the pot back to medium heat and the tomatoes to a boil, cooking for 15 minutes.
8. Stir in the paprika, pepper, and salt and then bring the temperature down to the lowest setting. Let it cook until it becomes thick, which is approximately 10 minutes.
9. Remove it from the heat while continuing to stir; add in white wine vinegar.

NUTRITION: Calories: 26 Carbs: 5.3g Proteins: 1.1g Fat: 0.6g

410. TASTY RANCH DRESSING/DIP

COOKING: 45' | **PREPARATION: 45'** | **SERVES: 15**

INGREDIENTS

- ½ cup soy milk, unsweetened
- 1 tablespoon dill, chopped
- 2 teaspoons parsley, chopped
- 1/4 teaspoon black pepper
- 1/2 teaspoon of the following: Onion powder Garlic powder
- 1 cup vegan mayonnaise

DIRECTIONS

1. In a medium bowl, whisk all theingredients together until smooth. If dressing is too thick, add 1/4 tablespoon of soy milk at a time until the desired consistency.
2. Transfer to an airtight container or jar and refrigerate for 1 hour.
3. Serve over leafy greens or as a dip.

NUTRITION: Calories: 93 Carbs: 0g Proteins: 0g Fat: 9g

THE PLANT BASED DIET COOKBOOK

CHAPTER 17: VEGETABLES RECIPES

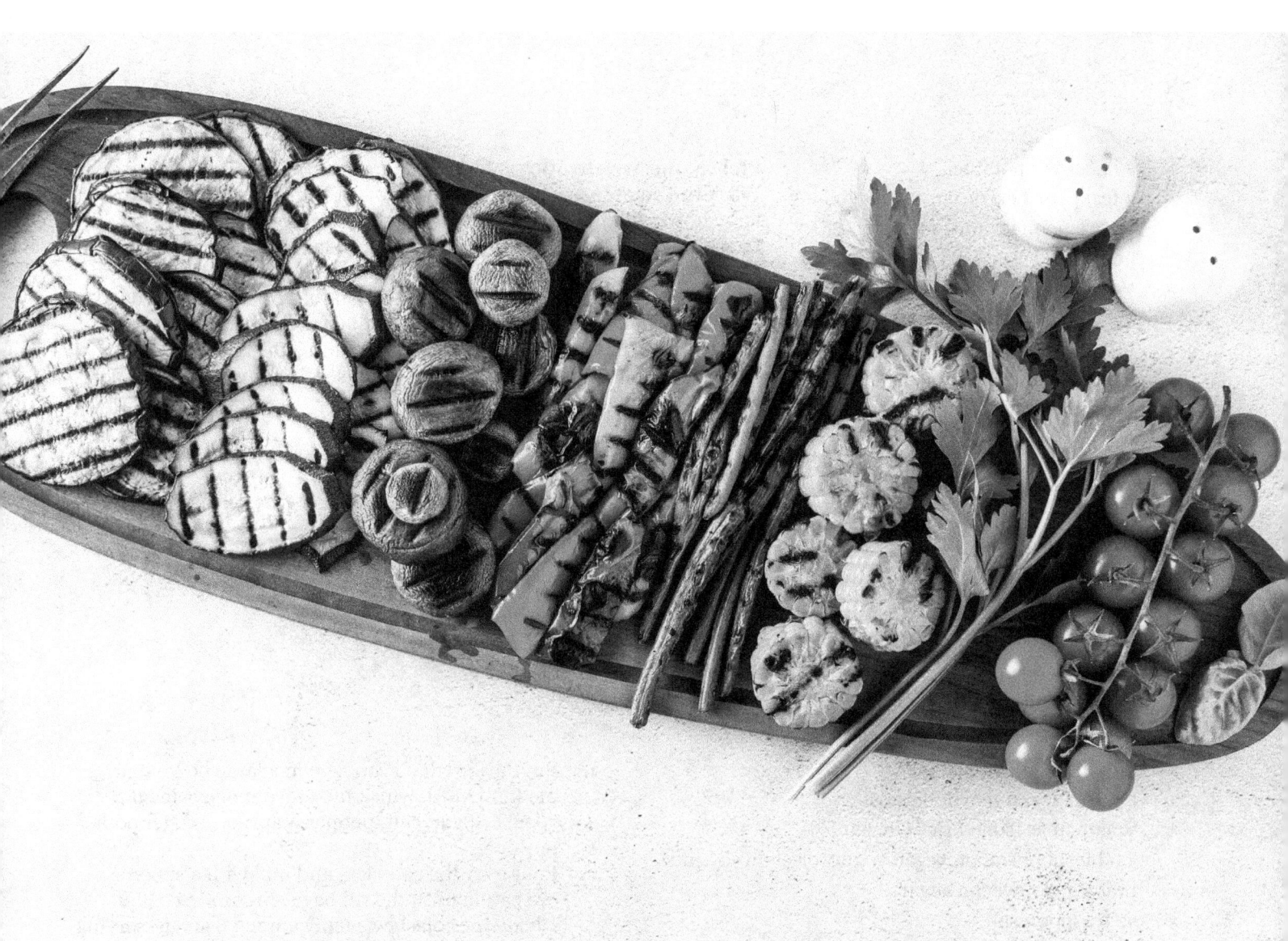

411. STEAMED CAULIFLOWER

COOKING: 10' **PREPARATION:** 5' **SERVES:** 6

INGREDIENTS

- 1 large head cauliflower
- 1 cup water
- ½ teaspoon salt
- 1 teaspoon red pepper flakes (optional)

DIRECTIONS

1. Remove any leaves from the cauliflower, and cut it into florets.
2. In a large saucepan, bring the water to a boil. Place a steamer basket over the water, and add the florets and salt. Cover and steam for 5 to 7 minutes, until tender. In a large bowl, toss the cauliflower with the red pepper flakes (if using). Transfer the florets to a large airtight container or 6 single-serving containers. Let cool before sealing the lids.

NUTRITION: Calories: 35, Fat: 0g, Protein: 3g, Carbs: 7g

412. CAJUN SWEET POTATOES

COOKING: 30' **PREPARATION:** 5' **SERVES:** 4

INGREDIENTS

- 2 lb.' sweet potatoes
- 2 teaspoons extra-virgin olive oil
- ½ teaspoon ground cayenne pepper
- ½ teaspoon smoked paprika
- ½ teaspoon dried oregano
- ½ teaspoon dried thyme
- ½ teaspoon garlic powder
- ½ teaspoon salt (optional)

DIRECTIONS

1. Preheat the oven to 400°F. Line a baking sheet with parchment paper.
2. Wash the potatoes, pat dry, and cut into ¾-inch cubes. Transfer to a large bowl, and pour the olive oil over the potatoes.
3. In a small bowl, combine the cayenne, paprika, oregano, thyme, and garlic powder. Sprinkle the spices over the potatoes and combine until the potatoes are well coated. Spread the potatoes on the prepared baking sheet in a single layer. Season with the salt (if using). Roast for 30 minutes, stirring the potatoes after 15 minutes.
4. Divide the potatoes evenly among 4 single-serving containers. Let cool completely before sealing.

NUTRITION: Calories: 219, Fat: 3g, Protein: 4g, Carbs: 46g

413. SMOKY COLESLAW

COOKING: 0' **PREPARATION:** 10' **SERVES:** 6

INGREDIENTS

- 1 pound shredded cabbage
- 1/3 cup vegan mayonnaise
- ¼ cup unseasoned rice vinegar
- 3 tablespoons plain vegan yogurt or plain soymilk
- 1 tablespoon vegan sugar
- ½ teaspoon salt
- ¼ teaspoon freshly ground black pepper
- ¼ teaspoon smoked paprika
- ¼ teaspoon chipotle powder

DIRECTIONS

1. Put the shredded cabbage in a large bowl. In a medium bowl, whisk the mayonnaise, vinegar, yogurt, sugar, salt, pepper, paprika, and chipotle powder.
2. Pour over the cabbage, and mix with a spoon or spatula until the cabbage shreds are coated. Divide the coleslaw evenly among 6 single-serving containers. Seal the lids.

NUTRITION: Calories: 73, Fat: 4g, Protein: 1g, Carbs: 8g

414. MEDITERRANEAN HUMMUS PIZZA

COOKING: 30' | **PREPARATION: 10'** | **SERVES: 2 PIZZAS**

INGREDIENTS

- ½ zucchini, thinly sliced
- ½ red onion, thinly sliced
- 1 cup cherry tomatoes, halved
- 2 to 4 tablespoons pitted and chopped black olives
- Pinch sea salt
- Drizzle olive oil (optional)
- 2 prebaked pizza crusts
- ½ cup Classic Hummus
- 2 to 4 tablespoons Cheesy Sprinkle

DIRECTIONS

1. Preheat the oven to 400°F. Place the zucchini, onion, cherry tomatoes, and olives in a large bowl, sprinkle them with the sea salt, and toss them a bit. Drizzle with a bit of olive oil (if using), seal in the flavor and keep them from drying out in the oven.
2. Lay the two crusts out on a large baking sheet. Spread half the hummus on each crust, and top with the veggie mixture and some Cheesy Sprinkle. Pop the pizzas in the oven for 20 to 30 minutes, or until the veggies are soft.

NUTRITION: Calories: 500, Fat: 25g, Carbs: 58g, Protein: 15g

---

415. BAKED BRUSSELS SPROUTS

COOKING: 10' | **PREPARATION: 40'** | **SERVES: 4**

INGREDIENTS

- 1 pound Brussels sprouts
- 2 teaspoons extra-virgin olive or canola oil
- 4 teaspoons minced garlic (about 4 cloves)
- 1 teaspoon dried oregano
- ½ teaspoon dried rosemary
- ½ teaspoon salt
- ¼ teaspoon freshly ground black pepper
- 1 tablespoon balsamic vinegar

DIRECTIONS

1. Preheat the oven to 400°F. Line a rimmed baking sheet with parchment paper. Trim and halve the Brussels sprouts. Transfer to a large bowl. Toss with the olive oil, garlic, oregano, rosemary, salt, and pepper to coat well.
2. Transfer to the prepared baking sheet. Bake for 35 to 40 minutes, shaking the pan occasionally to help with even browning, until crisp on the outside and tender on the inside. Remove from the oven and transfer to a large bowl. Stir in the balsamic vinegar, coating well.
3. Divide the Brussels sprouts evenly among 4 single-serving containers. Let cool before sealing the lids.

NUTRITION: Calories: 77, Fat: 3g, Protein: 4g, Carbs: 12g

---

416. BASIC BAKED POTATOES

COOKING: 60' | **PREPARATION: 5'** | **SERVES: 5**

INGREDIENTS

- 5 medium Russet potatoes or a variety of potatoes, washed and patted dry
- 1 to 2 tablespoons extra-virgin olive oil
- ¼ teaspoon salt
- ¼ teaspoon freshly ground black pepper

DIRECTIONS

1. Preheat the oven to 400°F. Pierce each potato several times with a fork or a knife. Brush the olive oil over the potatoes, then rub each with a pinch of the salt and a pinch of the pepper.
2. Place the potatoes on a baking sheet and bake for 50 to 60 minutes, until tender. Place the potatoes on a baking rack and cool completely. Transfer to an airtight container or 5 single-serving containers. Let cool before sealing the lids.

NUTRITION: Calories: 171, Fat: 3g, Protein: 4g, Carbs: 34g

THE PLANT BASED DIET COOKBOOK

417. MISO SPAGHETTI SQUASH

COOKING: 40' — **PREPARATION: 5'** — **SERVES: 5**

INGREDIENTS

- 1 (3-pound) spaghetti squash
- 1 tablespoon hot water
- 1 tablespoon unseasoned rice vinegar
- 1 tablespoon white miso

DIRECTIONS

1. Preheat the oven to 400°F. Line a rimmed baking sheet with parchment paper. Halve the squash lengthwise and place, cut-side down, on the prepared baking sheet.
2. Bake for 35 to 40 minutes, until tender. Cool until the squash is easy to handle. With a fork, scrape out the flesh, which will be stringy, like spaghetti. Transfer to a large bowl. In a small bowl, combine the hot water, vinegar, and miso with a whisk or fork. Pour over the squash. Gently toss with tongs to coat the squash. Divide the squash evenly among 4 single-serving containers. Let cool before sealing the lids.

NUTRITION: Calories: 117, Fat: 2g, Protein: 3g, Carbs: 25g,

418. GARLIC AND HERB NOODLES

COOKING: 10' — **PREPARATION: 40'** — **SERVES: 4**

INGREDIENTS

- 1 teaspoon extra-virgin olive oil or 2 tablespoons vegetable broth
- 1 teaspoon minced garlic (about 1 clove)
- 4 medium zucchini, spiral
- ½ teaspoon dried basil
- ½ teaspoon dried oregano
- ¼ to ½ teaspoon red pepper flakes, to taste
- ¼ teaspoon salt (optional)
- ¼ teaspoon freshly ground black pepper

DIRECTIONS

1. In a large skillet over medium-high heat, heat the olive oil.
2. Add the garlic, zucchini, basil, oregano, red pepper flakes, salt (if using), and black pepper. Sauté for 1 to 2 minutes, until barely tender. Divide the noodles evenly among 4 storage containers. Let cool before sealing the lids.

NUTRITION: Calories: 44, Fat: 2g, Protein: 3g, Carbs: 7g

419. THAI ROASTED BROCCOLI

COOKING: 5' — **PREPARATION: 15'** — **SERVES: 4**

INGREDIENTS

- 1 head broccoli, cut into florets
- 2 tablespoons olive oil
- 1 tablespoon soy sauce or gluten-free tamari

DIRECTIONS

1. Preheat the oven to 425°F. Line a baking sheet with parchment paper. In a large bowl, combine the broccoli, oil, and soy sauce. Toss well to combine.
2. Spread the broccoli on the prepared baking sheet. Roast for 10 minutes.
3. Toss the broccoli with a spatula and roast for an additional 5 minutes, or until the florets' edges begin to brown.
4. Toss the broccoli with a spatula and roast for an additional 5 minutes, or until the florets' edges begin to brown.

NUTRITION: Calories: 44, Fat: 2g, Protein: 3g, Carbs: 7g

420. COCONUT CURRY NOODLE

COOKING: 30'   **PREPARATION: 10'**   **SERVES: 4**

INGREDIENTS

- ½ tablespoon oil
- 3 garlic cloves, minced
- 2 tablespoons lemongrass, minced
- 1 tablespoon fresh ginger, grated
- 2 tablespoons red curry paste
- 1 (14 oz) can coconut milk
- 1 tablespoon brown sugar
- 2 tablespoons soy sauce
- 2 tablespoons fresh lime juice
- 1 tablespoon hot chili paste
- 12 oz. linguine
- 2 cups broccoli florets
- 1 cup carrots, shredded
- 1 cup edamame, shelled
- 1 red bell pepper, sliced

DIRECTIONS

1. Fill a suitably-sized pot with salted water and boil it on high heat.
2. Add pasta to the boiling water and cook until it is al dente then rinse under cold water.
3. Now place a medium-sized saucepan over medium heat and add oil.
4. Stir in ginger, garlic, and lemongrass, then sauté for 30 seconds.
5. Add coconut milk, soy sauce, curry paste, brown sugar, chili paste, and lime juice.
6. Stir this curry mixture for 10 minutes, or until it thickens.
7. Toss in carrots, broccoli, edamame, bell pepper, and cooked pasta.
8. Mix well, then serve warm.

NUTRITION: Calories: 44, Fat: 2g, Protein: 3g, Carbs: 7g

421. COLLARD GREEN PASTA

COOKING: 20'   **PREPARATION: 10'**   **SERVES: 4**

INGREDIENTS

- 2 tablespoons olive oil
- 4 garlic cloves, minced
- 8 oz. whole wheat pasta
- ½ cup panko bread crumbs
- 1 tablespoon nutritional yeast
- 1 teaspoon red pepper flakes
- 1 large bunch collard greens
- 1 large lemon, zest and juiced

DIRECTIONS

1. Fill a suitable pot with salted water and boil it on high heat.
2. Add pasta to the boiling water and cook until it is al dente, then rinse under cold water.
3. Reserve ½ cup of the cooking liquid from the pasta.
4. Place a non-stick pan over medium heat and add 1 tablespoon olive oil.
5. Stir in half of the garlic, then sauté for 30 seconds.
6. Add breadcrumbs and sauté for approximately 5 minutes.
7. Toss in red pepper flakes and nutritional yeast then mix well.
8. Transfer the breadcrumbs mixture to a plate and clean the pan.
9. Add the remaining tablespoon oil to the nonstick pan.
10. Stir in the garlic clove, salt, black pepper, and chard leaves.
11. Cook for 5 minutes until the leaves are wilted.
12. Add pasta along with the reserved pasta liquid.
13. Mix well, then add garlic crumbs, lemon juice, and zest.
14. Toss well, then serve warm.

NUTRITION: Calories: 245, Fat: 2.5g, Protein: 4g, Carbs: 12g

THE PLANT BASED DIET COOKBOOK

422. JALAPENO RICE NOODLES

COOKING: 25' **PREPARATION: 10'** **SERVES: 4**

INGREDIENTS

- ¼ cup soy sauce
- 1 tablespoon brown sugar
- 2 teaspoons sriracha
- 3 tablespoons lime juice
- 8 oz. rice noodles
- 3 teaspoons toasted sesame oil
- 1 package extra-firm tofu, pressed
- 1 onion, sliced
- 2 cups green cabbage, shredded
- 1 small jalapeno, minced
- 1 red bell pepper, sliced
- 1 yellow bell pepper, sliced
- 3 garlic cloves, minced
- 3 scallions, sliced
- 1 cup Thai basil leaves, roughly chopped
- Lime wedges for serving

DIRECTIONS

1. Fill a suitably-sized pot with salted water and boil it on high heat.
2. Add pasta to the boiling water and cook until it is al dente, then rinse under cold water.
3. Put lime juice, soy sauce, sriracha, and brown sugar in a bowl then mix well.
4. Place a large wok over medium heat then add 1 teaspoon sesame oil.
5. Toss in tofu and stir for 5 minutes until golden-brown.
6. Transfer the golden-brown tofu to a plate and add 2 teaspoons oil to the wok.
7. Stir in scallions, garlic, peppers, cabbage, and onion.
8. Sauté for 2 minutes, then add cooked noodles and prepared sauce.
9. Cook for 2 minutes, then garnish with lime wedges and basil leaves.
10. Serve fresh.

NUTRITION: Calories: 45, Fat: 2.5g, Protein: 4g, Carbs: 9g

423. RAINBOW SOBA NOODLES

COOKING: 20' **PREPARATION: 10'** **SERVES: 4**

INGREDIENTS

- 8 oz. tofu, pressed and crumbled
- 1 teaspoon olive oil
- ½ teaspoon red pepper flakes
- 10 oz. package buckwheat soba noodles, cooked
- 1 package broccoli slaw
- 2 cups cabbage, shredded
- ¼ cup very red onion, thinly sliced

Peanut Sauce

- ¼ cup peanut butter
- ¾ cup hot water
- 2 tablespoons apple cider vinegar
- 1 tablespoon maple syrup
- 1–2 garlic cloves, minced
- 1 lime, zest, and juice
- Salt and crushed red pepper flakes, to taste
- Cilantro, for garnish
- Crushed peanuts, for garnish

DIRECTIONS

1. Crumble tofu on a baking sheet and toss in 1 teaspoon oil and 1 teaspoon red pepper flakes.
2. Bake the tofu for 20 minutes at 400°F in a preheated oven.
3. Meanwhile, whisk peanut butter with hot water, garlic cloves, maple syrup, cider vinegar, lime zest, salt, lime juice, and pepper flakes in a large bowl.
4. Toss in cooked noodles, broccoli slaw, cabbages, and onion.
5. Mix well, then stir in tofu, cilantro, and peanuts. Enjoy.

NUTRITION: Calories: 45, Fat: 2.5g, Protein: 4g, Carbs: 9g

424. SPICY PAD THAI PASTA

COOKING: 10'   **PREPARATION: 10'**   **SERVES: 4**

INGREDIENTS

Spicy Tofu
- 1 lb extra-firm tofu, sliced
- 1 tablespoon peanut butter
- 3 tablespoons soy sauce
- 2 tablespoons Sriracha
- 2 tablespoons rice vinegar
- 2 teaspoons sesame oil
- 2 teaspoons ginger, grated

Pad Thai
- 8 oz. brown rice noodles
- 2 teaspoons coconut oil
- 1 red pepper, sliced
- ½ white onion, sliced
- 2 carrots, sliced
- 1 Thai chili, chopped
- ½ cup peanuts, chopped
- ½ cup cilantro, chopped

Spicy Pad Thai Sauce
- 3 tablespoons soy sauce
- 3 tablespoons fresh lime juice
- 1 tablespoon Sriracha
- 3 tablespoons brown sugar
- 3 tablespoons vegetable broth
- 1 teaspoon garlic-chili paste
- 2 garlic cloves, minced

DIRECTIONS

1. Fill a suitably-sized pot with water and soak rice noodles in it.
2. Press the tofu to squeeze excess liquid out of it.
3. Place a non-stick pan over medium-high heat and add tofu.
4. Sear the tofu for 2-3 minutes per side until brown.
5. Whisk all the ingredients for tofu crumbles in a large bowl.
6. Stir in tofu and mix well.
7. Separately mix the pad Thai sauce in a bowl and add to the tofu.
8. Place a wok over medium heat and add 1 teaspoon oil.
9. Toss in chili, carrots, onion, and red pepper, then sauté for 3 minutes.
10. Transfer the veggies to the tofu bowl.
11. Add more oil to the same pan and stir in drained noodles, then stir cook for 1 minute.
12. Transfer the noodles to the tofu and toss it all well.
13. Add cilantro and peanuts.
14. Serve fresh.

NUTRITION: Calories: 45, Fat: 2.5g, Protein: 4g, Carbs: 9g

425. LINGUINE WITH WINE SAUCE

COOKING: 18'   **PREPARATION: 10'**   **SERVES: 4**

INGREDIENTS

- 1 tablespoon olive oil
- 5 garlic cloves, minced
- 16 oz. shiitake, chopped
- ¼ teaspoon salt
- ¼ teaspoon ground pepper
- 1 pinch red pepper flakes
- ½ cup dry white wine
- 12 oz. linguine
- 2 teaspoons vegan butter
- ¼ cup Italian parsley, finely chopped

DIRECTIONS

1. Fill a suitably-sized pot with salted water and bring it to a boil on high heat.
2. Add pasta to the boiling water then cook until it is al dente, then rinse under cold water.
3. Place a non-stick skillet over medium-high heat then add olive oil.
4. Stir in garlic and sauté for 1 minute.
5. Stir in mushrooms and cook for 10 minutes.
6. Add salt, red pepper flakes, and black pepper for seasoning.
7. Toss in the cooked pasta and mix well.
8. Garnish with parsley and butter. Enjoy.

NUTRITION: Calories: 240 Fat: 2.0g Protein: 5g Carbs: 12g

THE PLANT BASED DIET COOKBOOK

426. CHEESY MACARONI WITH BROCCOLI

COOKING: 25' **PREPARATION: 10'** **SERVES: 6**

INGREDIENTS

- 1/3 cup melted coconut oil
- ¼ cup nutritional yeast
- 1 tablespoon tomato paste
- 1 tablespoon dried mustard
- 2 garlic cloves, minced
- 1 ½ teaspoons salt
- ½ teaspoon ground turmeric
- 4 ½ cups almond milk
- 3 cups cauliflower florets, chopped
- 1 cup raw cashews, chopped
- 1 lb shell pasta
- 1 tablespoon white vinegar
- 3 cups broccoli florets

DIRECTIONS

1. Place a suitably-sized saucepan over medium heat and add coconut oil.
2. Stir in mustard, yeast, garlic, salt, tomato paste, and turmeric.
3. Cook for 1 minute then add almond milk, cashews, and cauliflower florets.
4. Continue cooking for 20 minutes on a simmer.
5. Transfer the cauliflower mixture to a blender jug then blend until smooth.
6. Stir in vinegar and blend until creamy.
7. Fill a suitably-sized pot with salted water and bring it to a boil on high heat.
8. Add pasta to the boiling water.
9. Place a steamer basket over the boiling water and add broccoli to the basket.
10. Cook until the pasta is al dente. Drain and rinse the pasta and transfer the broccoli to a bowl.
11. Add the cooked pasta to the cauliflower-cashews sauce.
12. Toss in broccoli florets, salt, and black pepper. Mix well then serve.

NUTRITION: Calories: 40 Fat: 2.0g Protein: 5g Carbs: 7g Sodium: 18mg

427. SOBA NOODLES WITH TOFU

COOKING: 38' **PREPARATION: 10'** **SERVES: 4**

INGREDIENTS

Marinated Tofu
- 2 tablespoons olive oil
- 8 oz. firm tofu, pressed and drained
- ¼ cup cilantro, finely chopped
- ¼ cup mint, finely chopped
- 1-inch fresh ginger, grated

Soba Noodles
- 8 oz. soba noodles
- ¾ cup edamame
- 2 cucumbers, peeled and julienned
- 1 large carrot, peeled and julienned
- 2 tablespoons black sesame seeds
- 2 tablespoons white sesame seeds
- 2 scallions, chopped

Ginger-Soy Sauce
- 2 tablespoons fresh lime juice
- 2 tablespoons soy sauce
- 1 tablespoon brown sugar
- 1 tablespoon fresh ginger, grated
- 2 tablespoons sesame oil
- ½ tablespoon garlic chili sauce

DIRECTIONS

1. Blend herbs, ginger, salt, black pepper, and olive oil in a blender.
2. Add the spice mixture to the tofu and toss it well to coat.
3. Allow the tofu to marinate for 30 minutes at room temperature.
4. Fill a suitably-sized pot with salted water and bring it to a boil on high heat.
5. Add pasta to the boiling water then cook until it is al dente, then rinse under cold water.
6. Place a large wok over medium heat and add marinated tofu.
7. Sauté for 5–8 minutes until golden-brown, then transfer to a large bowl.
8. Add veggies to the same wok and stir until veggies are soft.
9. Transfer the veggies to the tofu and add cooked noodles.
10. Toss well, then serve warm. Enjoy!

NUTRITION: Calories: 30 Fat: 3.5.0g Protein: 6g Carbs: 6g Sodium: 18mg

428. PLANT BASED KETO LO MEIN

COOKING: 10' **PREPARATION: 10'** **SERVES: 2**

INGREDIENTS

- 2 tablespoons carrots, shredded
- 1 package kelp noodles, soaked in water
- 1 cup broccoli, frozen
- For the Sauce
- 1 tablespoon sesame oil
- 2 tablespoons tamari
- ½ teaspoon ground ginger
- ¼ teaspoon Sriracha
- ½ teaspoon garlic powder

DIRECTIONS

1. Put the broccoli in a saucepan on medium low heat and add the sauce ingredients.
2. Cook for about 5 minutes and add the noodles after draining water.
3. Allow to simmer about 10 minutes, occasionally stirring to avoid burning.
4. When the noodles have softened, mix everything well and dish out to serve.

NUTRITION: Calories: 30 Fat: 3.5.0g Protein: 6g Carbs: 6g

429. VEGETARIAN CHOW MEIN

COOKING: 30' **PREPARATION: 20'** **SERVES: 4**

INGREDIENTS

- ½ large onion, chopped
- ½ small leek, chopped
- ½ tablespoon ginger paste
- ½ tablespoon Worcester sauce
- ½ tablespoon Oriental seasoning
- ½ teaspoon parsley
- Salt and black pepper, to taste
- ½ pound noodles
- 2 large carrots, diced
- 2 celery sticks, chopped
- 1 tablespoon olive oil
- ½ teaspoon garlic paste
- 1½ tablespoons soy sauce
- 1 tablespoon Chinese five spice
- ½ teaspoon coriander
- 2 cups water

DIRECTIONS

1. Put olive oil, ginger, garlic paste, and onion in a pot on medium heat and sauté for about 5 minutes.
2. Stir in all the vegetables and cook for about 5 minutes.
3. Add rest of the ingredients and combine well.
4. Secure the lid and cook on medium heat for about 20 minutes, stirring occasionally.
5. Open the lid and dish out to serve hot.

NUTRITION: Calories: 30 Fat: 3.5.0g Protein: 6g Carbs: 6g

430. VEGGIE NOODLES

COOKING: 5'   **PREPARATION: 10'**   **SERVES: 2**

INGREDIENTS

- 2 tablespoons vegetable oil
- 4 spring onions, divided
- 1 cup snap pea
- 2 tablespoons brown sugar
- 9 oz. dried rice noodles, cooked
- 5 garlic cloves, minced
- 2 carrots, cut into small sticks
- 3 tablespoons soy sauce

DIRECTIONS

1. Heat vegetable oil in a skillet over medium heat and add garlic and 3 spring onions.
2. Cook for about 3 minutes and add the carrots, peas, brown sugar and soy sauce.
3. Add rice noodles and cook for about 2 minutes.
4. Season with salt and black pepper and top with remaining spring onion to serve.

NUTRITION: Calories: 25 Fat: 2.0g Protein: 5.2g Carbs: 5.3g

431. MINUTES VEGETARIAN PASTA

COOKING: 16'   **PREPARATION: 5'**   **SERVES: 4**

INGREDIENTS

- 3 shallots, chopped
- ¼ teaspoon red pepper flakes
- ¼ cup vegan parmesan cheese
- 2 tablespoons olive oil
- 2 garlic cloves, minced
- 8-oz. spinach leaves
- 8-oz. linguine pasta
- 1 pinch salt
- 1 pinch black pepper

DIRECTIONS

1. Boil salted water in a large pot and add pasta.
2. Cook for about 6 minutes and drain the pasta in a colander.
3. Heat olive oil over medium heat in a large skillet and add the shallots.
4. Cook for about 5 minutes until soft and caramelized and stir in the spinach, garlic, red pepper flakes, salt and black pepper.
5. Cook for about 5 minutes and add pasta and 2 spoons of pasta water.
6. Stir in the parmesan cheese and dish out in a bowl to serve.

NUTRITION: Calories: 25 Fat: 2.0g Protein: 5.2g Carbs: 5.3g

432. ASIAN VEGGIE NOODLES

COOKING: 20' **PREPARATION: 10'** **SERVES: 4**

INGREDIENTS

- ½ cup peas
- 1 teaspoon rice vinegar
- 3 carrots, chopped
- 1 small packet vermicelli
- 3 tablespoons sesame oil
- 1 red pepper, chopped in small cubes
- 1 can baby corn
- 1 clove garlic, chopped
- 2 tablespoons soy sauce
- 1 teaspoon ginger powder
- ½ teaspoon curry powder
- Salt and black pepper, to taste

DIRECTIONS

1. Take a bowl and add ginger powder, vinegar, soy sauce, curry powder, and a pinch of salt to it.
2. Cook the noodles according to the instructions and drain them.
3. Heat the sesame oil and cook vegetables in it for 10 minutes on medium heat.
4. Add noodles to it and cook for 3 more minutes.
5. Remove from heat and serve to enjoy.

NUTRITION: Calories: 25 Fat: 2.0g Protein: 5.2g Carbs: 5.3g

433. CAULIFLOWER LATKE

COOKING: 30' **PREPARATION: 15'** **SERVES: 4**

INGREDIENTS

- 12 oz. cauliflower rice, cooked
- 1 egg, beaten
- 1/3 cup cornstarch
- Salt and pepper to taste
- ¼ cup vegetable oil, divided
- Chopped onion chives

DIRECTIONS

1. Squeeze excess water from the cauliflower rice using paper towels.
2. Place the cauliflower rice in a bowl.
3. Stir in the egg and cornstarch.
4. Season with salt and pepper.
5. Fill 2 tablespoons of oil into a pan over medium heat.
6. Add 2 to 3 tablespoons of the cauliflower mixture into the pan.
7. Cook for 3 minutes each side.
8. Repeat until you've used up the rest of the batter.
9. Garnish with chopped chives.

NUTRITION: Calories: 209 Fat: 3.9g Carbs: 7g Protein: 3.4g

434. ROASTED BRUSSELS SPROUTS

COOKING: 20'   **PREPARATION: 30'**   **SERVES: 4**

INGREDIENTS

- 1 lb. Brussels sprouts, sliced in half
- 1 shallot, chopped
- 1 tablespoon olive oil
- Salt and pepper to taste
- 2 teaspoons balsamic vinegar
- ¼ cup pomegranate seeds
- ¼ cup goat cheese, crumbled

DIRECTIONS

1. Preheat your oven to 400°F.
2. Coat the Brussels sprouts with oil.
3. Sprinkle with salt and pepper.
4. Transfer to a baking pan.
5. Roast in the oven for 20 minutes.
6. Drizzle with the vinegar.
7. Sprinkle with the seeds and cheese before serving.

NUTRITION: Calories: 117 Fat: 6.8g Carbs: 5g Protein: 5.8g

435. BRUSSELS SPROUTS & CRANBERRIES

COOKING: 0'   **PREPARATION: 10'**   **SERVES: 6**

INGREDIENTS

- 3 tablespoons lemon juice
- ¼ cup olive oil
- Salt and pepper to taste
- 1 lb. Brussels sprouts, sliced thinly
- ¼ cup dried cranberries, chopped
- ½ cup pecans, toasted and chopped
- ½ cup Parmesan cheese, shaved

DIRECTIONS

1. Mix the lemon juice, olive oil, salt and pepper in a bowl.
2. Toss the Brussels sprouts, cranberries and pecans in this mixture.
3. Sprinkle the Parmesan cheese on top.

NUTRITION: Calories: 245 Fat: 7.8g Carbs: 8.9 Protein: 6.4g

436. POTATO LATKE

COOKING: 10'   **PREPARATION: 15'**   **SERVES: 6**

INGREDIENTS

- 3 eggs, beaten
- 1 onion, grated
- 1 ½ teaspoons baking powder
- Salt and pepper to taste
- 2 lb. potatoes, peeled and grated
- ¼ cup all-purpose flour
- 4 tablespoons vegetable oil
- Chopped onion chives

DIRECTIONS

1. Prep your oven to 400°F.
2. Scourge eggs, onion, baking powder, salt and pepper.
3. Squeeze moisture from the shredded potatoes using paper towel.
4. Add potatoes to the egg mixture.
5. Stir in the flour.
6. Fill oil into a pan over medium heat.
7. Cook a small amount of the batter for 3 to 4 minutes per side.
8. Repeat. Garnish with the chives.

NUTRITION: Calories: 266 Fat: 15.1g Carbs: 34.6g Protein: 7.6g

437. BROCCOLI RABE

COOKING: 15'   **PREPARATION: 15'**   **SERVES: 8**

INGREDIENTS

- 2 oranges, sliced in half
- 1 lb. broccoli rabe
- 2 tablespoons sesame oil, toasted
- Salt and pepper to taste
- 1 tablespoon sesame seeds, toasted

DIRECTIONS

1. Fill oil into a pan over medium heat.
2. Add the oranges and cook until caramelized.
3. Transfer to a plate.
4. Put the broccoli in the pan and cook for 8 minutes.
5. Squeeze the oranges to release juice in a bowl.
6. Stir in the oil, salt and pepper.
7. Coat the broccoli rabe with the mixture.
8. Sprinkle seeds on top.

NUTRITION: Calories: 59 Carbs: 4.1g Fat: 1.5g Protein: 2.2g

---

438. WHIPPED POTATOES

COOKING: 35'   **PREPARATION: 20'**   **SERVES: 10**

INGREDIENTS

- 4 cups water
- 3 lb. potatoes, sliced into cubes
- 3 cloves garlic, crushed
- 6 tablespoons butter
- 2 bay leaves
- 10 sage leaves
- ½ cup Greek yogurt
- ¼ cup low-Fat: milk

DIRECTIONS

1. Cook potatoes in water for 30 minutes. Drain.
2. Cook garlic in butter for 1 minute over medium heat.
3. Add the sage and cook for 5 more minutes. Discard the garlic.
4. Use a fork to mash the potatoes.
5. Whip using an electric mixer while gradually adding the butter, yogurt, and milk.
6. Season with salt.

NUTRITION: Calories: 169 Fat: 17.2g Carbs: 22g Protein: 4.2g

---

439. QUINOA AVOCADO SALAD

COOKING: 15'   **PREPARATION: 15'**   **SERVES: 6**

INGREDIENTS

- 2 tablespoons balsamic vinegar
- ¼ cup cream
- ¼ cup buttermilk
- 5 tablespoons lemon juice
- 1 clove garlic, grated
- 2 tablespoons shallot, minced
- Salt and pepper to taste
- 2 tablespoons avocado oil, divided
- 1 ¼ cups quinoa, cooked
- 2 heads endive, sliced
- 2 firm pears, sliced thinly
- 2 avocados, sliced
- ¼ cup fresh dill, chopped

DIRECTIONS

1. Combine the vinegar, cream, milk, 1 tablespoon lemon juice, garlic, shallot, salt and pepper in a bowl.
2. Pour 1 tablespoon oil into a pan over medium heat.
3. Heat the quinoa for 4 minutes.
4. Transfer quinoa to a plate.
5. Toss the endive and pears in a mixture of remaining oil, remaining lemon juice, salt and pepper.
6. Transfer to a plate.
7. Toss the avocado in the reserved dressing.
8. Add to the plate.
9. Top with the dill and quinoa.

NUTRITION: Calories: 431 Fat: 6g Carb: 18g Protein: 6.6g

THE PLANT BASED DIET COOKBOOK

440. ROASTED SWEET POTATOES

COOKING: 20' | **PREPARATION: 20'** | **SERVES: 4**

INGREDIENTS

- 2 potatoes, sliced into wedges
- 2 tablespoons olive oil, divided
- Salt and pepper to taste
- 1 red bell pepper, chopped
- ¼ cup fresh cilantro, chopped
- 1 garlic, minced
- 2 tablespoons almonds, toasted and sliced
- 1 tablespoon lime juice

DIRECTIONS

1. Preheat your oven to 425°F.
2. Toss the sweet potatoes in oil and salt.
3. Transfer to a baking pan.
4. Roast for 20 minutes.
5. In a bowl, combine the red bell pepper, cilantro, garlic and almonds.
6. In another bowl, mix the lime juice, remaining oil, salt and pepper.
7. Drizzle this mixture over the red bell pepper mixture.
8. Serve sweet potatoes with the red bell pepper mixture.

NUTRITION: Calories: 146 Fat: 9.9g Carbs: 19g Protein: 2.3g

441. CAULIFLOWER SALAD

COOKING: 15' | **PREPARATION: 20'** | **SERVES: 4**

INGREDIENTS

- 8 cups cauliflower florets
- 5 tablespoons olive oil, divided
- Salt and pepper to taste
- 1 cup parsley
- 1 clove garlic, minced
- 2 tablespoons lemon juice
- ¼ cup almonds, toasted and sliced
- 3 cups arugula
- 2 tablespoons olives, sliced
- ¼ cup feta, crumbled

DIRECTIONS

1. Preheat your oven to 425°F.
2. Toss the cauliflower in a mixture of 1 tablespoon olive oil, salt and pepper.
3. Place in a baking pan and roast for 15 minutes.
4. Put the parsley, remaining oil, garlic, lemon juice, salt and pepper in a blender.
5. Pulse until smooth.
6. Place the roasted cauliflower in a salad bowl.
7. Stir in the rest of the ingredients along with the parsley dressing.

NUTRITION: Calories: 198 Fiber: 4.1g Carbs: 14g Protein: 5.4g

442. GARLIC MASHED POTATOES & TURNIPS

COOKING: 30' | **PREPARATION: 20'** | **SERVES: 8**

INGREDIENTS

- 1 head garlic
- 1 teaspoon olive oil
- 1 lb. turnips, sliced into cubes
- 2 lb. potatoes, sliced into cubes
- ½ cup almond milk
- ½ cup Parmesan cheese, grated
- 1 tablespoon fresh thyme, chopped
- 1 tablespoon fresh chives, chopped
- 2 tablespoons butter

DIRECTIONS

1. Preheat your oven to 375°F.
2. Slice the tip off the garlic head.
3. Dash little oil and roast in the oven for 45 minutes.
4. Boil the turnips and potatoes in a pot of water for 30 minutes or until tender.
5. Incorporate all the ingredients to a food processor along with the garlic.
6. Pulse until smooth.

NUTRITION: Calories: 141 Fat: 12.1g Carbs: 18g Protein: 4.6g

443. GREEN BEANS

COOKING: 20' **PREPARATION: 15'** **SERVES: 8**

INGREDIENTS

- 1 shallot, chopped
- 24 oz. green beans
- Salt and pepper to taste
- ½ teaspoon smoked paprika
- 1 teaspoon lemon juice
- 2 teaspoons vinegar

DIRECTIONS

1. Preheat your oven to 450°F.
2. Stir in the shallot and beans.
3. Season with salt, pepper and paprika.
4. Roast for 10 minutes.
5. Drizzle with the lemon juice and vinegar.
6. Roast for another 2 minutes.

NUTRITION: Calories: 49 Fiber: 3g Carbs: 5g Protein: 2.9g

444. COCONUT BRUSSELS SPROUTS

COOKING: 10' **PREPARATION: 15'** **SERVES: 4**

INGREDIENTS

- 1 lb. Brussels sprouts, trimmed and sliced in half
- 2 tablespoons coconut oil
- ¼ cup coconut water
- 1 tablespoon soy sauce

DIRECTIONS

1. In skillet over medium heat, stir the coconut oil and cook the Brussels sprouts for 4 minutes.
2. Pour in the coconut water.
3. Cook for 3 minutes.
4. Add the soy sauce and cook for another 1 minute.

NUTRITION: Calories: 114 Fat: 6g Carbs: 6g Protein: 4g

445. CREAMY POLENTA

COOKING: 45' **PREPARATION: 5'** **SERVES: 8**

INGREDIENTS

- 1 1/3 cup cornmeal
- 6 cups water
- Salt to taste

DIRECTIONS

1. Incorporate all the ingredients in a pan over medium high heat.
2. Boil and then simmer for 5 minutes.
3. Reduce the heat to low.
4. Stir until creamy for 45 minutes.
5. Let sit before serving.

NUTRITION: Calories: 74 Fat: 9g Carbs: 30g Protein: 1.6g

THE PLANT BASED DIET COOKBOOK

446. SKILLET QUINOA

COOKING: 25'   **PREPARATION: 20'**   **SERVES: 4**

INGREDIENTS

- 1 cup sweet potato, cubed
- ½ cup water
- 1 tablespoon olive oil
- 1 onion, chopped
- 3 cloves garlic, minced
- 1 teaspoon ground cumin
- 1 teaspoon ground coriander
- ½ teaspoon chili powder
- ½ teaspoon dried oregano
- 15 oz. black beans, rinsed and drained
- 15 oz. roasted tomatoes
- 1 ¼ cups vegetable broth
- 1 cup frozen corn
- 1 cup quinoa (uncooked)
- Salt to taste
- ½ cup light sour cream
- ½ cup fresh cilantro leaves

DIRECTIONS

1. Add the water and sweet potato in a pan over medium heat.
2. Bring to a boil.
3. Decrease heat and cook sweet potatoes.
4. Add the oil and onion.
5. Cook for 3 minutes.
6. Cook garlic and spices for 1 minute.
7. Incorporate rest of the ingredients except the sour cream and cilantro.
8. Cook for 20 minutes.
9. Serve with sour cream and top with the cilantro before serving.

NUTRITION: Calories: 421 Fat: 12g Carbs: 28g Protein: 16g

447. GREEN BEANS WITH BALSAMIC SAUCE

COOKING: 15'   **PREPARATION: 10'**   **SERVES: 6**

INGREDIENTS

- 2 shallots, sliced
- 8 cups green beans, trimmed
- 2 tablespoons olive oil
- Salt and pepper to taste
- 2 tablespoons balsamic vinegar
- ¼ cup Parmesan cheese, grated

DIRECTIONS

1. Preheat your oven to 425°F.
2. Line your baking with foil.
3. In the pan, toss the shallots and beans in oil, salt and pepper.
4. Roast in the oven for 15 minutes.
5. Drizzle with the vinegar and top with cheese.

NUTRITION: Calories: 78 Fat: 4g Carbs: 6g Protein: 1.9g

448. GREEN BEANS GREMOLATA

COOKING: 5'   **PREPARATION: 15'**   **SERVES: 6**

INGREDIENTS

- 1-pound fresh green beans
- 3 garlic cloves, minced
- Zest of 2 oranges
- 3 tablespoons minced fresh parsley
- 2 tablespoons pine nuts
- 3 tablespoons olive oil
- Sea salt
- Freshly ground black pepper

DIRECTIONS

1. Boil water over high heat. Cook green beans for 3 minutes. Drain r and rinse with cold water to stop the cooking.
2. Blend garlic, orange zest, and parsley.
3. In a huge sauté pan over medium-high heat, toast the pine nuts in the dry, hot pan for 3 minutes. Remove from the pan and set aside.
4. Cook olive oil in the same pan until it shimmers. Add the beans and cook, stirring frequently, until heated through, about 2 minutes. Take pan away from the heat and add the parsley mixture and pine nuts. Season with salt and pepper. Serve immediately.

NUTRITION: Calories: 98 Fat: 9g Carbs: 7g Protein 3g

449. MINTED PEAS

COOKING: 5' — **PREPARATION: 5'** — **SERVES: 4**

INGREDIENTS

- 1 tablespoon olive oil
- 4 cups peas, fresh or frozen (not canned)
- ½ teaspoon sea salt
- Freshly ground black pepper
- 3 tablespoons chopped fresh mint

DIRECTIONS

1. In a large sauté pan, cook olive oil over medium-high heat until hot. Add the peas and cook, about 5 minutes. Remove the pan from heat. Stir in the salt, season with pepper, and stir in the mint. Serve hot.

NUTRITION: Calories: 90 Fat: 3g Carbs: 1.8g Protein: 8g

450. SWEET AND SPICY BRUSSELS SPROUT HASH

COOKING: 15' — **PREPARATION: 10'** — **SERVES: 4**

INGREDIENTS

- 3 tablespoons olive oil
- 2 shallots, thinly sliced
- 1½ lb. Brussel sprouts
- 3 tablespoons apple cider vinegar
- 1 tablespoon pure maple syrup
- ½ teaspoon sriracha sauce (or to taste)
- Sea salt
- Freshly ground black pepper

DIRECTIONS

1. In pan, cook olive oil over medium-high heat until it shimmers. Mix the shallots and Brussels sprouts and cook, stirring frequently, until the vegetables soften and begin to turn golden brown, about 10 minutes. Stir in the vinegar, using a spoon to scrape any browned bits from the pan's bottom. Stir in the maple syrup and Sriracha.
2. Simmer, stirring frequently, until the liquid reduces, 3 to 5 minutes. Season and serve immediately.

NUTRITION: Calories: 97 Fat: 4g Carbs: 7g Protein: 7g

451. GLAZED CURRIED CARROTS

COOKING: 15' — **PREPARATION: 5'** — **SERVES: 6**

INGREDIENTS

- 1-pound carrots
- 2 tablespoons olive oil
- 2 tablespoons curry powder
- 2 tablespoons pure maple syrup
- Juice of ½ lemon

DIRECTIONS

1. Cook carrots with water over medium-high heat for 10 minutes. Drain and return them to the pan over medium-low heat.
2. Stir in the olive oil, curry powder, maple syrup, and lemon juice. Cook, stirring constantly, until the liquid reduces, about 5 minutes. Season well and serve immediately.

NUTRITION: Calories: 91 Fat: 5g Carbs: 7g Protein: 9g

452. PEPPER MEDLEY

COOKING: 15' **PREPARATION: 10'** **SERVES: 4**

INGREDIENTS

- 3 tablespoons olive oil
- 1 red bell pepper, sliced
- 1 orange bell pepper, sliced
- 1 yellow bell pepper, sliced
- 1 green bell pepper, sliced
- 2 garlic cloves, minced
- 3 tablespoons red wine vinegar
- 2 tablespoons chopped fresh basil

DIRECTIONS

1. Warm up olive oil over medium-high heat. Stir in the bell peppers and cook, stir, for 7 to 10 minutes. Cook garlic for 30 seconds. Add the vinegar, using a spoon to scrape any browned bits off the bottom of the pan.
2. Simmer until the vinegar reduces, 2 to 3 minutes. Season. Stir in the basil and serve immediately.

NUTRITION: Calories: 96 Fat: 7g Carbs: 9g Protein: 5g

453. GARLICKY RED WINE MUSHROOMS

COOKING: 15' **PREPARATION: 10'** **SERVES: 4**

INGREDIENTS

- 3 tablespoons olive oil
- 2 cups sliced mushrooms
- 3 garlic cloves, minced
- ½ cup red wine
- 1 tablespoon dried thyme

DIRECTIONS

1. Cook olive oil over medium-high heat until it shimmers. Mix in the mushrooms and sit, untouched, until they release their liquid and begin to brown, about 5 minutes. Stir the mushrooms occasionally, cooking until softened and golden brown, about 5 minutes more. Cook garlic. Add the red wine and thyme, using a wooden spoon to scrape any browned bits off the pan's bottom.
2. Adjust heat to medium. Cook for 5 minutes. Season well and serve.

NUTRITION: Calories: 98 Fat: 4g Carbs: 3g Protein: 6g

454. SAUTÉED CITRUS SPINACH

COOKING: 10' **PREPARATION: 10'** **SERVES: 4**

INGREDIENTS

- 2 tablespoons olive oil
- 1 shallot, chopped
- 2 garlic cloves, minced
- 10 oz. baby spinach
- Zest and juice of 1 orange

DIRECTIONS

1. Cook olive oil over medium-high heat. Cook the shallot for 3 minutes. Cook garlic for 30 seconds.
2. Add the spinach, orange juice, and orange zest. Cook for 2 minutes. Season with salt and pepper. Serve warm.

NUTRITION: Calories: 91 Fat: 4g Carbs: 8g Protein: 7g

455. LEMON BROCCOLI RABE

COOKING: 10'   **PREPARATION: 10'**   **SERVES: 4**

INGREDIENTS

- 8 cups water
- Sea salt
- 2 bunches broccoli rabe, chopped
- 3 tablespoons olive oil
- 3 garlic cloves, minced
- Pinch of cayenne pepper
- Zest of 1 lemon

DIRECTIONS

1. Boil 8 cups of the water. Sprinkle a pinch of salt and the broccoli rabe. Cook until the broccoli rabe is slightly softened, about 2 minutes. Drain.
2. Heat olive oil over medium-high heat. Cook the garlic for 30 seconds. Stir in the broccoli rabe, cayenne, and lemon zest. Season with salt and black pepper. Serve immediately.

NUTRITION: Calories: 99 Fat: 3g Carbs: 8g Protein: 11g

---

456. SPICY SWISS CHARD

COOKING: 10'   **PREPARATION: 10'**   **SERVES: 4**

INGREDIENTS

- 2 tablespoons olive oil
- 1 onion, chopped
- 2 bunches Swiss chard
- 3 garlic cloves, minced
- ½ teaspoon red pepper flakes (or to taste)
- Juice of ½ lemon

DIRECTIONS

1. In a big pot, cook olive oil over medium-high heat until it shimmers. Cook the onion and chard stems for 5 minutes.
2. Cook chard leaves for 1 minute. Stir in the garlic and pepper flakes. Cover and cook for 5 minutes. Stir in the lemon juice. Season with salt and serve immediately.

NUTRITION: Calories: 94 Fat: 5g Carbs: 5g Protein: 7g

---

457. RED PEPPERS AND KALE

COOKING: 15'   **PREPARATION: 5'**   **SERVES: 4**

INGREDIENTS

- 2 bunches kale
- 3 tablespoons olive oil
- ½ onion, chopped
- 2 red bell peppers, cut into strips
- 3 garlic cloves, minced
- ¼ teaspoon red pepper flakes

DIRECTIONS

1. In steamer basket in a pan, steam the kale until it softens, 5 to 10 minutes. Remove from the heat and set aside.
2. Meanwhile, in a sauté pan, heat the olive oil over medium-high heat until it shimmers. Cook onion and bell peppers for 5 minutes. Cook garlic for 30 seconds. Take out from heat and stir in the kale and red pepper flakes. Season and serve immediately.

NUTRITION: Calories: 101 Fat: 5g Carbs: 4g Protein: 10g

THE PLANT BASED DIET COOKBOOK

458. MASHED CAULIFLOWER WITH ROASTED GARLIC

COOKING: 10' **PREPARATION: 5'** **SERVES: 4**

INGREDIENTS

- 2 heads cauliflower, cut into small florets
- 1 tablespoon olive oil
- 8 jarred roasted garlic cloves
- 2 teaspoons chopped fresh rosemary
- Sea salt
- Freshly ground black pepper
- 1 tablespoon chopped fresh chives

DIRECTIONS

1. Boil cauliflower florets for 9 minutes, then drain.
2. In a blender or food processor, combine the cauliflower, olive oil, garlic, and rosemary and process until smooth. Season with salt and pepper. Stir in the chives and serve hot.

NUTRITION: Calories: 88 Fat: 4.2g Carbs: 7g Protein: 2g

459. STEAMED BROCCOLI WITH WALNUT PESTO

COOKING: 10' **PREPARATION: 5'** **SERVES: 4**

INGREDIENTS

- 1-pound broccoli florets
- 2 cups chopped fresh basil
- ¼ cup olive oil
- 4 garlic cloves
- ½ cup walnuts
- Pinch of cayenne pepper

DIRECTIONS

1. Put the broccoli in a large pot and cover with water. Bring to a simmer over medium-high heat and cook until the broccoli is tender, about 5 minutes.
2. Process basil, olive oil, garlic, walnuts, and cayenne for ten 1-second pulses, scraping down the bowl halfway through processing.
3. Drain and put again to the pan. Toss with the pesto. Serve immediately.

NUTRITION: Calories: 101 Fat: 4g Carbs: 8g Protein: 5g

460. ROASTED ASPARAGUS WITH BALSAMIC REDUCTION

COOKING: 25' **PREPARATION: 10'** **SERVES: 4**

INGREDIENTS

- 1½ lb. asparagus, trimmed
- 2 tablespoons olive oil
- ½ teaspoon sea salt
- ¼ teaspoon freshly ground black pepper
- 1/3 cup balsamic vinegar
- Juice and zest of 1 Meyer lemon

DIRECTIONS

1. Preheat the oven to 375°F. On a large rimmed baking sheet, throw the asparagus with the olive oil, salt, and pepper and then spread the asparagus out into a single layer. Roast for 23 minutes.
2. While roasting, put the vinegar in a small saucepan and bring it to a boil over medium-high heat. Decrease heat to low and simmer for 8 minutes.
3. When the asparagus is roasted, remove the baking sheet from the oven. Stir lemon juice and zest to coat. Drizzle the balsamic reduction over the top. Serve immediately.

NUTRITION: Calories: 104 Fat: 4g Carbs: 5g Protein: 8g

461. SWEET AND SOUR TEMPEH

COOKING: 10'   **PREPARATION: 8'**   **SERVES: 4**

INGREDIENTS

- 1 cup pineapple juice
- 1 tablespoon unseasoned rice vinegar
- 1 tablespoon soy sauce
- 1 tablespoon cornstarch
- 2 tablespoons coconut oil
- 1-pound tempeh, cut into thin strips
- 6 green onions
- 1 green bell pepper, diced
- 4 garlic cloves, minced
- 2 cups prepared brown or white rice

DIRECTIONS

1. Blend pineapple juice, rice vinegar, soy sauce, and cornstarch and set aside.
2. In a wok or large sauté pan, heat the coconut oil over medium-high heat until it shimmers. Add the tempeh, green onions, and bell pepper and cook until vegetables soften, about 5 minutes.
3. Cook garlic. Stir in sauce and cook until it thickens. Serve over rice.

NUTRITION: Calories: 95 Fat: 4g Carbs: 9g Protein: 5g

---

462. FRIED SEITAN FINGERS

COOKING: 10'   **PREPARATION: 15'**   **SERVES: 4**

INGREDIENTS

- 1 cup all-purpose flour
- 1 teaspoon garlic powder
- 1 teaspoon onion powder
- Pinch of cayenne pepper
- 1 teaspoon dried thyme
- ½ teaspoon sea salt
- ½ teaspoon freshly ground black pepper
- 1 cup soy milk
- 1 tablespoon lemon juice
- 2 tablespoons baking powder
- 2 tablespoons olive oil
- 8 oz. Seitan

DIRECTIONS

1. In a shallow dish, incorporate flour, garlic powder, onion powder, cayenne, thyme, salt, and black pepper, whisking to mix thoroughly. In another shallow dish, whisk together the soy milk, lemon juice, and baking powder.
2. In sauté pan, cook the olive oil over medium-high heat. Dip each piece of seitan in the flour mixture, tapping off any excess flour. Next, dip the seitan in the soy milk mixture and then back in the flour mixture.
3. Fry for 4 minutes per side. Blot on paper towels before serving.

NUTRITION: Calories: 100 Fat: 12g Carbs: 13g Protein: 8g

---

463. VEGETABLE PIE

COOKING: 40'   **PREPARATION: 10'**   **SERVES: 6-8**

INGREDIENTS

- 1 red pepper (you can make it green)
- 1 bunch parsley
- 1/2 grated carrot
- 6 mushrooms cut it into slices
- 6 eggs
- 1 tablespoon oil
- 1 teaspoon salt, one pepper and a small cup of bread crumbs

DIRECTIONS

1. First of all, put to heat the oven to 180°F.
2. You must cut everything in small squares (parsley) the carrot, the mushrooms cut in sheets ah, and use natural, but everything is to your liking you can use the pot.
3. Once you have everything cut, put a small piece of oil and put it in a pan to brown (all the vegetables).
4. Once the vegetables are golden brown, put the six eggs in a bowl, salt, pepper, and bread crumbs.
5. Put the vegetables in the mold (or muffin molds) to taste and the time of each one, pour the ingredients of the bowl and put it in the oven for 35 or 40 minutes.
6. Serve and enjoy.

NUTRITION: Calories: 127 Protein: 7.81g Fat: 9.74g Carbs: 1.77g

THE PLANT BASED DIET COOKBOOK

464. COLLARD GREEN WRAP

COOKING: 0'   **PREPARATION: 10'**   **SERVES: 4**

INGREDIENTS

- ½ block feta, cut into 4 (1-inch thick) strips (4-oz)
- ½ cup purple onion, diced
- ½ medium red bell pepper, julienned
- 1 medium cucumber, julienned
- 4 large cherry tomatoes, halved
- 4 large collard green leaves, washed
- 8 whole kalamata olives, halved
- For the Sauce:
- 1 cup low-Fat: plain Greek yogurt
- 1 tablespoon white vinegar
- 1 teaspoon garlic powder
- 2 tablespoons minced fresh dill
- 2 tablespoons olive oil
- 2.5-oz. cucumber, seeded and grated (¼-whole)
- Salt and pepper to taste

DIRECTIONS

1. Make the sauce first: make sure to squeeze out all the excess liquid from the cucumber after grating. In a small bowl, put all together the sauce ingredients and mix thoroughly then refrigerate.
2. Prepare and slice all wrap ingredients.
3. On a flat surface, spread one collard green leaf. Spread 2 tablespoons of Tzatziki sauce in the middle of the leaf.
4. Layer ¼ of each of the tomatoes, feta, olives, onion, pepper, and cucumber. Place them on the center of the leaf, like piling them high instead of spreading them.
5. Fold the leaf-like you would a burrito. Repeat process for remaining ingredients.
6. Serve and enjoy.

NUTRITION: Calories: 463 Fat: 31g Carbs: 31g Protein: 20g

---

465. ZUCCHINI GARLIC FRIES

COOKING: 20'   **PREPARATION: 10'**   **SERVES: 6**

INGREDIENTS

- ¼ teaspoon garlic powder
- ½ cup almond flour
- 2 large egg whites, beaten
- 3 medium zucchinis, sliced into fry sticks
- Salt and pepper to taste

DIRECTIONS

1. Set the oven to 400°F.
2. Mix all together the ingredients in a bowl until the zucchini fries are well coated.
3. Place fries on the cookie sheet and spread evenly.
4. Put in the oven and cook for 20 minutes.
5. Halfway through cooking time, stir-fries.

NUTRITION: Calories: 11 Fat: 0.1g, Carbs: 1g Protein 1.5g

---

466. MASHED CAULIFLOWER

COOKING: 10'   **PREPARATION: 10'**   **SERVES: 3**

INGREDIENTS

- 1 cauliflower head
- 1 tablespoon olive oil
- ½ tsp salt
- ¼ tsp dill
- Pepper to taste
- 2 tbsp. low-Fat: milk

DIRECTIONS

1. Place a small pot of water to a boil.
2. Chop cauliflower in florets.
3. Add florets to boiling water and boil uncovered for 5 minutes. Turn off fire and let it sit for 5 minutes more.
4. In a blender, add all ingredients except for cauliflower and blend to mix well.
5. Drain cauliflower well and add it to a blender. Puree until smooth and creamy.
6. Serve and enjoy.

NUTRITION: Calories: 78 Fat: 5g Carbs: 6g Protein: 2g

467. STIR-FRIED EGGPLANT

COOKING: 10'   **PREPARATION: 10'**   **SERVES: 2**

INGREDIENTS

- 1 tablespoon coconut oil
- 2 eggplants, sliced into 3-inch in length
- 4 cloves of garlic, minced
- 1 onion, chopped
- 1 teaspoon ginger, grated
- 1 teaspoon lemon juice, freshly squeezed
- ½ tsp salt
- ½ tsp pepper

DIRECTIONS

1. Heat oil in a nonstick saucepan.
2. Pan-fry the eggplants for 2 minutes on all sides.
3. Add the garlic and onions until fragrant, around 3 minutes.
4. Stir in the ginger, salt, pepper, and lemon juice.
5. Add a ½ cup of water and bring to a simmer. Cook until eggplant is tender.

NUTRITION: Calories: 232 Fat: 8g Carbs: 41g Protein: 7g

---

468. SAUTÉED GARLIC MUSHROOMS

COOKING: 10'   **PREPARATION: 10'**   **SERVES: 4**

INGREDIENTS

- 1 tablespoon olive oil
- 3 cloves of garlic, minced
- 16 oz. fresh brown mushrooms, sliced
- 7 oz. fresh shiitake mushrooms, sliced
- ½ tsp salt
- ½ tsp pepper or more to taste

DIRECTIONS

1. Place a nonstick saucepan on medium-high fire and heat pan for a minute.
2. Add oil and heat for 2 minutes.
3. Stir in garlic and sauté for a minute.
4. Add remaining ingredients and stir fry until soft and tender, around 5 minutes.
5. Turn off fire, let mushrooms rest while the pan is covered for 5 minutes.
6. Serve and enjoy.

NUTRITION: Calories: 95 Fat: 4g Carbs: 14g Protein: 3g

---

469. STIR-FRIED ASPARAGUS AND BELL PEPPER

COOKING: 10'   **PREPARATION: 10'**   **SERVES: 6**

INGREDIENTS

- 1 tablespoon olive oil
- 4 cloves of garlic, minced
- 1-pound fresh asparagus spears, trimmed
- 2 large red bell peppers, seeded and julienned
- ½ teaspoon thyme
- 5 tablespoons water
- ½ tsp salt
- ½ tsp pepper or more to taste

DIRECTIONS

1. Place a nonstick saucepan on high fire and heat pan for a minute.
2. Add oil and heat for 2 minutes.
3. Stir in garlic and sauté for a minute.
4. Add remaining ingredients and stir fry until soft and tender, around 6 minutes.
5. Turn off fire, let veggies rest while the pan is covered for 5 minutes.

NUTRITION: Calories: 45 Fat: 2g Carbs: 5g Protein: 2g

THE PLANT BASED DIET COOKBOOK

470. WILD RICE WITH SPICY CHICKPEAS

COOKING: 60' **PREPARATION: 15'** **SERVES: 6-7**

INGREDIENTS

- 1 Cup basmati rice
- 1 Cup wild rice
- Salt & pepper to taste
- 4tbsp Olive oil
- 1tbsp Garlic powder
- 2tsp cumin powder
- ¼ Cup sunflower oil
- 3 Cups chickpeas
- 1tsp Flour
- 1tsp Curry powder
- 3tsp Paprika powder
- 1tsp Dill
- 3tbsp parsley (chopped)
- 1 Medium onion (thinly sliced)
- 2 Cups currants

DIRECTIONS

1. For cooking wild rice, fill the half pot with water and bring it to boil. Put the rice and let it simmer for at least 40 minutes.
2. Take olive in the pot and heat it on medium flame. Now add cumin powder, salt, and water and bring it to boil. Then add basmati rice and cook for 20 minutes.
3. Leave rice for cooking and prepare spicy chickpeas. Heat 2tbsp of olive oil in the pan and toss chickpeas, garlic powder, salt & pepper, cumin, and paprika powder in it.
4. In another pan, cook onion with sunflower oil until it is golden brown and add flour.
5. Mix flour and onion with your hands.
6. For serving, place both types of rice in a bowl with spicy chickpeas and fry the onion. Garnish it with parsley and herbs.

NUTRITION: Calories: 647 Protein: 25.43g Fat: 25.72g Carbs: 88.3g

471. CASHEW PESTO & PARSLEY WITH VEGGIES

COOKING: 10' **PREPARATION: 15'** **SERVES: 3-4**

INGREDIENTS

- 3 Zucchini (sliced)
- 8 Soaked bamboo skewers
- 2 Red capsicums
- ¼ Cup olive oil
- 750grams Eggplant
- 4 Lemon cheeks
- For Serving
- Couscous salad
- For Preparing Cashew Pesto
- ½ Cup cashew (roasted)
- ½ Cup parsley
- 2 Cup grated parmesan
- 2tbsp Lime juice
- ¼ Cup olive oil

DIRECTIONS

1. Toss capsicum, eggplant, and zucchini with oil and salt and thread it onto skewers.
2. Cook bamboo sticks for 6-8 minutes on a barbecue grill pan on medium heat.
3. Also, grill lemon cheeks from both sides.
4. For preparing cashew pesto, combine all ingredients in the food processor and blend.
5. For serving, place grill skewers in a plate with grill lemon slices and drizzle some cashew pesto over it.

NUTRITION: Calories: 666 Protein: 23.96g Fat: 48.04g Carbs: 41.4 g

472. SPICY CHICKPEAS WITH ROASTED VEGETABLES

COOKING: 25' **PREPARATION: 10'** **SERVES: 2-3**

INGREDIENTS

- 1 Large carrot (peeled)
- 2tbsp Sunflower oil
- 1 Cauliflower head
- 1tbsp ground cumin
- ½ Red onions (diced)
- 1 Red pepper (deseeded)
- 400g Can chickpeas

DIRECTIONS

1. Line a large baking tine in the preheated oven (at 240C).
2. Cut all the vegetables and toss with salt, pepper, and onion.
3. In a bowl, whisk olive oil, pepper, and cumin powder.
4. Add all veggies in the bowl and toss.
5. Transfer vegetables on baking tin and baked it almost for 15 minutes.
6. Now add chickpeas and stir.
7. Return to the oven and bake it for the next 10 minutes.
8. Serve it with toast bread.

NUTRITION: Calories: 348 Protein: 14.29g Fat: 15.88g Carbs: 40.65g

473. SPECIAL VEGETABLE KITCHREE

COOKING: 46' | **PREPARATION: 10'** | **SERVES: 5-6**

INGREDIENTS

- ½ Cup brown grain rice
- 1 Cup dry lentil or split peas
- 1tsp Sea salt, cumin powder, ground turmeric, ground fenugreek, and ground coriander
- 3tbsp Coconut oil
- 1tbsp Ginger
- 5 Cups vegetable stock
- 1 Cup baby spinach
- 1 Medium Zucchini (roughly chopped)
- 1 Small crown broccoli (chopped)
- Greek Yogurt (for serving)

DIRECTIONS

1. In a saucepan, warm the coconut oil on medium flame and add ginger, cumin, coriander, fennel seeds, fenugreek, and turmeric and cook it for 1 minute.
2. Now add lentils and brown rice in the spices and stir. Pour the vegetable stock in it and simmer for 40 minutes.
3. Add broccoli in the tender rice and lentils and cook for another 5 minutes. Now add other vegetables and stir for 10 minutes.
4. For serving, pour some Greek yogurt over vegetable kitcheree and serve hot.

NUTRITION: Calories: 1728 Protein: 4.13g Fat: 190.35g Carbs: 17.31g

474. MASHED SWEET POTATO BURRITOS

COOKING: 60' | **PREPARATION: 15'** | **SERVES: 4**

INGREDIENTS

- 4 Tortillas
- 1 Avocado
- 1tsp Capsicum, paprika powder, and oregano
- Salt & pepper as needed
- ½ Cup sour cream
- 1 Can diced tomato
- 2 Sweet Potatoes (mashed)
- 2 Garlic cloves (minced)
- 1tbsp Cumin powder
- Fresh cilantro or parsley

DIRECTIONS

1. Before mashing roast sweet potatoes for 45 minutes in an already preheated (320°F) oven.
2. Cook onion in a frying pan with oil on medium heat. Add garlic cloves and cook for 1 minute.
3. Add 1 tin of tomatoes and leave it to simmer for 10 minutes. In halfway through, add salt & pepper, paprika, cumin powder, and black beans.
4. After 5 minutes, add avocado in it.
5. Now make burritos, mix one scoop of mashed potatoes with avocado filling.
6. Wrap your tortilla and grill it in the oven at 400°F for 30seconds.
7. Serve it with sour cream and hot sauce.

NUTRITION: Calories: 442 Protein: 12.05g Fat: 15.43g Carbs: 66.85g

475. ZUCCHINI & PEPPER LASAGNA

COOKING: 60' | **PREPARATION: 10'** | **SERVES: 1**

INGREDIENTS

- ½ pack Soft Tofu
- ½ pack Firm Tofu
- ½ Box Wholegrain Lasagna Sheet
- 1 cup Baby spinach
- 1 cup Almond milk
- ¼ tsp. Garlic powder
- ½ cup Lemon Juice
- 1 ½ tbsp. Fresh basil, chopped
- 1 can Chopped Tomato
- Pinch ground black pepper
- 1 Zucchini, diced
- 1 Red pepper, diced (optional)

DIRECTIONS

1. Set the oven to 325°F.
2. In a blender, process the soft and firm tofu, garlic powder, almond milk, basil, lemon juice, and pepper until smooth.
3. Toss in the spinach and zucchini for the last 30 seconds.
4. Put about 1/3 of the chopped tomatoes at the bottom of an oven dish.
5. Top the sauce with 1/3 of the lasagna sheets and then 1/3 of the spinach/tofu mixture.
6. Repeat the layers finishing with the chopped tomatoes on top.
7. Cook for at least 1 hour, up to the pasta sheets are soft.
8. Serve with a lovely side salad and enjoy.

NUTRITION: Calories: 337 Protein: 19.17 g Fat: 15.29 g Carbs: 37.01 g

476. TOASTED CUMIN CRUNCH

COOKING: 1'   **PREPARATION: 10'**   **SERVES: 1**

INGREDIENTS

- 1 tbsp. Ground cumin seeds (Use pestle and mortar or Blender)
- 2 tbsp. Extra virgin olive oil
- 1 tsp. Crack black peppercorns
- ½ tsp. Cumin seeds, whole
- 1 tsp. Cilantro, finely chopped
- 1/2 Jalapeno, finely chopped
- 2 cups Green Cabbage, sliced
- 2 cups Carrots, grated
- ½ cup of Cilantro, chopped
- 3 tbsp. Lime Juice

DIRECTIONS

1. Get a large saucepan, and then heat the oil over medium heat.
2. Cook the peppercorns, coriander, and the whole cumin seeds for about a minute until browned.
3. Add in the jalapeno and then cook for another 45 seconds until tender.
4. Add in then the carrots and the cabbage, cooking for about 5 minutes or until the cabbage starts to soften.
5. Add in the crushed cumin seeds and cook for 30 seconds before taking off the heat and then stirring in the lime juice and the cilantro.
6. Serve warm.

NUTRITION: Calories: 377 Protein: 12.77 Fat: 20.54g Carbs: 41.82g

477. SPICY VEGETABLE BURGERS

COOKING: 15'   **PREPARATION: 2'**   **SERVES: 2**

INGREDIENTS

- 1 pack Extra firm tempeh
- 1 tsp. Red chili flakes
- 1 Red pepper, diced (optional)
- 1/2 Red Onion, diced
- 1/2 cup Baby spinach
- 1 tbsp. Olive Oil
- 2 100% Wholegrain Bun (optional)

DIRECTIONS

1. Heat the broiler on medium-high heat.
2. Marinate the tempeh in oil and red chilli flakes.
3. In a skillet, warm a little bit of oil on medium heat.
4. Sauté the onion in the skillet for 6-7 minutes or until caramelized.
5. Stir in the pepper and baby spinach for a further 3-4 minutes.
6. Broil the tempeh for around 4 minutes on each side.
7. Lay down the tempeh in the buns and then add the caramelized onion, spinach, and diced peppers.
8. Serve immediately while hot with a side of arugula.

NUTRITION: Calories: 833 Protein: 14.1g Fat: 54.47g Carbs: 73.01g

478. RATATOUILLE PASTA SHELLS

COOKING: 12' **PREPARATION: 30'** **SERVES: 4**

INGREDIENTS

- 16 Jumbo Pasta shells
- 1 tbsp. olive oil
- 1 tbsp. minced garlic
- ¾ cup onion, chopped
- 1.5 cups eggplant, diced
- 1 cup red bell pepper, diced
- ¾ cup zucchini, diced
- ¾ plum tomato, chopped
- ½ cup canned unsalted chickpeas
- 1.75 cups marinara sauce, low sodium
- 1 teaspoon ground black pepper
- ½ teaspoon kosher salt
- Cooking spray
- 4oz. shredded Italian 5-cheese blend

DIRECTIONS

1. Preheat the oven at 430°F
2. Boil water in a pot, cook pasta with no salt, drain
3. In a large skillet, heat oil over medium-high. Add garlic and onion; saute for 2 minutes.
4. Add bell pepper and eggplant. Cook for 4 minutes, stirring occasionally
5. Add chickpease, tomato and zucchini, cover pan and cook for 4 minutes
6. Remove skillet from heat, stir in ½ cup basil, salt, black pepper and 1 cup marinara
7. Spray a ceramic baking dish. Spread ¾ cup marinara over the dish. Stuff each pasta shell with ca 2 tbsp. vegetable mixture.
8. Lay filled shells in dish, sprinkle with cheese. Bake at 430°F for 12 minutes. Add basil at the end. Enjoy!

NUTRITION: Calories: 365 Protein: 14.6g Fat: 10.9g Carbs: 45g

479. LIGHT MUSHROOM RISOTTO

COOKING: 35' **PREPARATION: 10'** **SERVES: 4**

INGREDIENTS

- 18oz. medium potatoes
- 10oz. of mushrooms
- 8oz. of arborous rice or carnaroli
- 1 onion
- 1 clove garlic
- 1 l of vegetable broth
- 1 glass of white wine
- 2oz. of Parmesan cheese
- 4 tablespoons of olive oil
- A sprig of parsley
- Salt and pepper

DIRECTIONS

1. Heat the vegetable broth. Put the vegetable broth to heat. Wash the parsley, potatoes, dry it, reserve some whole leaves for decorating, and chopping the rest. Grate the Parmesan cheese.
2. Poach the garlic and onion. Peel and clean the garlic and onion and chop them. In a casserole with olive oil, beat them for about 5 minutes or so over low heat.
3. Skip the mushrooms. Meanwhile, clean the mushrooms. Leave a few whole pieces for decoration and the rest of the pieces in small pieces. Add them all to the casserole and sauté everything around five more minutes.
4. Incorporate the rice. Once you have sautéed the mushrooms with the onion and garlic, remove the ones that you had left whole and reserve them. Add the rice to the pan, arborous rice or carnaroli, and then sauté everything together for another 5 minutes, stirring constantly.
5. Make the risotto. Pour the glass of white wine and a broth of broth, and cook for 15 minutes, stirring frequently, and adding broth as the rice absorbs it.
6. Complete the risotto. After the indicated time, add the cheese, parsley, salt and pepper to taste, and the rest of the broth and cook for three more minutes, stirring vigorously. Let stand for 2 minutes and serve.

NUTRITION: Calories: 111 Fat: 2g Carbs: 19g Protein: 13.7g

THE PLANT BASED DIET COOKBOOK

CHAPTER 18: APPETIZER AND SNACK

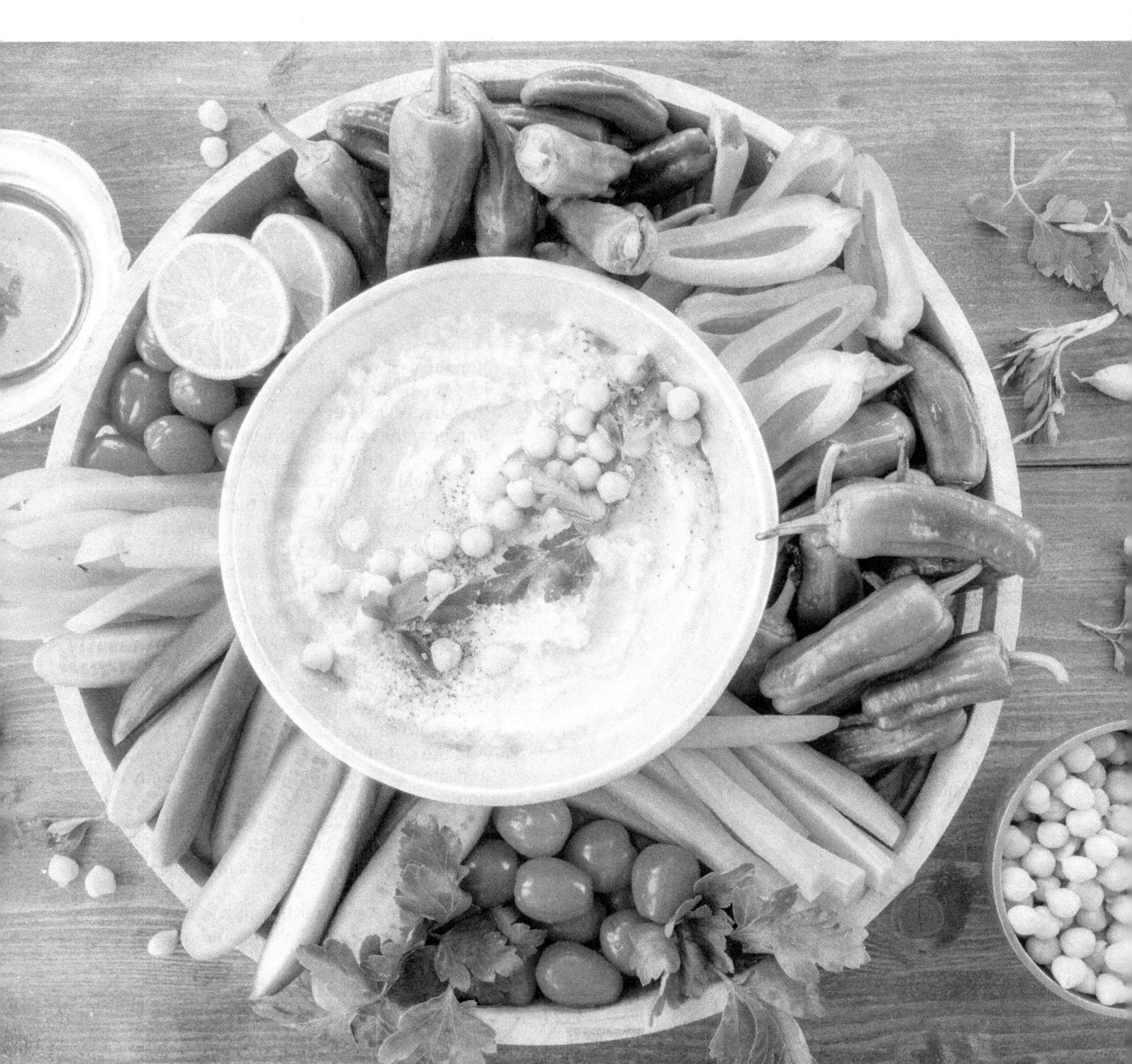

480. ALMOND VANILLA POPCORN

COOKING: 10'   **PREPARATION: 5'**   **SERVES: 4**

INGREDIENTS

- ½ cup popcorn kernels
- 2 Medjool dates
- 2 tablespoons coconut oil
- 2 tablespoons slivered almonds
- 2 teaspoons vanilla
- 1 tablespoon water

DIRECTIONS

1. Prep the oven to 325°F and prepare baking sheets with parchment paper.
2. Pop the popcorn.
3. Combine the dates, coconut, almonds, vanilla and water in a food processor and process until smooth, scraping down the sides a few times.
4. Pour the sauce into the popcorn and mix to be sure it is all well coated.
5. Spread out the popcorn out on the parchment paper, it will be wet, so you'll need baking sheets with shallow sides.
6. Bake for 9 minutes, stirring with a wooden spoon every two minutes.

NUTRITION: Calories: 97 Fat: 10 Cabrs: 12g Protein: 0.9g

481. CARROT HOTDOGS WITH RED CABBAGE

COOKING: 63'   **PREPARATION: 10'**   **SERVES: 4**

INGREDIENTS

- 4 carrots
- ¼ cup tamari sauce
- 1 tablespoon maple syrup
- ¼ cup water
- 1 tablespoon liquid smoke
- 1 teaspoon garlic powder
- 1 tablespoon paprika
- 2 tablespoons nutritional yeast
- 3 tablespoons olive oil
- 1 small onion, sliced
- 2 apples
- 2 more tablespoons maple syrup
- 1 small head red cabbage
- 2 tablespoons apple cider vinegar
- 1 more cup water
- 1 more tablespoons olive oil
- 4 whole-grain hot dog buns

DIRECTIONS

1. Boil the carrots for 12 to 14 minutes or until tender, in enough salt water to cover them. Drain and set the carrots aside to cool.
2. Combine the tamari, a tablespoon of maple syrup, the water, liquid smoke, garlic powder, paprika and nutritional yeast in a shallow dish. After they are cool, add the carrots, cover them, and place them in the refrigerator for 24 hours to marinate.
3. Make the red cabbage slaw by heating the three tablespoons of olive oil in a Dutch oven and adding the onion. Sauté until translucent.
4. Add the apple slices and the remaining two tablespoons of maple syrup, then sauté for four to five minutes until the apples are tender
5. Cut the cabbage into strips and combine them with the apple cider vinegar in another pot on the stove. Cover and simmer for 10 minutes.
6. Add the salt and pepper to taste with the water. Stir and simmer for 30 minutes. Drain out any leftover liquid.
7. Place the final tablespoon of olive oil in a skillet over medium heat and fry the carrots on all sides, cooking them for two to three minutes on each side.
8. Slice the buns, add a little cabbage slaw and a carrot and serve with ketchup and mustard.

NUTRITION: Calories: 473 Fat: 13.5g Carbs: 59.9g Protein: 10.2g

482. BROCCOLI SLAW STIR-FRY WITH TOFU

COOKING: 6'   **PREPARATION: 5'**   **SERVES: 6**

INGREDIENTS

For tofu:
- 28 oz. extra firm tofu
- 4 cloves garlic, sliced
- ½ cup rice wine
- 2 tablespoons soy sauce

For the stir-fry:
- 1 large onion, sliced
- 1 red bell pepper, sliced
- 12-oz., broccoli slaw
- ¼ cup water
- 4 cloves garlic, sliced
- 2 teaspoons minced ginger
- ¼ teaspoon red chili flakes
- 1 teaspoon sesame oil
- 2 tablespoons soy sauce

DIRECTIONS

1. Add tofu, garlic, rice wine and soya sauce into a large zip lock plastic bag. Seal the bag and turn the bag around a few times to coat well. Set aside for an hour
2. Place a large nonstick skillet over medium high heat. Remove tofu from the bag and add to the skillet. Pour rest of marinade into a large bowl.
3. Cook tofu until brown. Remove and place in the bowl of marinade. Cover and keep warm.
4. Add onions into the same skillet and sauté for a couple of minutes. Add rest of the ingredients except water and sesame oil and sauté for 2-3 minutes.
5. Add water, cover and cook for 2-3 minutes until the broccoli slaw is tender and crisp.
6. Add the tofu and marinade. Mix well and heat thoroughly. Serve immediately.

NUTRITION: Calories: 39 Fat: 12g Carbs: 18g Protein: 29.3g

483. EGGPLANT AND SESAME STIR-FRY

COOKING: 10'   **PREPARATION: 5'**   **SERVES: 4**

INGREDIENTS

- 2 tablespoons sesame oil
- 4 spring onions, sliced
- 2 red chilies, deseeded, sliced
- 2 tablespoons soy sauce
- 2 tablespoons mirin
- 2 teaspoons sesame seeds
- 6 cloves garlic, crushed
- 4 inches' piece's ginger, shredded
- 8 baby eggplant, cut into wedges
- 2 tablespoons rice wine vinegar
- 2 teaspoons cornstarch

DIRECTIONS

1. Place a wok over medium-high heat. Add oil. Once hot, add garlic and sauté for about a minute until aromatic.
2. Stir in the spring onions, chili and ginger and sauté for a couple of minutes.
3. Stir in the eggplant and sprinkle some water. Lower the heat and cook until soft.
4. Raise the heat to high heat. Add soy sauce, vinegar and mirin and cook until slightly thick.
5. Mix cornstarch with 1-2 tablespoons of water and add into the wok, stirring constantly.
6. Cook for 10 minutes until thick.
7. Serve over hot steamed rice. Sprinkle sesame seeds and a few chili slices. Also garnish with some spring onions and serve.

NUTRITION: Calories: 557 Fat: 11.4g Carbs: 11g Protein: 15.6g

THE PLANT BASED DIET COOKBOOK

484. VEGETABLE TERIYAKI STIR-FRY

COOKING: 15'   **PREPARATION: 4'**   **SERVES: 3**

INGREDIENTS

For stir-fry:
- 1 tablespoon olive oil
- 2 cloves garlic, minced
- 1 small onion, diced
- ½ tablespoon minced ginger
- ½ cup sliced bell pepper
- ¾ cup sugar snap peas
- 6 tablespoons roasted salted cashews
- 1 green onion
- 1 heaping cup carrot
- 1 medium head broccoli
- 1 cup quinoa
- ½ cup edamame

For sauce:
- ½ can pineapple chunks
- 1 tablespoon stevia
- ½ tablespoon chia seeds
- 2 tablespoons soy sauce
- ½ tablespoon seasoned rice vinegar
- 1 teaspoon Sriracha sauce

DIRECTIONS

1. Add all the ingredients for sauce into a blender and blend until smooth.
2. To make stir-fry: Place a large skillet or wok over medium heat. Add oil. When its heated, cook onion.
3. Cook ginger and garlic for 5 minutes.
4. Add all the vegetables except edamame and cook until tender.
5. Stir in rice, edamame and cashews and heat thoroughly for 10 minutes
6. Add sauce and mix well. Add salt and pepper to taste.
7. Sprinkle spring onions and cashews on top and serve.

NUTRITION: Calories: 546 Fat: 12 Carbs: 8g Protein: 16.8g

---

485. CHICKPEA BURGERS

COOKING: 6'   **PREPARATION: 5'**   **SERVES: 8**

INGREDIENTS

- 1 15-oz. can chickpeas
- ½ cup green onions, finely chopped
- 1/3 cup fresh dill, finely chopped
- 2 tablespoons dry whole-wheat breadcrumbs
- 2 tablespoons lemon juice
- ½ teaspoon salt
- ¼ teaspoon pepper
- ¼ teaspoon ground cumin
- 2 tablespoons tahini
- ¼ cup vegetable oil

DIRECTIONS

1. Pour have the chickpeas in a bowl and mash with a potato masher.
2. Add the green onions, dill, bread crumbs and lemon juice and mix well.
3. Situate rest of the chickpeas in a food processor and add the salt, pepper, cumin and tahini. Process until smooth.
4. Add to the mashed chickpeas in the bowl and mix well, using your hands. Shape them into six to eight patties.
5. Heat a 12-inch skillet over medium heat and pour in the vegetable oil. Let it heat up, then add the patties and cook them until crispy and dark golden on both sides, for about six minutes. Only flip them once.
6. Drain and serve with condiments.

NUTRITION: Calories: 291 Fat: 7.8g Carbs: 3.6g Protein: 11.7g

486. CHICKPEA CRUST PIZZA WITH VEGGIE TOPPING

COOKING: 15' **PREPARATION: 4'** **SERVES: 3**

INGREDIENTS

- 1 cup chickpea flour
- 1 cup unsweetened soy milk
- 1 tablespoon apple cider vinegar
- 1 tablespoon tahini
- ¼ teaspoon baking powder
- ¼ teaspoon sea salt
- 1/8 teaspoon ground pepper
- 1 zucchini, diced
- 1 red bell pepper
- ½ cup cauliflower florets
- 1 cup marinara sauce
- ¼ teaspoon crushed red pepper flakes

DIRECTIONS

1. Blend chickpea flour, soy milk, apple cider vinegar, tahini, baking powder, salt and pepper.
2. Grease skillet with nonstick spray and cook the batter over medium heat for 20 minutes. Use a wide spatula to flip the crust over and cook for another 10 minutes. Transfer to a cooling rack. Cool completely before topping.
3. Prepare the oven to 350°F and line a baking sheet with parchment paper. Make the topping.
4. Spray another skillet with butter flavored nonstick spray and sauté the zucchini, bell pepper and cauliflower for five to seven minutes until tender crisp. Add a little water if they start to burn or stick.
5. Top the crust with marinara sauce and spread the topping over it.
6. Bake for 15 minutes.

NUTRITION: Calories: 627 Fat: 12.3g Carbs: 9.6g Protein: 29.6g

487. DARK CHOCOLATE HAZELNUT POPCORN

COOKING: 0' **PREPARATION: 7'** **SERVES: 5**

INGREDIENTS

- 3 tablespoons coconut oil, divided
- ¼ cup unpopped popcorn kernels
- 2 tablespoons cocoa powder
- ½ cup unsweetened coconut flakes
- ½ cup chopped hazelnuts
- 2 tablespoons maple syrup
- ¼ teaspoon kosher salt

DIRECTIONS

1. Place two tablespoons of the coconut oil in a large pot with a lid.
2. Add the popcorn kernels, heat, shake and allow them to pop.
3. Once all the corn has popped, remove the pan from the heat and stir in the cocoa powder, coconut, hazelnuts, maple syrup and salt.
4. Mix well; spread the kernels out on a baking sheet until they are dry.

NUTRITION: Calories: 203 Fat: 23.7 Carbs: 21g Protein: 2.9g

THE PLANT BASED DIET COOKBOOK

488. GREEK PIZZA

COOKING: 20' **PREPARATION: 7'** **SERVES: 1**

INGREDIENTS

- ½ to 1 cup hummus
- 1 handful sliced Kalamata olives
- ½ red pepper, seeded and sliced
- ½ small red onion, diced
- 8 to 10 fresh basil leaves

DIRECTIONS

1. Preheat the oven to 375°F.
2. Spread hummus on the crust to about a half inch from the edge.
3. Sprinkle on the olives, red pepper and onion evenly over the surface of the pizza.
4. Place the basil leaves evenly on the pizza.
5. Bake for about 20 minutes. Check after 15 minutes and the pizza is done when the crust turns a light golden brown and the vegetables are cooked through.

NUTRITION: Calories: 246 Fat: 9.1g Carbs: 11.3g Protein: 11g

489. MEXICAN PIZZA

COOKING: 20' **PREPARATION: 5'** **SERVES: 4**

INGREDIENTS

- 1 cup refried beans
- ½ package mild taco seasoning
- ½ cup salsa
- ½ small yellow onion
- 1 handful black olives
- 1 tomato
- 1 handful fresh spinach leaves
- ¼ cup fresh cilantro

DIRECTIONS

1. Preheat the oven to 375°F.
2. In a small bowl, mix the cold refried beans with the taco seasoning and spread over the pizza crust to within a half inch of the edge.
3. Spread the salsa on top
4. Sprinkle the onion and olives over the surface of the pizza.
5. Place the thin slices of tomato over the surface of the pizza and top with spinach leaves and cilantro.
6. Cook for 15 to 20 minutes. The refried beans and salsa should be bubbly hot too.

NUTRITION: Calories: 93 Fat: 21g Carbs: 41g5.2g Protein

THE PLANT BASED DIET COOKBOOK

490. PLANT BASED CRISPY FALAFEL

COOKING: 30'   **PREPARATION: 20'**   **SERVES: 8**

INGREDIENTS

- 1 tbsp. extra-virgin olive oil
- 1 cup dried chickpeas soaked for 24 hours in the refrigerator
- 1 cup cauliflower, chopped
- ½ cup red onion, chopped
- ½ cup packed fresh parsley
- 2 cloves garlic, quartered
- 1 tsp. sea salt
- ½ tsp. ground black pepper
- ½ tsp. ground cumin
- ¼ tsp. ground cinnamon

DIRECTIONS

1. Preheat oven to 375°F.
2. In a food processor, mix chickpeas, cauliflower, onion, parsley, garlic, salt, pepper, cumin seeds, cinnamon, and olive oil until mixture is smooth.
3. Take 2 tbsps. of mixture and make the falafel into small patties.
4. Keep falafel on greased baking tray.
5. Bake falafel for about 25 to 30 minutes in preheated oven until golden brown from both sides.
6. Once cooked remove from oven.

NUTRITION: Calories 289, Fat: 9g, Carbs: 6g, Protein: 21g

491. CINNAMON ROLL POPCORN

COOKING: 10'   **PREPARATION: 0'**   **SERVES: 3**

INGREDIENTS

- 2 teaspoons vegetable oil
- 1/3 cup popcorn kernels
- 2 tablespoons coconut palm sugar
- ½ teaspoon ground cinnamon
- 2 tablespoons vegan butter
- 1 tablespoon maple syrup

DIRECTIONS

1. Use the vegetable oil in a large pan with a lid to make the popcorn according to package instructions.
2. Once the popcorn is popped, place the coconut palm sugar, cinnamon, butter and maple syrup in a saucepan over medium high heat. Stir constantly until everything melts and is well combined.
3. Place the popcorn in a large bowl and drizzle the sauce over the top. Toss with two large spoons to combine and let it cool before serving.

NUTRITION: Calories: 195 Fat: 12.1g Carbs:14g Protein: 2.5g

THE PLANT BASED DIET COOKBOOK

492. PUMPKIN FLAVORED POPCORN

COOKING: 10' **PREPARATION:** 5' **SERVES:** 10

INGREDIENTS

- 10 cups popped popcorn
- 2 tablespoons maple syrup
- 2 tablespoons coconut oil, melted
- 1 tablespoon pumpkin puree
- ¼ teaspoon cinnamon
- ½ teaspoon salt

DIRECTIONS

1. Make the popcorn and place it in a large bowl, reserving two cups of the popcorn to be placed in a four-cup measuring cup.
2. Preheat the oven to 325°F.
3. In a small saucepan, combine the maple syrup, coconut oil, puree, cinnamon and salt and put over medium heat. Stir constantly while it cooks, for about two minutes.
4. Put all the popcorn except the reserved two cups into a large roasting pan lined with aluminum foil.
5. Drizzle sauce over the popcorn in the roasting pan and stir until it is all coated.
6. Place in the oven for eight minutes, stirring every two or three minutes.
7. Remove from oven and let it cool; the popcorn will harden.
8. Pour the two cups of plain popcorn on top and stir to break up the hardened popcorn and incorporate them.

NUTRITION: Calories: 66 Fat: 21g Carbs: 31g Protein: 1.1g

493. QUINOA TACOS

COOKING: 1H **PREPARATION:** 10' **SERVES:** 6

INGREDIENTS

- 1 cup quinoa
- ¾ cup water
- 1 cup vegetable broth
- 1 tablespoon nutritional yeast
- ½ cup salsa
- ½ teaspoon garlic powder
- 2 teaspoons chili powder
- 2 teaspoon cumin
- ½ teaspoon sea salt
- ½ teaspoon ground pepper
- 1 tablespoon olive oil

DIRECTIONS

1. Rinse the quinoa and drain.
2. Preheat saucepan over medium heat and toast the quinoa for about four minutes stirring constantly.
3. Boil water and vegetable broth.
4. Simmer, cover and cook for 17 minutes. Fluff with a fork, put the lid back on and set to cool 10 minutes.
5. Prepare the oven to 375°F and cover a shallow sided baking sheet with aluminum foil.
6. Place the cooled quinoa in a mixing bowl and add the nutritional yeast, salsa, garlic powder, chili powder, cumin, salt, pepper and oil and stir to combine.
7. Spread on prepared baking sheet and bake 20 minutes, stir around in the pan and bake another 20 minutes.
8. Serve in taco shells or on tostadas.

NUTRITION: Calories: 149 Fat: 13g Carbs: 32g Protein: 6.2g

494. VEGAN CARAMEL POPCORN

COOKING: 1H   **PREPARATION: 5'**   **SERVES: 8**

INGREDIENTS

- 8 cups popped popcorn
- ½ cup vegan butter
- 2/3 cups brown sugar
- 2 tablespoons agave nectar
- ¼ teaspoon baking soda
- 1 pinch salt
- 1 teaspoon vanilla

DIRECTIONS

1. Prep the oven to 250°F and line a baking sheet with parchment paper.
2. Spread the popped popcorn on the baking sheet and set it aside.
3. Over medium heat, cook the butter in pan.
4. Add the brown sugar and whisk constantly until it starts to bubble.
5. Add the agave nectar, baking soda, salt and vanilla and stir.
6. Once the foaming stops, pour it onto the popcorn and use a spatula to turn the popcorn while drizzling in a stream. Make sure all the corn is coated and pat smooth.
7. Bake for one hour, stirring it up every 15 minutes.

NUTRITION: Calories: 180 Fat: 11g Carbs: 24g Protein: 1.2g

495. ZUCCHINI NUGGETS

COOKING: 40'   **PREPARATION: 5'**   **SERVES: 8**

INGREDIENTS

- 7 small potatoes
- 2 medium zucchinis, grate
- ½ teaspoon sweet paprika
- ¼ teaspoon salt
- ¼ teaspoon ground pepper

DIRECTIONS

1. Cook the potatoes in boiling water. Drain and let them cool so they can be handled.
2. Ready the oven to 425°F and line two baking sheets with parchment paper. It is hard to get them all on one baking sheet, but the second may only be half full.
3. Grid the zucchini and squeeze out the liquid by wrapping it in a clean kitchen towel and twisting and squeezing. Place in a medium bowl.
4. Grate the cooked potatoes and place them in the bowl with the zucchini.
5. Add the paprika, salt and pepper, adjusting to your taste and mix with your hands.
6. Scoop out 1½ to two tablespoons of the mixture at a time and shape them into nuggets or tot shapes. Brush each one with olive oil on all sides. Place on baking sheets.
7. Bake for 35 to 40 minutes.

NUTRITION: Calories: 111 Fat: 7g Carbs: 31g Protein: 2.8g

496. SUNFLOWER SEED BITES

COOKING: 0'   **PREPARATION: 10'**   **SERVES: 4**

INGREDIENTS

- ¾ cup of sunflower seeds
- ½ cup of dates (pitted)
- 3 tbsp of raw cacao
- 2 tbsp of agave
- 1 tbsp of coconut oil
- ½ tsp of cinnamon
- ¼ tsp of nutmeg
- ¼ tsp of Himalayan salt

DIRECTIONS

1. Add the sunflower seeds to a blender and blend it on medium-high speed until it is a fine meal consistency. Don't over-blend the sunflower seeds, as it will turn into butter.
2. Add the raw cacao, dates, coconut oil, agave, cinnamon, nutmeg, and Himalayan salt until you've reached a dough consistency.
3. Form the dough by rolling it into 2 ½ to 3-inch balls. Once done, place all the bites on a board, and refrigerate it for 30 minutes.

NUTRITION: Calories 48 Fat: 5 Carbs: 2g Protein: 1.1g

---

497. SWEET NUT BARS

COOKING: 15'   **PREPARATION: 5'**   **SERVES: 4**

INGREDIENTS

- 1 ½ cups of mixed raw nuts
- 1 cup of coconut flakes
- ½ cup of hemp seeds
- ½ cup of pumpkin seeds
- ½ cup of sesame seeds
- ½ cup of cranberries
- ½ cup of almond butter
- 4 tbsp of agave
- 1 tsp of cinnamon
- 1 tsp of vanilla extract

DIRECTIONS

1. Preheat the oven to 350°F.
2. Line an oven tin with parchment paper.
3. Mix coconut flakes, nuts, cranberries, sesame seeds, hemp seeds, cinnamon, and pumpkin seeds in a bowl to combine.
4. Add the almond butter and agave to the bowl, and mix well. Then, add the vanilla extract and stir once more.
5. Add the bowl mixture to a non-stick pan, and stir everything until well combined.
6. Transfer the mixture to the oven tin, and press it to form an even layer.
7. Bake the bars for 15 minutes before removing it from the oven to cool down.
8. Once cooled, cut it into 10 to 12 bars.

NUTRITION: Calories: 340 Fat: 22g Carbs: 19g Protein: 10.2g

498. PEANUT BUTTER CRUNCH RICE CAKES

COOKING: 0' **PREPARATION: 5'** **SERVES: 4**

INGREDIENTS
- 8 medium rice cakes (gluten-free)
- 5 to 6 tbsp of crunchy peanut butter (natural)
- ½ cup of raisins
- ¼ cup of agave

DIRECTIONS
1. Plate 2 rice cakes per serving, and spread ½ to 1 tbsp of crunchy peanut butter evenly on top.
2. Add some raisins, and a drizzle of agave (optional).
3. Place the 3 to 4 ingredients in small separate containers, and prep per serving.

NUTRITION: Calories: 265 Fat: 12 Carbs: 2.6g Protein: 7g

---

499. SPICY EDAMAME

COOKING: 0' **PREPARATION: 5'** **SERVES: 4**

INGREDIENTS
- 2 cups of edamame
- ½ tsp. of Aleppo pepper
- ¼ tsp of black pepper

DIRECTIONS
1. Steam the edamame according to its package instructions, remove, and allow it to cool down. Transfer to a bowl.
2. Sprinkle Aleppo pepper and black pepper on top, and shake the bowl for the spice to cover all the edamame.

NUTRITION: Calories: 100 Fat: 1g Carbs: 9.3g Protein: 8g

---

500. SWEET PISTACHIO BITES

COOKING: 0' **PREPARATION: 10'** **SERVES: 4**

INGREDIENTS
- 2 cups of dates
- 1 cup of cranberries
- 1 cup of pistachios
- 1 tsp of pumpkin seeds
- ¼ tsp of black pepper

DIRECTIONS
1. Blend dates, cranberries, pistachios, pumpkin seeds, and black pepper to a high-performance food processor.
2. Roll the date dough into 2 ½ to 3-inch round balls, usually 1 tbsp each.

NUTRITION: Calories: 70 Fat: 22g Carbs: 13.2g Protein: 1.2g

---

501. BAGEL POPCORN

COOKING: 5' **PREPARATION: 0'** **SERVES: 4**

INGREDIENTS
- 6 tbsp of popcorn kernels
- 2 tsp of sesame seeds
- 2 tsp of poppy seeds
- ½ tsp of garlic powder
- ½ tsp of onion powder
- 4 tsp of olive oil
- ½ tsp of salt

DIRECTIONS
1. Add the popcorn kernels to a paper bag.
2. Fold over the top of the bag up to three times to seal the bag.
3. Microwave the bag until the kernels stop popping, usually for 1 to 2 minutes.
4. Add the olive oil, salt, garlic powder, onion powder, sesame seeds, and poppy seeds to the popcorn in the bag.
5. Fold the bag once more and shake it to coat.

NUTRITION: Calories: 140 Fat: 15g Carbs: 20.1g Protein: 3.5g

THE PLANT BASED DIET COOKBOOK

502. CRISPY CHICKPEAS

COOKING: 10'   **PREPARATION: 5'**   **SERVES: 4**

INGREDIENTS

- 1 15 oz. of chickpeas
- 2 lime wedges
- 1 tsp of olive oil
- ¼ tsp of paprika
- ¼ tsp of red chili flakes
- 1/8 tsp of salt

DIRECTIONS

1. Spread the chickpeas on paper towels, and top them with paper towels, covering them to pat them dry.
2. Add the oil and chickpeas to a bowl and combine. Add the paprika, red chili flakes, and salt to the bowl, and mix the ingredients well.
3. Add parchment paper to a baking sheet, spreading the chickpeas onto the sheet evenly.
4. Drizzle 1 tsp of olive oil onto the chickpeas, and cook them at °F for 10 minutes.
5. Drizzle lime juice on top and serve immediately.

NUTRITION: Calories: 130 Fat: 2g Carbs: 12g Protein: 4.5g

---

503. FRUIT AND NUT BARS

COOKING: 1H   **PREPARATION: 15'**   **SERVES: 4**

INGREDIENTS

- ¾ cup of dates
- ¾ cup of coconut flakes
- ½ cup of raw cashews
- ½ cup of almonds
- ¼ cup of cherries
- 1/8 tsp of salt

DIRECTIONS

1. Soak the dates in lukewarm-hot water in a bowl for up for at least 10 minutes, and drain.
2. Prepare the loaf pan with parchment paper, and ensure it overlaps over all four sides of the pan. Coat the loaf pan with a light layer of cooking spray.
3. Add the soaked dates, cherries, cashews, almonds, coconut, and salt to a food processor, and process on high speed for 30 seconds.
4. Add the nut mixture to the loaf pan, and spread it evenly, pressing it down into an even layer.
5. Refrigerate the pan for 1 hour. Once done, remove the fruit and nut loaf from the pan. Slice it into 6 to 8 individual bars.

NUTRITION: Calories: 320 Fat: 11g Carbs: 15.2g Protein: 3.2g

504. CREAMY LOG BOATS

COOKING: 0' PREPARATION: 5' SERVES: 4

INGREDIENTS

- 8 celery sticks
- 4 tbsp of smooth peanut butter
- 4 tbsp of dried cranberries

DIRECTIONS

1. Spread each celery stick with smooth ½ tbsp peanut butter.
2. Top the celery sticks with ½ tbsp of dried cranberries each, and serve 2 celery sticks per serving.

NUTRITION: Calories: 140 Fat: 9 Carbs: 12g Protein: 4g

505. VEGGIE STICKS AND DIP

COOKING: 0' PREPARATION: 5' SERVES: 4

INGREDIENTS

- 2 red bell peppers
- 2 green bell peppers
- 1 cup of baby carrots
- 1 cup of hummus
- ½ tsp of black pepper

DIRECTIONS

1. Prep the red and green bell peppers by washing, coring, and seeding them.
2. Chop them into thin stick shapes.
3. Divide the bell peppers and carrots between 4 servings, and place them into 4 separate containers.
4. Serve each serving with ¼ cup of hummus and a pinch of black pepper.

NUTRITION: Calories: 160 Fat: 4g Carbs: 21g Protein: 5.2g

506. TRAIL MIX

COOKING: 0' PREPARATION: 5' SERVES: 4

INGREDIENTS

- ¼ cup of almonds
- ¼ cup of cashews
- ¼ cup of dried apricots
- ¼ cup of dried cranberries
- ¼ cup of pitted dates

DIRECTIONS

1. Combine the almonds, cashews, cranberries, apricots, and dates in a bowl.

NUTRITION: Calories: 130 Fat: 15 Carbs: 14.2g Protein: 3.4g

THE PLANT BASED DIET COOKBOOK

507. VEGGIE CRISPS

COOKING: 20' | **PREPARATION: 5'** | **SERVES: 4**

INGREDIENTS
- 2 medium carrots
- 1 medium beetroot
- 1 medium baby marrow
- 1 small sweet potato
- 1 small turnip
- 1-2 tsp of olive oil
- ½ tsp of black pepper
- ½ tsp of Himalayan salt

DIRECTIONS
1. Preheat the oven to 350-400°F. In a baking tray, lay out parchment paper.
2. Slice the vegetables each into 1-inch slices with a sharp knife, and place them in a bowl.
3. Mix in olive oil and season the vegetables, coat well.
4. Arrange vegetables onto the baking sheet, and bake them for 10 minutes on one side. Then, turn over, and bake them for 6-8 minutes.
5. Remove the vegetable crisps from the oven, and allow them to cool down.

NUTRITION: Calories: 78 Fat: 11g Carbs: 34g Protein: 2.4g

---

508. VEGAN CHEESE SQUARES

COOKING: 15' | **PREPARATION: 12'** | **SERVES: 4**

INGREDIENTS
- 2/3 cups AP flour
- 1 cup of oat flour
- 3 tbsp of cornmeal
- 3 tbsp of vegan butter
- 3 tbsp of water
- 2 tbsp of nutritional yeast
- ½ tsp of Himalayan salt
- ½ tsp of onion powder
- ¼ tsp of baking powder

DIRECTIONS
1. Heat the oven to 375-400°F.
2. Prep a baking sheet with parchment paper.
3. Add oat flour, all-purpose flour, cornmeal, nutritional yeast, onion powder, baking powder, and Himalayan salt to the food processor. Process the ingredients until properly combined.
4. Add cold water to the mixture, 1 tbsp at a time, mixing it until the dough reaches a more paste-like texture.
5. Pull out dough mixture from the food processor. Form into a ball. Then, place the dough ball onto a floured surface (ideally you can add flour to parchment paper), and dust the dough with flour. Flatten the dough, rolling it into a 1/8-inch-thick pastry layer.
6. Slice dough into squares, about 2 ½ inches long and wide to form mini crackers.
7. Spread the mini dough crackers onto the baking sheet, and bake them for 12 minutes in the oven.

NUTRITION: Calories: 80 Fat: 12g Carbs: 9g Protein: 1.7g

---

509. TAMARI ALMONDS

COOKING: 20' | **PREPARATION: 5'** | **SERVES: 4**

INGREDIENTS
- 14 oz. of raw almonds
- ¼ cup of tamari sauce
- ¼ tsp of sea salt

DIRECTIONS
1. Heat the oven to 180°F, and line a baking tray with parchment paper.
2. Spread the almonds onto the baking tray, drizzle the tamari sauce over the nuts, and add the sea salt.
3. Bake the almonds in the oven for 25 minutes, moving them around every 5 to 10 minutes until the nuts absorb the tamari sauce.

NUTRITION: Calories: 115 Fat: 1g Carbs: 2.1g Protein: 2.1g

510. SWEET TIFFIN

COOKING: 2H — **PREPARATION: 15'** — **SERVES: 4**

INGREDIENTS

- 1 cup of dark chocolate (vegan)
- 2/3 cups of macadamia nuts
- 1/3 cup of dried cranberries
- 1/3 cup of coconut oil
- ¼ cup of pistachios
- 2 tbsp of maple syrup

DIRECTIONS

1. Spray a brownie tin with cooking spray. Layer the tin with a single sheet of parchment paper.
2. Add the chocolate and maple syrup to a microwaveable bowl, and microwave it for 30 seconds or until you reach a smooth consistency.
3. Crush the nuts into smaller pieces in a bowl. Add the cranberries and pistachios. Mix the ingredients to combine, and add the chocolate mixture to the bowl. Mix once more, then pour the mixture into the brownie tin.
4. Press the mixture with the back of a spoon to ensure it creates a flat, even layer. Refrigerate it for 2 hours, before cutting it into squares, about 4-inches in length and width.

NUTRITION: Calories: 130 Fat: 11g Carbs: 10g Protein: 1.1g

511. BLACK BEAN BALLS

COOKING: 0' — **PREPARATION: 20'** — **SERVES: 3**

INGREDIENTS

- 15 oz. can black beans
- 3 oz. raw cacao powder
- 1 oz. almond butter
- 15 ml maple syrup

DIRECTIONS

1. In a food processor, combine black beans, cacao powder, almond butter, and maple syrup.
2. Process until the mixture is well combined.
3. Shape the mixture into 12 balls.
4. Roll the balls through remaining cacao powder.
5. Place the balls in a refrigerator for 10 minutes. Serve.

NUTRITION: Calories: 1.1g Fat: 6g Carbs: 31g Protein: 13.1g

512. CHIA SOY PUDDING

COOKING: 0' — **PREPARATION: 5'** — **SERVES: 2**

INGREDIENTS

- 1.5 oz. almond butter
- 15ml maple syrup
- ¼ teaspoon vanilla paste
- 235ml soymilk
- 1.5 oz. chia seeds
- 1 small banana, sliced
- .5 oz. crushed almonds

DIRECTIONS

1. Combine almond butter, maple syrup, vanilla, and soymilk in a jar.
2. Stir in chia seeds.
3. Cover and refrigerate 3 hours.
4. After 3 hours, open the jar.
5. Top the chia pudding with banana and crushed almonds. Serve.

NUTRITION: Calories: 298 Carbs 11g Fat: 9g Protein: 10g

THE PLANT BASED DIET COOKBOOK

513. BLUEBERRY ICE CREAM

COOKING: 0'   **PREPARATION: 10'**   **SERVES: 2**

INGREDIENTS

- 5 oz. raw cashews
- 4 oz. silken tofu
- 8 oz. fresh blueberries
- .1 oz. lemon zest
- 100ml maple syrup
- 100ml coconut oil
- .5 oz. almond butter

DIRECTIONS

1. Rinse and drain cashews.
2. Place the cashews, blueberries, pale syrup, coconut oil, and almond butter in a food processor.
3. Process until smooth.
4. Transfer the mixture into the freezer-friendly container.
5. Seal with plastic foil and freeze for 4 hours.
6. Remove the ice cream from the fridge 15 minutes before serving.

NUTRITION: Calories: 544 Fat: 6.7g Carbs: 3g Protein: 8.1g

514. CHICKPEA CHOCO SLICES

COOKING: 50'   **PREPARATION: 10'**   **SERVES: 2**

INGREDIENTS

- 14 oz. can chickpeas
- 9 oz. almond butter
- 70ml maple syrup
- 15ml vanilla paste
- 1 pinch salt
- 2g baking powder
- 2g baking soda
- 1.5 oz. vegan chocolate chips

DIRECTIONS

1. Preheat oven to 350°F.
2. Grease large baking pan with coconut oil.
3. Combine chickpeas, almond butter, maple syrup, vanilla, salt, baking powder, and baking soda in a food blender.
4. Blend until smooth. Stir in half the chocolate chips-
5. Arrange batter into the prepared baking pan.
6. Sprinkle with reserved chocolate chips.
7. Bake for 45-50 minutes.
8. Set aside on wire rack for 20 minutes. slice and serve.

NUTRITION: Calories: 426 Fat: 4.9g Carbs: 21g Protein: 10g

515. SWEET GREEN COOKIES

COOKING: 30'   **PREPARATION: 10'**   **SERVES: 3**

INGREDIENTS

- 6 oz. green peas
- 3 oz. chopped Medjool dates
- 2 oz. silken tofu, mashed
- 3.5 oz. almond flour
- 1 teaspoon baking powder
- 12 almonds

DIRECTIONS

1. Preheat oven to 350°F.
2. Combine peas and dates in a food processor.
3. Process until the thick paste is formed.
4. Transfer the pea mixture into a bowl. Stir in tofu, almond flour, and baking powder.
5. Shape the mixture into 12 balls.
6. Arrange balls onto baking sheet, lined with parchment paper. Flatten each ball with oiled palm.
7. Insert an almond into each cookie. Bake the cookies for 25-30 minutes.

NUTRITION: Calories: 221 Carbs: 15g Fat: 6g Protein: 8.2g

516. CHOCOLATE ORANGE MOUSSE

COOKING: 0' **PREPARATION: 10'** **SERVES: 4**

INGREDIENTS

- 16 oz. can black beans
- 2 oz. dates
- 30 ml coconut oil
- 110 ml maple syrup
- 60 ml soymilk
- 1 orange

DIRECTIONS

1. Place the black bean in a food processor.
2. Add drained dates and process until smooth.
3. Add coconut oil, maple syrup, and soymilk. Process for 1 minute.
4. Finally, stir in lemon zest.
5. Spoon the mixture into four dessert bowls.
6. Chill for 1 hour before serving.

NUTRITION: Calories: 375 Carbs: 11g Fat: 8g Protein: 11.3g

517. EASY MANGO TOFU CUSTARD

COOKING: 0' **PREPARATION: 15'** **SERVES: 2**

INGREDIENTS

- 3.5 oz. mango puree
- 10.5 oz. soft tofu
- 15ml lime juice
- 15ml maple syrup
- 2g baking soda
- 1.5 oz. vegan chocolate chips

DIRECTIONS

1. Combine all ingredients in a food blender.
2. Divide among two serving bowls.
3. Refrigerate 30 minutes. Serve.

NUTRITION: Calories: 148 Carbs: 3g Fat: 2g Protein: 10.2g

518. CHICKPEA COOKIE DOUGH

COOKING: 0' **PREPARATION: 10'** **SERVES: 4**

INGREDIENTS

- 14 oz. can chickpeas
- 4.5 oz. smooth peanut butter
- 10 ml vanilla extract
- ½ teaspoon cinnamon
- 10g chia seeds
- 1.5 oz. quality dark Vegan chocolate chips

DIRECTIONS

1. Drain chickpeas in a colander.
2. Remove the skin from the chickpeas.
3. Place chickpeas, peanut butter, vanilla, cinnamon, and chia in a food blender.
4. Stir in chocolate chips and divide among four serving bowls.

NUTRITION: Calories: 376 Carbs: 18g Fat: 5g Protein: 14.2g

519. CACAO THIN MINTS

COOKING: 0' | **PREPARATION: 10'** | **SERVES: 2**

INGREDIENTS

- 2 oz. rice Protein: powder
- 1 oz. cacao powder
- 5 ml vanilla extract
- 5 ml peppermint extract
- ½ teaspoon liquid stevia
- 90 ml melted and cooled coconut oil
- 1.5 oz. ground almonds

DIRECTIONS

1. Combine Protein: powder and cacao powder in a bowl.
2. Mix vanilla, peppermint extract, stevia, and coconut oil.
3. Mix in liquid ingredients into the dry ones.
4. Line small cookie sheet with parchment paper.
5. Drop 10 mounds of prepared batter onto the cookie sheet.
6. Sprinkle the cookies with ground almonds.
7. Place in a freezer for 20 minutes. Serve.

NUTRITION: Calories: 251 Carbs: 6g Fat: 15g Protein: 12g

520. BANANA BARS

COOKING: 30' | **PREPARATION: 10'** | **SERVES: 8**

INGREDIENTS

- oz. smooth peanut butter
- 60ml maple syrup
- 1 banana, mashed
- 45ml water
- .5 oz. ground flax seeds
- 3 oz. cooked quinoa
- 1 oz. chia seeds
- 5ml vanilla
- 3 oz. quick cooking oats
- 2 oz. whole-wheat flour
- 5g baking powder
- 5g cinnamon
- 1 pinch salt
- Topping:
- 5ml melted coconut oil
- 1 oz. vegan chocolate, chopped

DIRECTIONS

1. Preheat oven to 350°F.
2. Line 16cm baking dish with parchment paper.
3. Mix flax seeds and water. Place aside 10 minutes.
4. In a separate bowl, incorporate peanut butter, maple syrup, and banana. Fold in the flax seed's mixture.
5. Once smooth, stir in quinoa, chia seeds, vanilla extract, oat, whole-wheat flour, baking powder, cinnamon, and salt.
6. Pour the batter into prepared baking dish. Cut into 8 bars.
7. Bake the bars for 30 minutes.
8. In the meantime, make the topping; combine chocolate and coconut oil in a heat-proof bowl. Set over simmering water, until melted.
9. Remove the bars from the oven. Cool on wire rack for 15 minutes.
10. Drizzle with chocolate topping. Serve.

NUTRITION: Calories: 278 Fat: 7g Carbs: 12g Protein: 9.4g

521. PUMPKIN PUDDING

COOKING: 0' | **PREPARATION: 5'** | **SERVES: 4**

INGREDIENTS

- 470ml soymilk
- 8.5oz. organic pumpkin puree
- 30ml maple syrup
- ½ teaspoon cinnamon
- ¼ teaspoon ground ginger
- ¼ teaspoon ground nutmeg
- 2oz. vanilla flavored brown rice Protein: powder

DIRECTIONS

1. Blend all ingredients, until smooth.
2. Divide between four dessert glasses and chill for 30 minutes before serving.

NUTRITION: Calories: 163 Carbs: 17g Fat: 5g Protein: 15g

522. SWEET HUMMUS

COOKING: 0' PREPARATION: 10' SERVES: 4

INGREDIENTS

- 60ml vanilla soymilk
- 30ml maple syrup
- 14oz. can chickpeas
- 4.5oz. pumpkin puree
- 5ml vanilla extract
- 7oz. fresh blueberries
- 2 carrots, finely grated

DIRECTIONS

1. Combine soymilk, maple syrup, chickpeas, pumpkin puree, vanilla, and carrots in a food processor.
2. Serve, topped with fresh blueberries.

NUTRITION: Calories: 252 Fat: 4g Carbs: 15g Protein: 10.3g

523. LENTIL BALLS

COOKING: 0' PREPARATION: 10' SERVES: 2

INGREDIENTS

- 5oz. cooked green lentils
- 10ml coconut oil
- 5g coconut sugar
- 6 oz. quick cooking oats
- 1.5oz. unsweetened coconut
- 1.5oz. raw pumpkin seeds
- 4oz. peanut butter
- 40ml maple syrup

DIRECTIONS

1. Combine all ingredients.
2. Shape the mixture into 16 balls.
3. Arrange the balls onto a plate, lined with parchment paper.
4. Refrigerate 30 minutes. Serve.

NUTRITION: Calories: 305 Carbs: 12g Fat: 9.5g Protein: 12.6g

524. HOMEMADE GRANOLA

COOKING: 24' PREPARATION: 10' SERVES: 8

INGREDIENTS

- 10oz. rolled oats
- 3.5oz. coconut flakes
- 1.5oz. pumpkin seeds
- 3oz. hemp seeds
- 30ml coconut oil
- 70ml maple syrup
- 2oz. Goji berries

DIRECTIONS

1. Incorporate all ingredients on baking sheet.
2. Preheat oven to 350°F.
3. Bake the granola for 12 minutes. Remove from the oven and stir.
4. Bake an additional 12 minutes.
5. Serve at room temperature.

NUTRITION: Calories: 344 Fat: 5.8 Carbs: 18g Protein: 9.9g

525. PEANUT BUTTER QUINOA CUPS

COOKING: 0'   **PREPARATION: 10'**   **SERVES: 6**

INGREDIENTS

- 4oz. puffed quinoa
- 2oz. smooth peanut butter
- 1.5oz. coconut butter
- 30ml coconut oil
- 25ml maple syrup
- 5ml vanilla extract

DIRECTIONS

1. Combine peanut butter, coconut butter, and coconut oil in a microwave-safe bowl.
2. Microwave on high until melted, in 40-second intervals.
3. Stir in the puffed quinoa. Stir gently to combine.
4. Divide the mixture among 12 paper cases. Freeze for 1 hour

NUTRITION: Calories: 231 Carbs: 12g Fat: 9g Protein: 6.3g

CHAPTER 19: DESSERTS

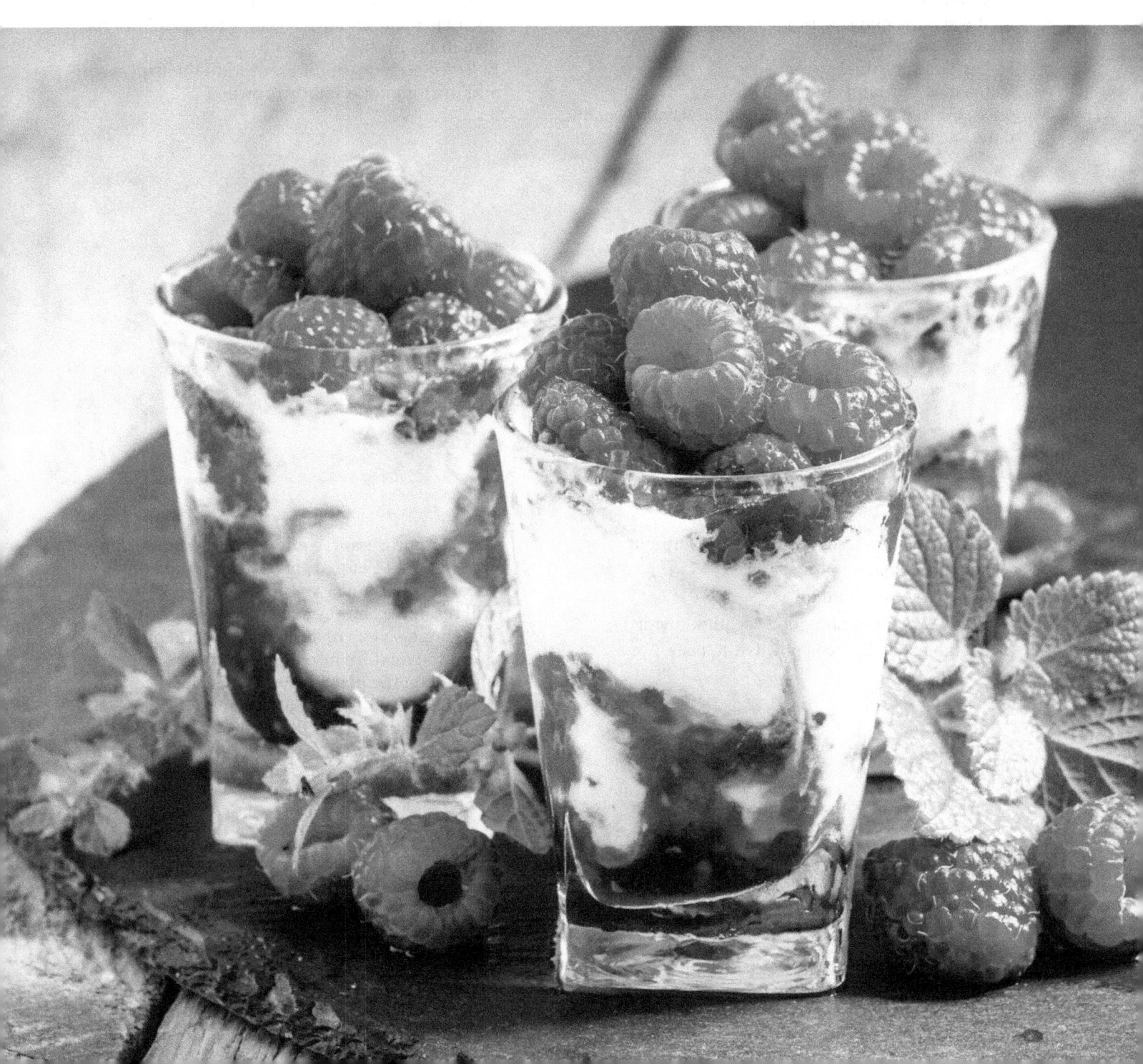

526. APPLE CRUMBLE

COOKING: 25'   **PREPARATION: 20'**   **SERVES: 6**

INGREDIENTS

For the filling
- 4 to 5 apples, cored and chopped (about 6 cups)
- ½ cup unsweetened applesauce, or ¼ cup water
- 2 to 3 tablespoons unrefined sugar (coconut, date, sucanat, maple syrup)
- 1 teaspoon ground cinnamon
- Pinch sea salt
- For the crumble
- 2 tablespoons almond butter, or cashew or sunflower seed butter
- 2 tablespoons maple syrup
- 1½ cups rolled oats
- ½ cup walnuts, finely chopped
- ½ teaspoon ground cinnamon
- 2 to 3 tablespoons unrefined granular sugar (coconut, date, sucanat)

DIRECTIONS

1. Preheat the oven to 350°F. Put the apples and applesauce in an 8-inch-square baking dish, and sprinkle with the sugar, cinnamon, and salt. Toss to combine.
2. In a medium bowl, mix the nut butter and maple syrup until smooth and creamy. Add the oats, walnuts, cinnamon, and sugar and stir to coat, using your hands if necessary. (If you have a small food processor, pulse the oats and walnuts together before adding them to the mix.)
3. Sprinkle the topping over the apples, and put the dish in the oven.
4. Bake for 20 to 25 minutes, or until the fruit is soft and the topping is lightly browned.

NUTRITION: Calories: 195 Fat: 7g Carbs: 6g Sugar 4g Protein: 24g

527. CASHEW-CHOCOLATE TRUFFLES

COOKING: 0'   **PREPARATION: 15'**   **SERVES: 12**

INGREDIENTS

- 1 cup raw cashews, soaked in water overnight
- ¾ cup pitted dates
- 2 tablespoons coconut oil
- 1 cup unsweetened shredded coconut, divided
- 1 to 2 tablespoons cocoa powder, to taste

DIRECTIONS

1. In a food processor, combine the cashews, dates, coconut oil, ½ cup of shredded coconut, and cocoa powder. Pulse until fully incorporated; it will resemble chunky cookie dough. Spread the remaining ½ cup of shredded coconut on a plate.
2. Form the mixture into tablespoon-size balls and roll on the plate to cover with the shredded coconut. Transfer to a parchment paper–lined plate or baking sheet. Repeat to make 12 truffles.
3. Place the truffles in the refrigerator for 1 hour to set. Transfer the truffles to a storage container or freezer-safe bag and seal.

NUTRITION: Calories: 160 Fat: 1g Carbs: 1g Sugar 2.5g Protein: 22g

528. BANANA CHOCOLATE CUPCAKES

COOKING: 20'   **PREPARATION: 20'**   **SERVES: 1**

INGREDIENTS

- 3 medium bananas
- 1 cup non-dairy milk
- 2 tablespoons almond butter
- 1 teaspoon apple cider vinegar
- 1 teaspoon pure vanilla extract
- 1¼ cups whole-grain flour
- ½ cup rolled oats
- ¼ cup coconut sugar (optional)
- 1 teaspoon baking powder
- ½ teaspoon baking soda
- ½ cup unsweetened cocoa powder
- ¼ cup chia seeds, or sesame seeds
- Pinch sea salt
- ¼ cup dark chocolate chips, dried cranberries, or raisins (optional)

DIRECTIONS

1. Preheat the oven to 350°F. Lightly grease the cups of two 6-cup muffin tins or line with paper muffin cups.
2. Put the bananas, milk, almond butter, vinegar, and vanilla in a blender and purée until smooth. Or stir together in a large bowl until smooth and creamy.
3. Put the flour, oats, sugar (if using), baking powder, baking soda, cocoa powder, chia seeds, salt, and chocolate chips in another large bowl, and stir to combine. Mix the wet and dry ingredients, stirring as little as possible. Spoon into muffin cups, and bake for 20 to 25 minutes. Take the cupcakes out of the oven and let them cool fully before taking out of the muffin tins, since they'll be very moist.

NUTRITION: Calories: 295 Fat: 17g Carbs: 4g Sugar 4.1g Protein: 29g

529. MINTY FRUIT SALAD

COOKING: 5'   **PREPARATION: 15'**   **SERVES: 4**

INGREDIENTS

- ¼ cup lemon juice (about 2 small lemons)
- 4 teaspoons maple syrup or agave syrup
- 2 cups chopped pineapple
- 2 cups chopped strawberries
- 2 cups raspberries
- 1 cup blueberries
- 8 fresh mint leaves

DIRECTIONS

1. Beginning with 1 mason jar, add the ingredients in this order:
2. 1 tablespoon of lemon juice, 1 teaspoon of maple syrup, ½ cup of pineapple, ½ cup of strawberries, ½ cup of raspberries, ¼ cup of blueberries, and 2 mint leaves.
3. Repeat to fill 3 more jars. Close the jars tightly with lids.
4. Place the airtight jars in the refrigerator for up to 3 days.

NUTRITION: Calories: 339 Fat: 17.5g Carbs: 2g Sugar 6g Protein: 44g

THE PLANT BASED DIET COOKBOOK

530. MANGO COCONUT CREAM PIE

COOKING: 30'   **PREPARATION: 20'**   **SERVES: 8**

INGREDIENTS

- For the crust
- ½ cup rolled oats
- 1 cup cashews
- 1 cup soft pitted dates
- For the filling
- 1 cup canned coconut milk
- ½ cup water
- 2 large mangos, peeled and chopped, or about 2 cups frozen chunks
- ½ cup unsweetened shredded coconut

DIRECTIONS

1. Put all the crust ingredients in a food processor and pulse until it holds together. If you don't have a food processor, chop everything as finely as possible and use ½ cup cashew or almond butter in place of half the cashews. Press the mixture down firmly into an 8-inch pie or springform pan.
2. Put the all filling ingredients in a blender and purée until smooth (about 1 minute). It should be very thick, so you may have to stop and stir until it's smooth.
3. Pour the filling into the crust, use a rubber spatula to smooth the top, and put the pie in the freezer until set, about 30 minutes. Once frozen, it should be set out for about 15 minutes to soften before serving.
4. Top with a batch of Coconut Whipped Cream scooped on top of the pie once it's set. Finish it off with a sprinkling of toasted shredded coconut.

NUTRITION: Calories: 545 Fat: 39.6g Carbs: 9.5g Sugar 7.1g Protein: 43g

531. CHERRY-VANILLA RICE PUDDING (PRESSURE COOKER)

COOKING: 30'   **PREPARATION: 5'**   **SERVES: 4-6**

INGREDIENTS

- 1 cup short-grain brown rice
- 1¾ cups nondairy milk, plus more as needed
- 1½ cups water
- 4 tablespoons unrefined sugar or pure maple syrup (use 2 tablespoons if you use a sweetened milk), plus more as needed
- 1 teaspoon vanilla extract (use ½ teaspoon if you use vanilla milk)
- Pinch salt
- ¼ cup dried cherries or ½ cup fresh or frozen pitted cherries

DIRECTIONS

1. Preparing the Ingredients. In your electric pressure cooker's cooking pot, combine the rice, milk, water, sugar, vanilla, and salt.
2. High pressure for 30 minutes. Close and lock the lid, and select High Pressure for 30 minutes.
3. Pressure Release. Once the cooking is complete, let the pressure release naturally, about 20 minutes. Unlock and remove the lid. Stir in the cherries and put the lid back on loosely for about 10 minutes. Serve, adding more milk or sugar, as desired.

NUTRITION: Calories: 420 Fat: 27.4g Carbs: 2g Sugar 12.3g Protein: 46.3g

532. LIME IN THE COCONUT CHIA PUDDING

COOKING: 20'   **PREPARATION: 10'**   **SERVES: 4**

INGREDIENTS

- Zest and juice of 1 lime
- 1 (14-oz.) can coconut milk
- 1 to 2 dates, or 1 tablespoon coconut or other unrefined sugar, or 1 tablespoon maple syrup, or 10 to 15 drops pure liquid stevia
- 2 tablespoons chia seeds, whole or ground
- 2 teaspoons matcha green tea powder (optional)

DIRECTIONS

1. Blend all the ingredients in a blender until smooth. Chill in the fridge for about 20 minutes, then serve topped with one or more of the topping ideas.
2. Try blueberries, blackberries, sliced strawberries, Coconut Whipped Cream, or toasted unsweetened coconut.

NUTRITION: Calories: 381 Fat: 17.1g Carbs: 4.1g Sugar 11.6g Protein: 50.6g

533. MINT CHOCOLATE CHIP SORBET

COOKING: 0'   **PREPARATION: 5'**   **SERVES: 1**

INGREDIENTS

- 1 frozen banana
- 1 tablespoon almond butter, or peanut butter, or other nut or seed butter
- 2 tablespoons fresh mint, minced
- ¼ cup or less non-dairy milk (only if needed)
- 2 to 3 tablespoons non-dairy chocolate chips, or cocoa nibs
- 2 to 3 tablespoons goji berries (optional)

DIRECTIONS

1. Put the banana, almond butter, and mint in a food processor or blender and purée until smooth.
2. Add the non-dairy milk if needed to keep blending (but only if needed, as this will make the texture less solid). Pulse the chocolate chips and goji berries (if using) into the mix so they're roughly chopped up.

NUTRITION: Calories: 299 Fat: 16g Carbs: 3g Sugar 6g Protein: 38g

THE PLANT BASED DIET COOKBOOK

534. PEACH-MANGO CRUMBLE (PRESSURE COOKER)

COOKING: 6'   **PREPARATION: 10'**   **SERVES: 4-6**

INGREDIENTS

- 3 cups chopped fresh or frozen peaches
- 3 cups chopped fresh or frozen mangos
- 4 tablespoons unrefined sugar or pure maple syrup, divided
- 1 cup gluten-free rolled oats
- ½ cup shredded coconut, sweetened or unsweetened
- 2 tablespoons coconut oil or vegan margarine

DIRECTIONS

1. Preparing the Ingredients. In a 6- to 7-inch round baking dish, toss together the peaches, mangos, and 2 tablespoons of sugar. In a food processor, combine the oats, coconut, coconut oil, and remaining 2 tablespoons of sugar. Pulse until combined. (If you use maple syrup, you'll need less coconut oil. Start with just the syrup and add oil if the mixture isn't sticking together.) Sprinkle the oat mixture over the fruit mixture.
2. Cover the dish with aluminum foil. Put a trivet in the bottom of your electric pressure cooker's cooking pot and pour in a cup or two of water. Using a foil sling or silicone helper handles, lower the pan onto the trivet.
3. High pressure for 6 minutes. Close and lock the lid, and select High Pressure for 6 minutes.
4. Pressure Release. Once the cooking is complete, quick release the pressure. Unlock and remove the lid.
5. Let cool for a few minutes before carefully lifting out the dish with oven mitts or tongs. Scoop out portions to serve.

NUTRITION: Calories: 275 Fat: 19g Carbs: 19g Sugar 12g Protein: 14g

535. ZESTY ORANGE-CRANBERRY ENERGY BITES

COOKING: 15'   **PREPARATION: 10'**   **SERVES: 12**

INGREDIENTS

- 2 tablespoons almond butter, or cashew or sunflower seed butter
- 2 tablespoons maple syrup, or brown rice syrup
- ¾ cup cooked quinoa
- ¼ cup sesame seeds, toasted
- 1 tablespoon chia seeds
- ½ teaspoon almond extract, or vanilla extract
- Zest of 1 orange
- 1 tablespoon dried cranberries
- ¼ cup ground almonds

DIRECTIONS

1. In a medium bowl, mix the nut or seed butter and syrup until smooth and creamy. Stir in the rest of the ingredients, and mix to ensure the consistency is holding together in a ball. Form the mix into 12 balls.
2. Place them on a baking sheet lined with parchment or waxed paper and put in the fridge to set for about 15 minutes.
3. If your balls aren't holding together, it's likely because of the moisture content of your cooked quinoa. Add more nut or seed butter mixed with syrup until it all sticks together.

NUTRITION: Calories: 493 Fat: 33g Carbs: 8g Sugar 18g Protein: 47g

536. ALMOND-DATE ENERGY BITES

COOKING: 15' **PREPARATION: 5'** **SERVES: 24**

INGREDIENTS

- 1 cup dates, pitted
- 1 cup unsweetened shredded coconut
- ¼ cup chia seeds
- ¾ cup ground almonds
- ¼ cup cocoa nibs, or non-dairy chocolate chips

DIRECTIONS

1. Purée everything in a food processor until crumbly and sticking together, pushing down the sides whenever necessary to keep it blending. If you don't have a food processor, you can mash soft Medjool dates. But if you're using harder baking dates, you'll have to soak them and then try to purée them in a blender.
2. Form the mix into 24 balls and place them on a baking sheet lined with parchment or waxed paper. Put in the fridge to set for about 15 minutes. Use the softest dates you can find. Medjool dates are the best for this purpose. The hard dates you see in the baking aisle of your supermarket will take a long time to blend up. If you use those, try soaking them in water for at least an hour before you start, and then draining.

NUTRITION: Calories: 171 Fat: 4 g Carbs: 7 g Sugar 7 g Protein: 22 g

537. PUMPKIN PIE CUPS (PRESSURE COOKER)

COOKING: 6' **PREPARATION: 5'** **SERVES: 4-6**

INGREDIENTS

- 1 cup canned pumpkin purée
- 1 cup nondairy milk
- 6 tablespoons unrefined sugar or pure maple syrup (less if using sweetened milk), plus more for sprinkling
- ¼ cup spelt flour or whole-grain flour
- ½ teaspoon pumpkin pie spice
- Pinch salt

DIRECTIONS

1. Preparing the Ingredients. In a medium bowl, stir together the pumpkin, milk, sugar, flour, pumpkin pie spice, and salt. Pour the mixture into 4 heat-proof ramekins. Sprinkle a bit more sugar on the top of each, if you like. Put a trivet in the bottom of your electric pressure cooker's cooking pot and pour in a cup or two of water. Place the ramekins onto the trivet, stacking them if needed (3 on the bottom, 1 on top).
2. High pressure for 6 minutes. Close and lock the lid, and select High Pressure for 6 minutes.
3. Pressure Release. Once the cooking is complete, quick release the pressure. Unlock and remove the lid. Let cool for a few minutes before carefully lifting out the ramekins with oven mitts or tongs. Let cool for at least 10 minutes before serving.

NUTRITION: Calories: 152 Fat: 4g Carbs: 4g Sugar 8g Protein: 18g

538. COCONUT AND ALMOND TRUFFLES

COOKING: 0'   **PREPARATION: 15'**   **SERVES: 8**

INGREDIENTS

- 1 cup pitted dates
- 1 cup almonds
- ½ cup sweetened cocoa powder, plus extra for coating
- ½ cup unsweetened shredded coconut
- ¼ cup pure maple syrup
- 1 teaspoon vanilla extract
- 1 teaspoon almond extract
- ¼ teaspoon sea salt

DIRECTIONS

1. In the bowl of a food processor, combine all the ingredients and process until smooth. Chill the mixture for about 1 hour.
2. Roll the mixture into balls and then roll the balls in cocoa powder to coat.
3. Serve immediately or keep chilled until ready to serve.

NUTRITION: Calories: 126 Fat: 5g Carbs: 13g Sugar 7g Protein: 5g

539. FUDGY BROWNIES (PRESSURE COOKER)

COOKING: 5'   **PREPARATION: 10'**   **SERVES: 4-6**

INGREDIENTS

- 3 oz. dairy-free dark chocolate
- 1 tablespoon coconut oil or vegan margarine
- ½ cup applesauce
- 2 tablespoons unrefined sugar
- 1/3 cup whole-grain flour
- ½ teaspoon baking powder
- Pinch salt

DIRECTIONS

1. Put a trivet in your electric pressure cooker's cooking pot and pour in a cup or two of two of water. Select Sauté or Simmer. In a large heat-proof glass or ceramic bowl, combine the chocolate and coconut oil. Place the bowl over the top of your pressure cooker, as you would a double boiler. Stir occasionally until the chocolate is melted, then turn off the pressure cooker. Stir the applesauce and sugar into the chocolate mixture. Add the flour, baking powder, and salt and stir just until combined. Pour the batter into 3 heat-proof ramekins. Put them in a heat-proof dish and cover with aluminum foil. Using a foil sling or silicone helper handles, lower the dish onto the trivet. (Alternately, cover each ramekin with foil and place them directly on the trivet, without the dish.)
2. High pressure for 6 minutes. Close and lock the lid, and select High Pressure for 5 minutes.
3. Pressure Release. Once the cooking is complete, quick release the pressure. Unlock and remove the lid.
4. Let cool for a few minutes before carefully lifting out the dish, or ramekins, with oven mitts or tongs. Let cool for a few minutes more before serving.
5. Top with fresh raspberries and an extra drizzle of melted chocolate.

NUTRITION: Calories: 256 Fat: 29g Carbs: 1g Sugar 0.5g Protein: 11g

540. CHOCOLATE MACAROONS

COOKING: 15' **PREPARATION: 10'** **SERVES: 8**

INGREDIENTS

- 1 cup unsweetened shredded coconut
- 2 tablespoons cocoa powder
- 2/3 cup coconut milk
- ¼ cup agave
- pinch of sea salt

DIRECTIONS

1. Preheat the oven to 350°F. Line a baking sheet with parchment paper. In a medium saucepan, cook all the ingredients over medium-high heat until a firm dough is formed. Scoop the dough into balls and place on the baking sheet.
2. Bake for 15 minutes, remove from the oven, and let cool on the baking sheet.
3. Serve cooled macaroons or store in a tightly sealed container for up to

NUTRITION: Calories: 371 Fat: 15g Carbs: 7g Sugar 2g Protein: 41g

541. CHOCOLATE PUDDING

COOKING: 0' **PREPARATION: 5'** **SERVES: 1**

INGREDIENTS

- 1 banana
- 2 to 4 tablespoons nondairy milk
- 2 tablespoons unsweetened cocoa powder
- 2 tablespoons sugar (optional)
- ½ ripe avocado or 1 cup silken tofu (optional)

DIRECTIONS

1. In a small blender, combine the banana, milk, cocoa powder, sugar (if using), and avocado (if using). Purée until smooth. Alternatively, in a small bowl, mash the banana very well, and stir in the remaining ingredients.

NUTRITION: Calories: 537 Fat: 26g Carbs: 13g Sugar 16g Protein: 54g

THE PLANT BASED DIET COOKBOOK

542. LIME AND WATERMELON GRANITA

COOKING: 0' **PREPARATION: 15'** **SERVES: 4**

INGREDIENTS

- 8 cups seedless watermelon chunks
- juice of 2 limes, or 2 tablespoons prepared lime juice
- ½ cup. brown sugar
- strips of lime zest, for garnish

DIRECTIONS

1. In a blender or food processor, combine the watermelon, lime juice, and sugar and process until smooth. You may have to do this in two batches. After processing, stir well to combine both batches.
2. Pour the mixture into a 9-by-13-inch glass dish. Freeze for 2 to 3 hours. Remove from the freezer and use a fork to scrape the top layer of ice. Leave the shaved ice on top and return to the freezer.
3. In another hour, remove from the freezer and repeat. Do this a few more times until all the ice is scraped up. Serve frozen, garnished with strips of lime zest.

NUTRITION: Calories: 281 Fat: 20g Carbs: 14g Sugar 9g Protein: 11g

543. COCONUT-BANANA PUDDING

COOKING: 5' **PREPARATION: 4'** **SERVES: 4**

INGREDIENTS

- 3 bananas, divided
- 1 (13.5-oz.) can full-Fat: coconut milk
- ¼ cup organic cane sugar
- 1 tablespoon cornstarch
- 1 teaspoon vanilla extract
- 2 pinches sea salt
- 6 drops natural yellow food coloring (optional)
- Ground cinnamon, for garnish

DIRECTIONS

1. Combine 1 banana, the coconut milk, sugar, cornstarch, vanilla, and salt in a blender. Blend until smooth and creamy. If you're using the food coloring, add it to the blender now and blend until the color is evenly dispersed.
2. Transfer to a saucepot and bring to a boil over medium-high heat. Immediately reduce to a simmer and whisk for 3 minutes, or until the mixture thickens to a thin pudding and sticks to a spoon.
3. Transfer the mixture to a container and allow to cool for 1 hour. Cover and refrigerate overnight to set. When you're ready to serve, slice the remaining 2 bananas and build individual servings as follows: pudding, banana slices, pudding, and so on until a single-serving dish is filled to the desired level. Sprinkle with ground cinnamon.

NUTRITION: Calories: 170 Fat: 4g Carbs: 34 Sugar 14g Protein: 9g

544. SPICED APPLE CHIA PUDDING

COOKING: 0' | **PREPARATION: 5'** | **SERVES: 1**

INGREDIENTS

- ½ cup unsweetened applesauce
- ¼ cup nondairy milk or canned coconut milk
- 1 tablespoon chia seeds
- 1½ teaspoons sugar
- Pinch ground cinnamon or pumpkin pie spice

DIRECTIONS

1. In a small bowl, stir together the applesauce, milk, chia seeds, sugar, and cinnamon. Enjoy as is, or let sit for 30 minutes so the chia seeds soften and expand.

NUTRITION: Calories: 145 Fat: 4g Carbs: 19g Sugar 9g Protein: 2 g

545. CARAMELIZED PEARS WITH BALSAMIC GLAZE

COOKING: 15' | **PREPARATION: 5'** | **SERVES: 4**

INGREDIENTS

- 1 cup balsamic vinegar
- ¼ cup plus 3 tablespoons brown sugar
- ¼ teaspoon grated nutmeg
- pinch of sea salt
- ¼ cup coconut oil
- 4 pears, cored and cut into slices

DIRECTIONS

1. In a medium saucepan, heat the balsamic vinegar, ¼ cup of the brown sugar, the nutmeg, and salt over medium-high heat, stirring to thoroughly incorporate the sugar. Allow to simmer, stirring occasionally, until the glaze reduces by half, 10 to 15 minutes.
2. Meanwhile, heat the coconut oil in a large sauté pan over medium-high heat until it shimmers. Add the pears to the pan in a single layer. Cook until they turn golden, about 5 minutes. Add the remaining 3 tablespoons brown sugar and continue to cook, stirring occasionally, until the pears caramelize, about 5 minutes more.
3. Place the pears on a plate. Drizzle with balsamic glaze and serve.

NUTRITION: Calories: 237 Fat: 5g Carbs: 7g Sugar 12.4g Protein: 31g

546. SALTED COCONUT-ALMOND FUDGE

COOKING: 12' **PREPARATION: 5'** **SERVES: 12**

INGREDIENTS

- ¾ cup creamy almond butter
- ½ cup maple syrup
- 1/3 cup coconut oil, softened or melted
- 6 tablespoons fair-trade unsweetened cocoa powder
- 1 teaspoon coarse or flaked sea salt

DIRECTIONS

1. Line a loaf pan with a double layer of plastic wrap. Place one layer horizontally in the pan with a generous amount of overhang, and the second layer vertically with a generous amount of overhang.
2. In a medium bowl, gently mix the almond butter, maple syrup, and coconut oil until well combined and smooth. Add the cocoa powder and gently stir it into the mixture until well combined and creamy.
3. Pour the mixture into the prepared pan and sprinkle with the sea salt. Bring the overflowing edges of the plastic wrap over the top of the fudge to completely cover it. Place the pan in the freezer for at least 1 hour or overnight, until the fudge is firm.
4. Remove the pan from the freezer and lift the fudge out of the pan using the plastic-wrap overhangs to pull it out. Transfer to a cutting board and cut into 1-inch pieces.

NUTRITION: Calories: 297 Fat: 20.3g Carbs: 4g Sugar 6g Protein: 21g

547. CARAMELIZED BANANAS

COOKING: 10' **PREPARATION: 5'** **SERVES: 2**

INGREDIENTS

- 2 tablespoons vegan margarine or coconut oil
- 2 bananas, peeled, halved crosswise and then lengthwise
- 2 tablespoons dark brown sugar, demerara sugar, or coconut sugar
- 2 tablespoons spiced apple cider
- Chopped walnuts, for topping

DIRECTIONS

1. Melt the margarine in a nonstick skillet over medium heat. Add the bananas, and cook for 2 minutes. Flip, and cook for 2 minutes more.
2. Sprinkle the sugar and cider into the oil around the bananas, and cook for 2 to 3 minutes, until the sauce thickens and caramelizes around the bananas. Carefully scoop the bananas into small bowls, and drizzle with any remaining liquid in the skillet. Sprinkle with walnuts.

NUTRITION: Calories: 413 Fat: 13g Carbs: 64g Sugar: 21g Protein: 37g

548. MIXED BERRIES AND CREAM

COOKING: 0' **PREPARATION:** 10' **SERVES:** 4

INGREDIENTS

- 2 15-oz. cans full-Fat: coconut milk
- 3 tablespoons agave
- ½ teaspoon vanilla extract
- 1 pint fresh blueberries
- 1 pint fresh raspberries
- 1 pint fresh strawberries, sliced

DIRECTIONS

1. Refrigerate the coconut milk overnight. When you open the can, the liquid will have separated from the solids. Spoon out the solids and reserve the liquid for another purpose.
2. In a medium bowl, whisk the agave and vanilla extract into the coconut solids. Divide the berries among four bowls. Top with the coconut cream. Serve immediately.

NUTRITION: Calories: 468 Fat: 19g Carbs: 53g Sugar: 21g Protein: 23g

549. "RUGGED" COCONUT BALLSGLAZE

COOKING: 0' **PREPARATION:** 15' **SERVES:** 8

INGREDIENTS

- 1/3 cup coconut oil melted
- 1/3 cup coconut butter softened
- 2 oz. coconut, finely shredded, unsweetened
- 4 tbsp coconut palm sugar
- 1/2 cup shredded coconut

DIRECTIONS

1. Combine all ingredients in a blender.
2. Blend until soft and well combined.
3. Form small balls from the mixture and roll in shredded coconut.
4. Place on a sheet lined with parchment paper and refrigerate overnight.
5. Keep coconut balls into sealed container in fridge up to one week.

NUTRITION: Calories: 247 Fat: 7g Carbs: 33g Sugar: 18g Protein: 12g

550. ALMOND - CHOCO CAKE

COOKING: 32'   **PREPARATION: 45'**   **SERVES: 8**

INGREDIENTS

- 1 1/2 cups of almond flour
- 1/3 cup almonds finely chopped
- 1/4 cup of cocoa powder unsweetened
- Pinch of salt
- 1/2 tsp baking soda
- 2 Tbsp almond milk
- 1/2 cup Coconut oil melted
- 2 tsp pure vanilla extract
- 1/3 cup brown sugar (packed)

DIRECTIONS

1. Preheat oven to 350°F.
2. Line 9" cake pan with parchment paper, and grease with a little melted coconut oil; set aside.
3. Stir the almond flour, chopped almonds, cocoa powder, salt, and baking soda in a bowl.
4. In a separate bowl, stir the remaining ingredients.
5. Combine the almond flour mixture with the almond milk mixture and stir well.
6. Place batter in a prepared cake pan.
7. Bake for 30 to 32 minutes.
8. Remove from the oven, allow it to cool completely.
9. Store the cake-slices a freezer, tightly wrapped in a double layer of plastic wrap and a layer of foil. It will keep on this way for up to a month.

NUTRITION: Calories: 460 Fat: 32g Saturated Fat: 23g Carbs: 16g Sugar: 21g Protein: 29g

551. BANANA-ALMOND CAKE

COOKING: 45'   **PREPARATION: 15'**   **SERVES: 8**

INGREDIENTS

- 4 ripe bananas in chunks
- 3 Tbsp honey or maple syrup
- 1 tsp pure vanilla extract
- 1/2 cup almond milk
- 3/4 cup of self-rising flour
- 1 tsp cinnamon
- 1 tsp baking powder
- 1 pinch of salt
- 1/3 cup of almonds finely chopped
- Almond slices for decoration

DIRECTIONS

1. Preheat the oven to 400°F (air mode).
2. Oil a cake mold; set aside.
3. Add bananas into a bowl and mash with the fork.
4. Add honey, vanilla, almond, and stir well.
5. In a separate bowl, stir flour, cinnamon, baking powder, salt, the almonds broken, and a spoon mix.
6. Combine the flour mixture with the banana mixture, and stir until all ingredients combined well.
7. Transfer the mixture to prepared cake mold and sprinkle with sliced almonds.
8. Bake for 40-45 minutes or until the toothpick inserted comes out clean.
9. Remove from the oven, and allow the cake to cool completely.
10. Cut cake into slices, place in tin foil, or an airtight container, and refrigerate up to one week.

NUTRITION: Calories: 301 Fat: 8g Carbs: 21g Sugar: 18g Protein: 26g

552. BANANA-COCONUT ICE CREAM

COOKING: 0'   **PREPARATION: 15'**   **SERVES: 6**

INGREDIENTS

- 1 cup coconut cream
- 1/2 cup Inverted sugar
- 2 large frozen bananas (chunks)
- 3 Tbsp honey extracted
- 1/4 tsp cinnamon powder

DIRECTIONS

1. In a bowl, whip the coconut cream with the inverted sugar.
2. In a separate bowl, beat the banana with honey and cinnamon.
3. Incorporate the coconut whipped cream and banana mixture; stir well.
4. Cover the bowl and let cool in the refrigerator over the night.
5. Stir the mixture 3 to 4 times to avoid crystallization.
6. Keep frozen 1 to 2 months.

NUTRITION: Calories: 257 Fat: 4g Carbs: 37g Sugar: 23g Protein: 20g

553. COCONUT BUTTER CLOUDS COOKIES

COOKING: 10'   **PREPARATION: 15'**   **SERVES: 8**

INGREDIENTS

- 1/2 cup coconut butter softened
- 1/2 cup peanut butter softened
- 1/2 cup of granulated sugar
- 1/2 cup of brown sugar
- 2 Tbsp chia seeds soaked in 4 tablespoons water
- 1/2 tsp pure vanilla extract
- 1/2 tsp baking soda
- 1/4 tsp salt
- 1 cup of all-purpose flour

DIRECTIONS

1. Preheat oven to 360°F.
2. Add coconut butter, peanut butter, and both sugars in a mixing bowl.
3. Beat with a mixer until soft and sugar combined well.
4. Add soaked chia seeds and vanilla extract; beat.
5. Add baking soda, salt, and flour; beat until all ingredients are combined well.
6. With your hands, shape dough into cookies.
7. Arrange your cookies onto a baking sheet, and bake for about 10 minutes.
8. Remove cookies from the oven and allow to cool completely.
9. Sprinkle with icing sugar and enjoy your cookies.
10. Place cookies in an airtight container and keep refrigerated up to 10 days.

NUTRITION: Calories: 731 Fat: 26g Carbs: 56g Fat: 34g Protein: 45g

554. CHOCOMINT HAZELNUT BARS

COOKING: 15' **PREPARATION: 5'** **SERVES: 8**

INGREDIENTS

- 1/2 cup coconut oil, melted
- 4 Tbsp cocoa powder
- 1/4 cup almond butter
- 3/4 cup brown sugar - (packed)
- 1 tsp vanilla extract
- 1 tsp pure peppermint extract
- pinch of salt
- 1 cup shredded coconut
- 1 cup hazelnuts sliced

DIRECTIONS

1. Chop the hazelnuts in a food processor; set aside.
2. Fill the bottom of a double boiler with water and place it on low heat.
3. Put the coconut oil, cacao powder, almond butter, brown sugar, vanilla, peppermint extract, and salt in the top of a double boiler over hot (not boiling) water and constantly stir for 10 minutes.
4. Add hazelnuts and shredded coconut to the melted mixture and stir together.
5. Pour the mixture in a dish lined with parchment and freeze for several hours.
6. Remove from the freezer and cut into bars.
7. Store in airtight container or freezer bag in a freezer.
8. Let the bars at room temperature for 10 to 15 minutes before eating.

NUTRITION: Calories: 186 Fat: 4g Carbs: 23g Sugar: 18g Protein: 19g

555. COCO-CINNAMON BALLS

COOKING: 5' **PREPARATION: 10'** **SERVES: 12**

INGREDIENTS

- 1 cup coconut butter softened
- 1 cup coconut milk canned
- 1 tsp pure vanilla extract
- 3/4 tsp cinnamon
- 1/2 tsp nutmeg
- 2 Tbsp coconut palm sugar (or granulated sugar)
- 1 cup coconut shreds

DIRECTIONS

1. Combine all ingredients (except the coconut shreds) in a heated bath - bain-marie.
2. Cook and stir until all ingredients are soft and well combined.
3. Remove bowl from heat, place into a bowl, and refrigerate until the mixture firmed up.
4. Form cold coconut mixture into balls, and roll each ball in the shredded coconut.
5. Store into a sealed container, and keep refrigerated up to one week.

NUTRITION: Calories: 213 Fat: 6g Fiber: 13g Carbs: 16g Sugar: 18g Protein: 22g

556. WAFFLES WITH ALMOND FLOUR

COOKING: 15'   **PREPARATION: 15'**   **SERVES: 4**

INGREDIENTS

- 1 cup almond milk
- 2 tbsps. chia seeds
- 2 tsp lemon juice
- 4 tbsps. coconut oil
- 1/2 cup almond flour
- 2 tbsps. maple syrup
- Cooking spray or cooking oil

DIRECTIONS

1. Mix coconut milk with lemon juice in a mixing bowl.
2. Leave it for 5-8 minutes on room temperature to turn it into butter milk.
3. Once coconut milk is turned into butter milk, add chai seeds into milk and whisk together.
4. Add other ingredients in milk mixture and mix well.
5. Preheat a waffle iron and spray it with coconut oil spray.
6. Pour 2 tbsp. of waffle mixture into the waffle machine and cook until golden.
7. Top with some berries and serve hot.

NUTRITION: Calories: 332 Fat: 8g Carbs: 16g Sugar: 17g Protein: 19g

557. SIMPLE BANANA FRITTERS

COOKING: 15'   **PREPARATION: 15'**   **SERVES: 8**

INGREDIENTS

- 4 Bananas
- 3 Tbsps. Maple Syrup
- ¼ Tsp. Cinnamon Powder
- ¼ Tsp. Nutmeg
- 1 Cup Coconut Flour

DIRECTIONS

1. Preheat oven to 350°F.
2. Mash the bananas in a large mixing bowl and maple syrup, cinnamon, nutmeg powder and coconut flour.
3. Mix all the ingredients well.
4. Take 2 tbsps. mixture and make small 1-inch-thick patties from this mixture.
5. Place cakes in greased baking tray.
6. Bake patties in preheated oven for about 10-15 minutes until golden from both sides.
7. Once done, take them out of the oven.
8. Serve with coconut cream.

NUTRITION: Calories: 415 Fat: 18g Carbs: 18g Sugar: 21g Protein: 18g

558. COCONUT AND BLUEBERRIES ICE CREAM

COOKING: 0' | **PREPARATION: 5'** | **SERVES: 4**

INGREDIENTS

- 1/4 Cup Coconut Cream
- 1 Tbsp. Maple Syrup
- ¼ Cup Coconut Flour
- 1 Cup Blueberries
- ¼ Cup Blueberries for Topping

DIRECTIONS

1. Put ingredients into food processor and mix well on high speed.
2. Pour mixture in silicon molds and freeze in freezer for about 2-4 hours.
3. Once balls are set remove from freezer.
4. Top with berries.

NUTRITION: Calories: 315 Fat: 13g Carbs: 6g Sugar: 18g Protein: 9g

559. PEACH CROCKPOT PUDDING

COOKING: 4H | **PREPARATION: 15'** | **SERVES: 6**

INGREDIENTS

- 2 Cups Sliced Peaches
- 1/4 Cup Maple Syrup
- 1/2 Tsp. Cinnamon Powder
- 2 Cups Coconut Milk
- For Serving
- ½ Cup Coconut Cream
- 1 Oz. Coconut Flakes

DIRECTIONS

1. Lightly grease the crockpot and place peaches in the bottom.
2. Add maple syrup, cinnamon powder and milk.
3. Cover and cook on high for 4 hours.
4. Once cooked remove from crockpot.
5. For serving pour coconut cream.
6. Top with coconut flakes.

NUTRITION: Calories: 433 ,Fat: 18g, Carbs: 21g, Sugar: 19g, Protein: 12g

560. RASPBERRIES & CREAM ICE CREAM

COOKING: 0' | **PREPARATION: 5'** | **SERVES: 4**

INGREDIENTS

- 2 Cups Raspberries
- 8 Oz. Coconut Cream
- 2 Tbsps. Coconut Flour
- 1 Tsp Maple Syrup
- 4-8 Raspberries for Filling

DIRECTIONS

1. Mix all ingredients in food processor and blend until well combined.
2. Spoon mixture into silicone mold and with raspberries and freeze for about 4 hours.
3. Remove balls from freezer and pop them out of the molds.

NUTRITION: Calories: 263 ,Fat: 19g, Carbs: 16g, Sugar: 17g, Protein: 9g

561. HEALTHY CHOCOLATE MOUSSE

COOKING: 0' | **PREPARATION: 5'** | **SERVES: 2**

INGREDIENTS
- 1/2 Cup Coconut Milk
- 1 Tsp. Maple Syrup
- 1-3 Tbsps. Cocoa Powder
- Pinch Instant Coffee
- 2 Tbsps. Coconut Cream
- Blackberries for Topping

DIRECTIONS
1. Heat coconut milk and maple syrup until it just begins to simmer.
2. Add cocoa and coffee in milk mixture.
3. Add cream to same mixture and whip until relatively stiff peaks form.
4. Transfer to a serving glass.
5. Chill the mousse in freezer for 2-3 hours.
6. Top with some berries and spoon of coconut cream.

NUTRITION: Calories: 258, Fat: 11g, Carbs: 15g, Sugar: 14g, Protein: 8g

562. FRUITS, PINE NUTS AND MINT SALAD

COOKING: 0 | **PREPARATION: 5'** | **SERVES: 2**

INGREDIENTS
- 2 yellow kiwis
- 2 green kiwis
- 2 tangerines
- 2 teaspoons honey
- 2 teaspoons lemon juice
- pine nuts
- sprig of mint
- cinnamon

DIRECTIONS
1. Wash and clean kiwis. Cut cubes and transfer them into a deep saucer.
2. Peel the tangerine. Divide into slices, then cut. Add tangerines to kiwi.
3. Mix honey, lemon juice and cinnamon in the separate container. Mix well and dress fruit with sauce.
4. Finally, add cedar nuts and mint leaves to the dish to taste.

NUTRITION: Calories: 216, Fat: 2g, Carbs: 45g, Sugar 19g, Protein: 3g

563. VEGAN MINI GINGERBREAD LOAVES

COOKING: 30' | **PREPARATION: 15'** | **SERVES: 8**

INGREDIENTS

For Gingerbread
- 3 cups gluten-free flour
- 2 teaspoons baking powder
- 1 teaspoon baking soda
- 1 1/2 teaspoons cinnamon
- 1 1/2 teaspoons ground ginger
- 1 cup coconut milk, unsweetened
- 1 cup coconut sugar
- ½ cup unsweetened applesauce
- ½ cup pumpkin puree
- 2/3 cup canola oil
- ½ cup molasses
- 1 teaspoon vanilla extract

For the Ginger Vanilla Glaze
- 1 1/2 cup powdered sugar
- 3 tablespoon coconut milk
- ½ teaspoon ground ginger
- ½ teaspoon pure vanilla extract

DIRECTIONS

For Gingerbread
1. Preheat oven to 350°F.
2. Spray small loaf pans with cooking spray or line with parchment paper.
3. Sift together flour, baking powder, soda, cinnamon, salt, and ginger. Mix well.
4. Mix coconut milk, applesauce, pumpkin puree, vanilla, oil, and molasses.
5. Add liquid ingredients to the dry mixture, and stir to combine.
6. Pour batter into the small loaf pans.
7. Bake for 30 minutes until a toothpick inserted into the center of the gingerbread comes out clean.
8. Cool desserts for 10 minutes before removing from pan.

For Glaze
9. Mix powdered sugar, coconut milk, vanilla, and ginger in a blender.
10. Drizzle glaze over cooled gingerbread.

NUTRITION: Calories: 579, Fat: 26g, Carbs: 99g, Sugar: 24g, Protein: 5g

THE PLANT BASED DIET COOKBOOK

564. VEGAN CHOCOLATE TURRON

COOKING: 5' — **PREPARATION: 10'** — **SERVES: 16**

INGREDIENTS

- ½ lb dark chopped chocolate
- 2 tablespoons melted coconut oil
- 2 oz. unsalted raw hazelnuts

DIRECTIONS

1. Place dark chocolate in a saucepan. Cook over medium heat, stirring occasionally until chocolate is melted.
2. Remove chocolate from the heat. Add hazelnuts, and combine well.
3. Pour the chocolate-hazelnuts mixture into lined rectangular dish.
4. Cool to room temperature. Chop the turron.
5. If it's too hot in the room, keep turron in the fridge.

NUTRITION: Calories: 120, Protein: 2g, Fat: 10g, Sugar 8g, Carbs: 10g

565. VEGAN CHOCOLATE ORANGE TRUFFLES

COOKING: 0 — **PREPARATION: 15'** — **SERVES: 16**

INGREDIENTS

- ½ lb pitted dates
- 2 oz. almond meal
- 2 tablespoons unsweetened cocoa powder
- 2 teaspoons cocoa powder (for rolling the balls)
- 2 tablespoons orange juice
- 1 lemon peel

DIRECTIONS

1. Place pitted dates, almond meal, cocoa powder, orange juice, and lemon zest in a food processor or a powerful blender. Mix well.
2. Make the mixture into balls using your hands. Make 16 truffles.
3. Roll the candies in cocoa powder to taste.

NUTRITION: Calories: 58, Protein: 1g, Fat: 2g, Sugar 3g, Carbs: 11g

566. GLUTEN-FREE CHOCOLATE ORANGE VEGAN CAKE

COOKING: 40' — **PREPARATION: 10'** — **SERVES: 8**

INGREDIENTS

For the Cake
- 3 tablespoons flax seeds
- 6 tablespoons water
- 4 oz. gluten-free oat flour
- 2 oz. unsweetened cocoa powder
- 4 oz. brown sugar
- 1 teaspoon baking soda
- 1 teaspoon baking powder
- ½ cup agave syrup
- 1 cup orange juice
- 2 tablespoons extra virgin olive oil
- 1 tablespoon orange marmalade

For Chocolate Frosting
- 125 ml water
- ½ lb dates
- 2 tablespoons unsweetened cocoa powder
- 4 tablespoons orange juice
- 1 tablespoon orange marmalade

DIRECTIONS

For the Cake
1. Preheat the oven to 355ºF.
2. Place flax seeds and water in a blender. Blend well.
3. Mix chickpea flour, cocoa powder, sugar, oat flour, baking powder, and soda in a bowl.
4. Mix blended flax seeds, agave syrup, orange juice, marmalade, and oil in another bowl.
5. Mix wet and dry ingredients until smooth.
6. Put parchment paper on a bottom of the sheet Pour the mixture into a deep baking dish. Bake for 40 minutes.

For the Frosting
7. Mix all the ingredients with a blender until smooth.
8. Spread the mixture over the cooled cake.

NUTRITION: Calories: 200, Protein: 3g, Fat 4g, Sugar 5g, Carbs: 40g

567. COCONUT SNOWBALLS

COOKING: 0' **PREPARATION:** 20' + 1 WEEK FOR FREEZING **SERVES:** 10

INGREDIENTS

- 3 oz. shredded coconut
- 1-oz. almond flour
- 3 oz. agave syrup

DIRECTIONS

1. Mix shredded coconut, flour, and syrup in a food processor until well combined.
2. Make 10 balls using your hands.
3. Roll the balls in 1 oz. shredded coconut.
4. You can keep these balls in a sealed container in a fridge for one week.

NUTRITION: Calories: 88, Protein: 1g, Fat 5g, Sugar: 4g, Carbs: 9g

568. CHAMPAGNE JELLY WITH FRUITS AND BERRIES

COOKING: 0' **PREPARATION:** 20' **SERVES:** 4

INGREDIENTS

- 500 ml semi-sweet champagne
- 1/3-oz. agar-agar powder
- 1 medium pear
- 1 medium peach
- 1 medium nectarine
- 2-3 apricots
- 5 oz. seedless grapes
- 5 oz. sweet cherries
- 5 oz. strawberries

DIRECTIONS

1. Wash fruits and berries well.
2. Peel the fruits and berries. Cut into pieces. Leave the grapes and other small berries for decorating.
3. Pour agar-agar into the champagne in a deep saucepan and place on low heat. Stir until the gelatin dissolves. Remove from heat.
4. Line the jelly containers with plastic wrap.
5. Place the fruits and berries in a container. Pour champagne over fruit.
6. Refrigerate for 5-6 hours. Turn the container over and remove the plastic wrap.

NUTRITION: Calories: 134, Protein: 2g, Fat 1g, Sugar 5g, Carbs: 32

569. ORANGES WITH CINNAMON AND HONEY

COOKING: 15' **PREPARATION:** 5' **SERVES:** 4

INGREDIENTS

- 10 1/2 oz. orange
- 4 tablespoons honey
- 1 teaspoon cinnamon
- 1 oz. walnuts

DIRECTIONS

1. Peel the oranges, divide into slices.
2. Place the slices on a baking dish.
3. Chop the nuts.
4. Mix honey with cinnamon and nuts.
5. Sprinkle honey-nut mixture on oranges slices.
6. Preheat the oven to 390 ºF. Then place the baking sheet in the oven and bake for 15 minutes.
7. You can eat orange slices cool or warm.

NUTRITION: Calories: 179, Protein: 2g, Fat: 5g, Sugar: 5g, Carbs: 32g

570. GREEN BUCKWHEAT COFFEE CAKE

COOKING: 30'   **PREPARATION: 20'**   **SERVES: 10**

INGREDIENTS

For the Cake Base
- 15 bright dates
- 2 tablespoons cocoa
- 1 cup walnuts (or other to your taste)

For the Filling
- 1/8 cup green buckwheat
- 1 cup plain milk
- 15 dates
- 3 teaspoons chicory
- 2 teaspoons cocoa
- ½-1 cup milk (additional)

DIRECTIONS

For the Base
1. Soak dates overnight to soften. Remove the pits from the dates and blend them in a food processor.
2. Peel the walnuts, and grind nuts into crumbs.
3. Add cocoa to the nuts.
4. Mix half the dates, nuts and cocoa with a fork until smooth. Make into balls with wet hands. If the dough is too thin, add cocoa or nuts.
5. Spread the dough on the bottom of a medium middle baking sheet.

For the Filling
6. Grind the green buckwheat into flour using a coffee grinder.
7. Place the buckwheat flour in a saucepan. Add a little milk and stir well until no lumps remain.
8. Warm up the mixture and boil until it thickens (for 5-10 minutes).
9. Place the second half of the dates, chicory, cocoa and a little milk in a food processor. Beat into thick, homogeneous cream. Add milk as needed.
10. Place the mixture on top of the base. Freeze cake for 2-3 hours. If the cake is too frozen, let it stand at room temperature for 15-20 minutes.
11. Coat the cake with the melted chocolate or icing.

NUTRITION: Calories: 328, Protein: 8g, Fat: 19g, Sugar: 10g, Carbs: 33g

571. SWEET CHOCOLATE HUMMUS

COOKING: 5'   **PREPARATION: 10'**   **SERVES: 3**

INGREDIENTS

- 2 tablespoons boiled chickpeas
- 4 full tablespoons cocoa
- 4 tablespoons honey
- 1 tablespoon orange juice
- 5 tablespoons oil, coconut or peanut
- 1/5 teaspoon cinnamon, nutmeg or vanilla (optional)

DIRECTIONS

1. Boil the chickpeas. After cooking rinse and drain excess liquid.
2. Put chickpeas, honey, cocoa, softened butter and spices in a blender bowl. Pour in 2/3 cups of milk. If necessary, mix by hand, folding from the bottom up.
3. If it is hard for the blender to mix, add a little milk to get a smooth chocolate mixture without grains.
4. If hummus is not sweet enough, add honey or syrup.

NUTRITION: Calories: 432, Protein: 7g, Fat: 29g, Sugar: 10g, Carbs: 35g

572. FRUITS AND BERRIES IN ORANGE JUICE SALAD

COOKING: 0'   **PREPARATION: 10'**   **SERVES: 2**

INGREDIENTS

- 1 cup strawberries
- 1 cup sweet cherries
- 1/2 cup of blueberries
- 1 red apple
- 1 peach
- 1 kiwi
- 1 cup of orange juice
- 2 tablespoons lemon juice

DIRECTIONS

1. Wash and halve the cherries. Remove the pits. Put cherries on a deep plate.
2. Then, wash and cut strawberries into quarters. Add strawberries to the cherries.
3. Add washed blueberries.
4. Wash, cut, and peel the apple, peach, and kiwi. Add the pieces to the other ingredients.
5. Mix all fruits and berries. Pour orange juice over fruit mixture.
6. Add two tablespoons of lemon juice. Let the salad soak up the citrus, and then drain the juice. Eat chilled.

NUTRITION: Calories: 342, Protein: 3g, Fat: 1g, Carbs: 52g

573. TROPICAL FRUITS SALAD

COOKING: 0' **PREPARATION: 10'** **SERVES: 2**

INGREDIENTS

- 1 pineapple
- 2 mangoes
- 2 bananas
- 1/2 cup pomegranate seeds
- 2 tablespoons sweet coconut shavings

DIRECTIONS

1. Wash, peel and cut pineapple, mango and bananas into medium cubes. Put fruits in a deep plate.
2. Add the pomegranate seeds to the dish, mix and let stand for several hours in the refrigerator.
3. Sprinkle with coconut flakes before eating.

NUTRITION: Calories: 297, Protein: 5g, Fat: 6g, Sugar: 8g, Carbs: 10g

574. PEANUT PASTE (HALVA)

COOKING: 10' **PREPARATION: 0'** **SERVES: 10**

INGREDIENTS

- 7 oz. peanuts
- 40 ml sunflower oil
- 1/3 cup sugar
- 70 ml water
- 1/3 cup wheat flour
- 1 teaspoon vanilla sugar

DIRECTIONS

1. Peel the peanuts. Fry in a clean and dry pan for 3-5 minutes, stirring constantly.
2. Pour the wheat flour into another pan, stirring with a spoon. Fry until creamy.
3. Remove from the heat.
4. Grind the peanuts in food processers as finely as possible.
5. Pour the fried flour in the food processor. Grind for 2 minutes.
6. Place sugar, vanilla sugar and water in a small saucepan. Bring to a boil. Boil the syrup for one minute. Add vegetable oil, mix the ingredients, and remove from heat.
7. Pour the syrup into the peanut mixture. Mix well. The mass thickens quite quickly.
8. Put the mass into the mold. Line the form with parchment paper for easy removal. Leave the halva to cool completely.
9. The paste is ready. Cut into pieces and try! Halva can be from golden to brown, depending on the degree the flour and peanuts are roasted.

NUTRITION: Calories: 197, Protein: 6g, Fat: 13g, Sugar: 11g, Carbs: 11g

575. BLACK BEAN ORANGE MOUSSE

COOKING: 15' **PREPARATION: 5'** **SERVES: 5-6**

INGREDIENTS

- 4 tbsp. Cashew Milk
- 15 oz. Black beans
- Zest of 1 Orange
- oz. Dates, pitted
- 5 tbsp. Cacao Powder, raw
- 2 tbsp. Coconut oil, melted
- 8 tbsp. Brown Rice Syrup

DIRECTIONS

1. First, place the black beans and dates in the food processor.
2. Process them for 2 to 3 minutes or until finely grated.
3. Next, add all the remaining ingredients to the food processor and process it again.
4. Finally transfer the mixture to the serving bowls and sprinkle it with cacao nibs.

NUTRITION: Calories: 486 Proteins: 22.4g Carbs: 82.4g Sugar: 21g Fat: 8.4g

THE PLANT BASED DIET COOKBOOK

576. CASHEW PUDDING

COOKING: 25'   **PREPARATION: 10'**   **SERVES: 2**

INGREDIENTS

- ¼ cup Cocoa Powder, unsweetened
- 1 cup Cashews, raw
- Dash of Sea Salt
- 4 tbsp. Almond Milk, unsweetened
- 2 Medjool Dates
- 1 tbsp. Maple Syrup
- 1 tbsp. Coconut Oil

DIRECTIONS

1. First, place the cashews in a medium bowl along with hot water. Soak it for one hour.
2. Next, transfer the soaked cashews into a high-speed blender along with the remaining ingredients.
3. Blend for 2 minutes or until you get a smooth and creamy mixture.
4. Now, return the pudding to the bowl and cover it with a plastic wrap.
5. Finally, keep the bowl in the refrigerator for 2 to 3 hours or until set.
6. Serve and enjoy.

NUTRITION: Calories: 459 Proteins: 13.8g Carbs: 49.4g Sugar: 21g Fat: 28.6g

577. VANILLA MUG CAKE

COOKING: 4'   **PREPARATION: 1'**   **SERVESV: 1**

INGREDIENTS

- ¼ cup Cashew Milk
- 1 scoop Vanilla Protein Powder
- ¼ tsp. Vanilla Extract
- 1 tsp. Chocolate Chips
- ½ tsp. Baking Powder
- 1 tbsp. Granulated Sweetener of your choice
- 1 tbsp. Coconut Flour

DIRECTIONS

1. Start by applying baking spray all over a microwave-safe mug.
2. To this, stir in the Protein: powder, coconut flour, baking powder, and granulated sweetener. Mix well.
3. Now, pour the cashew milk into the flour mixture along with vanilla extract. Tip: At this point, if the combination seems crumbly, add more milk to it until you get a thick batter.
4. Next, cook in the microwave for 1 minute or until the center is set and cooked.
5. Serve and enjoy.

NUTRITION: Calories: 170 Proteins: 29g Carbs: 7g Sugar: 5g Fat: 6g

578. FRUITS AND SPROUTS BUCKWHEAT SALAD

COOKING: 0'   **PREPARATION: 10'**   **SERVES: 2**

INGREDIENTS

- 1 banana
- 1 orange
- 1 carrot
- 4 oz. green buckwheat
- 1 oz. raisins
- 1 oz. nuts

DIRECTIONS

For Buckwheat
1. Put green buckwheat in a deep dish and barely cover it with room temperature water. Cover container with the damp paper towel and set aside for a few days.
2. Check the grouts several times a day. Mix and, if necessary, additionally moisten or change the paper.
3. Sprouts usually appear on the third day, but it is better to wait five or six days. Buckwheat sprouts are not acceptable until they have green leaves.
4. After sprouting, rinse well with cold water. Drain, and place sends buckwheat sprouts on a deep plate.

For Salad
5. Wash and clean vegetables and fruits.
6. Cut carrots and banana into rounds. Feel free to experiment with their shape. Add them to the seedlings.
7. Clean the orange on a plate to collect the juice. Then press gently and cut into circles. Add orange slices to the other ingredients.
8. Add raisins and your choice of nuts. Dress salad with orange juice.

NUTRITION: Calories: 303, Protein: 9g, Fat: 7g, Sugar: 13g, Carbs: 69g

579. JUST APPLE SLICES

COOKING: 10' | **PREPARATION: 10'** | **SERVES: 4**

INGREDIENTS

- 1 cup of coconut oil
- ¼ cup date paste
- 2 tablespoons ground cinnamon
- 4 granny smith apples, peeled and sliced, cored

DIRECTIONS

1. Take a large-sized skillet and place it over medium heat
2. Add oil and allow the oil to heat up
3. Stir in cinnamon and date paste into the oil
4. Add cut up apples and cook for 5-8 minutes until crispy
5. Serve and enjoy!

NUTRITION: Calories: 368 Fat: 13g Protein: 1g Sugar: 8g, Carbs: 2g

580. THE CLASSIC RICE PUDDING

COOKING: 30' | **PREPARATION: 10'** | **SERVES: 8**

INGREDIENTS

- 1 cup of brown rice (uncooked)
- 1 teaspoon vanilla extract
- ½ teaspoon salt
- ½ teaspoon cinnamon
- ¼ teaspoon nutmeg
- 3 egg
- 3 cups coconut milk, light
- 2 cups brown rice, cooked

DIRECTIONS

1. Take a bowl and mix in all ingredients, stir well
2. Preheat your oven to 300°F
3. Transfer mixture to a baking dish and put the dish into the oven
4. Bake for 90 minutes
5. Serve and enjoy!

NUTRITION: Calories: 330 Fat: 10g Carbs: 15g Sugar: 12g Protein: 5g

581. CINNAMON AND PUMPKIN FUDGE

COOKING: 0' | **PREPARATION: 25'** | **SERVES: 4**

INGREDIENTS

- 1 teaspoon ground cinnamon
- 1 cup pumpkin puree
- ¼ teaspoon nutmeg, ground
- 1 ¾ cups of coconut butter, melted
- 1 tablespoon coconut oil

DIRECTIONS

1. Take a bowl and mix in pumpkin spices, coconut butter, coconut oil and whisk well
2. Spread mixture into pan and cover with foil, press it down well
3. Discard the foil
4. Let it chill for 2 hours
5. Chop into squares, serve and enjoy!

NUTRITION: Calories: 110 Fat: 10g Carbs: 11g Sugar: 9g Protein: 12g

582. BLUEBERRY AND PECAN BAKE

COOKING: 30' **PREPARATION: 10'** **SERVES: 4**

INGREDIENTS

- 14 oz. blueberries
- 1 tablespoon lemon juice, fresh
- 1 ½ teaspoons Stevia powder
- 3 tablespoons chia seeds
- 2 cups almond flour, blanched
- ¼ cup pecans, chopped
- 5 tablespoons coconut oil
- 2 tablespoons cinnamon

DIRECTIONS

1. Take a bowl and mix in blueberries, Stevia, chia seeds, lemon juice, and stir
2. Take an iron skillet and place it over heat, add mixture and stir
3. Take a bowl and mix in remaining ingredients, spread mixture over blueberries
4. Preheat your oven to 400°F
5. Transfer baking dish to your oven, bake for 30 minutes
6. Serve and enjoy!

NUTRITION: Calories: 380 Fat: 32g Carbs: 25g Sugar: 18g Protein: 10g

583. FANTASTIC STICKY MANGO RICE

COOKING: 25' **PREPARATION: 10'** **SERVES: 4**

INGREDIENTS

- 1/2 cup sugar
- 1 mango, sliced
- 14 oz. coconut milk, canned
- 1/2 cup basmati rice

DIRECTIONS

1. Cook the rice according to the package instructions, and add half of the sugar while cooking rice. Make sure to substitute half of the required water with coconut milk
2. Take another skillet and boil remaining coconut milk with sugar. Once the mixture is thick, add rice and gently stir
3. Add mango slices and serve
4. Enjoy!

NUTRITION: Calories: 550 Fat: 30g Carbs: 23g Sugar: 18g Protein: 6g

584. SESAME COOKIES

COOKING: 75' **PREPARATION: 10'** **SERVES: 20'**

INGREDIENTS

- 1 cup sesame seeds
- 1 cup sunflower seeds
- 1 cup flaxseeds
- ½ cup hulled hemp seeds
- 3 tablespoons Psyllium husk
- 1 teaspoon salt
- 1 teaspoon baking powder
- 2 cups of water

DIRECTIONS

1. Pre-heat your oven to a temperature of 350°F
2. Take your blender and add seeds, baking powder, salt, and Psyllium husk
3. Blend well until a sand-like texture appears
4. Stir in water and mix until a batter forms
5. Allow the batter to rest for 10 minutes until a dough-like thick mixture forms
6. Pour the dough onto a cookie sheet lined with parchment paper
7. Spread it evenly, making sure that it has a ¼ inch thickness all around
8. Bake for 75 minutes in the oven
9. Remove and cut up into 20 pieces
10. Allow them to cool for 30 minutes and enjoy!

NUTRITION: Calories: 156 Fat: 6g Carbs: 9g Sugar: 3g Protein: 5g

585. COOL AVOCADO PUDDING

COOKING: 0'   **PREPARATION: 3H**   **SERVES: 4**

INGREDIENTS

- 1 cup almond milk
- 2 avocados, peeled and pitted
- ¾ cup cocoa powder
- 1 teaspoon vanilla extract
- 2 tablespoons Stevia
- ¼ teaspoon cinnamon
- Walnuts, chopped for serving

DIRECTIONS

1. Add avocados to a blender and pulse well
2. Add cocoa powder, almond milk, Stevia, vanilla bean extract and pulse the mixture well
3. Pour into serving bowls and top with walnuts
4. Chill for 2-3 hours and serve!

NUTRITION: Calories: 221 Fat: 8g Carbs: 11g Sugar: 8g Protein: 3g

---

586. THE NO-BAKE FAUX CHEESECAKE

COOKING: 0'   **PREPARATION: 120'**   **SERVES: 10**

INGREDIENTS

For Crust
- 2 tablespoons ground flaxseeds
- 2 tablespoons desiccated coconut
- 1 teaspoon cinnamon

For Filling
- 4 oz. vegan cream cheese
- 1 cup cashews, soaked
- ½ cup frozen blueberries
- 2 tablespoons coconut oil
- 1 tablespoon lemon juice
- 1 teaspoon vanilla extract
- Liquid Stevia

DIRECTIONS

1. Take a container and mix in the crust ingredients, mix well
2. Flatten the mixture at the bottom to prepare the crust of your cheesecake
3. Take a blender/food processor and add the filling ingredients, blend until smooth
4. Gently pour the batter on top of your crust and chill for 2 hours
5. Serve and enjoy!

NUTRITION: Calories: 182 Fat: 16g Carbs: 16g Sugar: 9g Protein: 3g

---

587. BERRY POPSICLES

COOKING: 0'   **PREPARATION: 2H**   **SERVES: 2**

INGREDIENTS

- ½ can coconut cream, canned
- 2 teaspoons natural sweetener, such as Stevia
- ¼ cup mixed blackberries and blueberries

DIRECTIONS

1. Blend the listed ingredients in a blender until smooth
2. Pour mix into popsicle molds and let them chill for 2 hours
3. Serve and enjoy!

NUTRITION: Calories: 165 Fat: 5g Carbs: 2g Sugar: 4g Protein: 1g

588. GINGERBREAD MUFFINS

COOKING: 15' **PREPARATION: 10'** **SERVES: 6**

INGREDIENTS

- 1 tablespoon ground flaxseed
- 6 tablespoons coconut milk
- 1 tablespoon apple cider vinegar
- ½ cup peanut butter
- 2 tablespoons gingerbread spice blend
- 1 teaspoon baking powder
- 1 teaspoon vanilla extract
- 2 tablespoons Swerve

DIRECTIONS

1. Preheat your oven to 350°F
2. Take a bowl and add flaxseed, salt, vanilla, sweetener, spices, and non-dairy milk
3. Keep it on the side
4. Add peanut butter, baking powder and keep mixing
5. Stir well
6. Spoon batter into muffin liners and bake for 30 minutes
7. Let them cool and serve

NUTRITION: Calories: 283 Fat: 23g Carbs: 14g Sugar: 11g Protein: 11g

589. BAKE-FREE FUDGE

COOKING: 5' **PREPARATION: 15'** **SERVES: 25**

INGREDIENTS

- 1 ¾ cups of coconut butter
- 1 cup pumpkin puree
- 1 teaspoon ground cinnamon
- ¼ teaspoon ground nutmeg
- 1 tablespoon coconut oil

DIRECTIONS

1. Take an 8x8 inch square baking pan and line it with aluminum foil
2. Take a spoon and scoop out coconut butter into a heated pan and allow the butter to melt
3. Keep stirring well and remove the heat once fully melted
4. Add spices and pumpkin and keep straining until you have a grain-like texture
5. Add coconut oil and keep stirring to incorporate everything
6. Scoop the mixture into your baking pan and evenly distribute it
7. Place wax paper on top of the mixture and press gently to straighten the top
8. Remove the paper and discard
9. Allow it to chill for 1-2 hours
10. Once chilled, take it out and slice it up into pieces

NUTRITION: Calories: 120 Fat: 10g Carbs: Sugar: 7g Protein: 1.2g

590. TASTY ZUCCHINI BROWNIES

COOKING: 45' **PREPARATION: 5'** **SERVES: 4**

INGREDIENTS

- 2 cups flour
- 1 ½ cups vegan sugar
- 1 teaspoon baking soda
- 1 teaspoon salt
- ½ cup cocoa, unsweetened
- 2 tablespoons vanilla extract
- ½ cup oil
- 2 cups zucchini, peeled and grated

DIRECTIONS

1. Pre-heat your oven to 350°F
2. Take a bowl and sift in cocoa, salt, flour, sugar, and baking soda
3. Stir well
4. Add oil, vanilla, zucchini mix well until you have a nice batter
5. Pour mixture into a baking dish and transfer to the oven
6. Bake for 30-45 minutes until done

NUTRITION: Calories: 138 Fat: 5g Carbs: 11g Sugar: 7g Protein: 1.5g

591. GREAT CHIA AND BLACKBERRY PUDDING

COOKING: 0'   **PREPARATION: 45'**   **SERVES: 2**

INGREDIENTS

- ¼ cup chia seeds
- ½ cup blackberries, fresh
- 1 teaspoon liquid sweetener
- 1 cup coconut milk, full Fat: and unsweetened
- 1 teaspoon vanilla extract

DIRECTIONS

1. Take the vanilla, liquid sweetener and coconut milk and add to blender
2. Process until thick
3. Add in blackberries and process until smooth
4. Divide the mixture between cups and chill for 30 minutes
5. Serve and enjoy!

NUTRITION: Calories: 437 Fat: 18g Carbs: 16g Sugar: 14g Protein: 8g

THE PLANT BASED DIET COOKBOOK

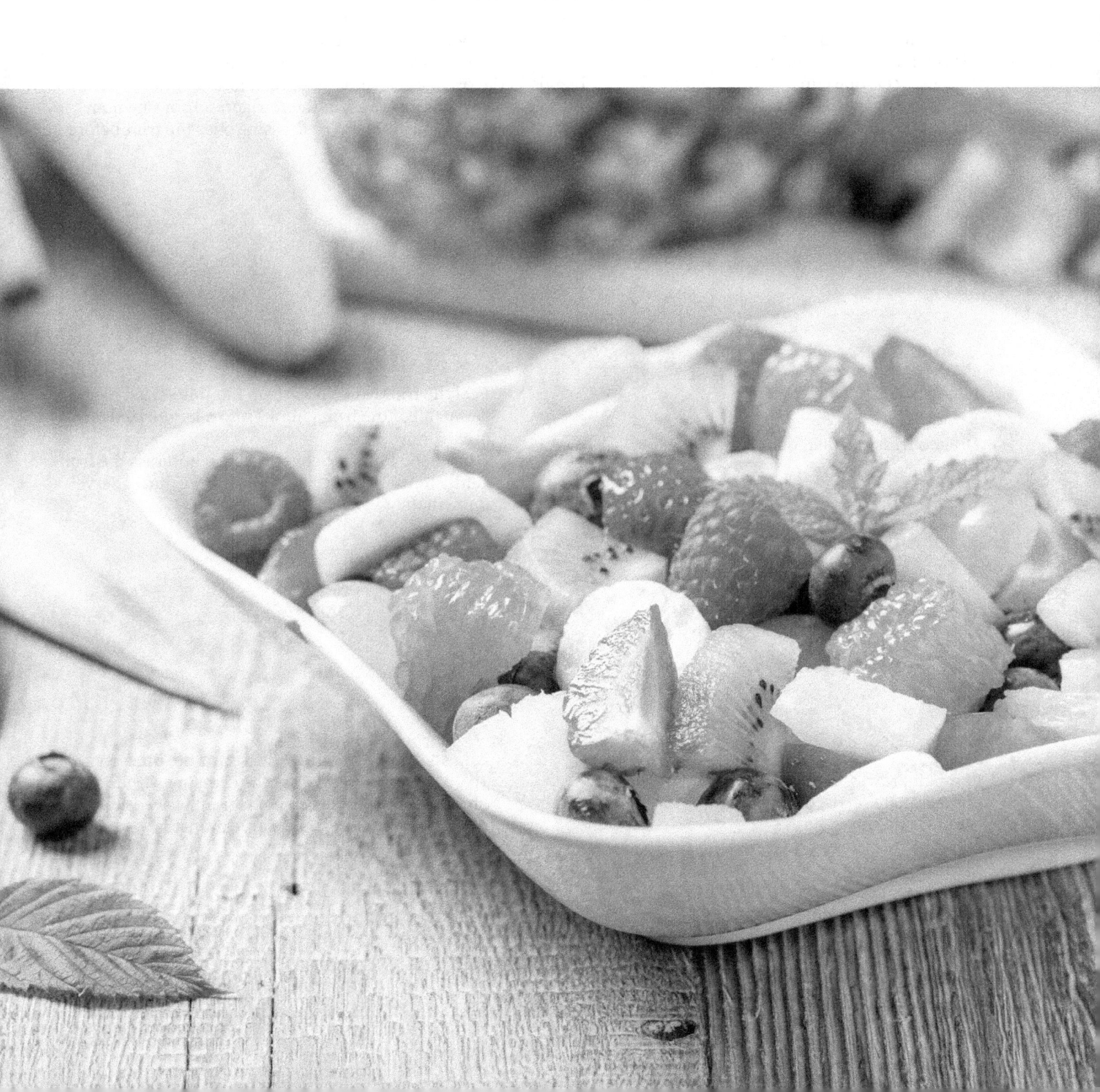

CHAPTER 10:
FRUIT SALAD

- » Orange zest, two teaspoons
- » Tofu, soft, pureed, one half cup
- » Orange juice, three tablespoons
- » Lemon juice, one third cup
- » Cornstarch, one tablespoon
- » Coconut, unsweetened shredded, one half cup
- » Grapes, one cup
- » Sugar, three tablespoons
- » Strawberries, sliced, one cup
- » Orange slices, one cup
- » Apples, fresh sliced, one cup
- » Pineapple, fresh chopped, one cup

1. Use a large-sized bowl to assemble the fruits and put it in the refrigerator.
2. In a small saucepan, mix the lemon juice with the cornstarch and keep stirring until they are well mixed.
3. Add in the orange juice and the sugar and place the saucepan over medium-high heat. Cook the mix for five to ten minutes while the mixture gets thicker. Keep stirring constantly.
4. When the mixture is thick, then take the saucepan off of the heat and let it get completely cool.
5. When the saucepan's mixture has cooled completely, then blends in the orange zest and the pureed tofu.
6. Allow this bowl of mix to rest in the refrigerator for one hour until it becomes chilled. Pour the dressing over the fruit before serving.

Calories: 257 Protein: 8g Fat: 8g Carbs: 44g

- » Lime juice, one tablespoon
- » Kiwi, two
- » Dragon fruit, one half of one
- » Strawberries, twelve
- » Mango, one half of one

1. Peel the fruits and chop them into bite-sized pieces. Dump all of the fruit chunks into a large-sized mixing bowl.
2. Drizzle the lime juice over the fruit and toss the fruit gently to coat all of the pieces with the juice. Serve immediately

Calories: 154 Protein: 2g Fat: 1g Carbs: 37g

- » Salad
- » Pumpkin, raw, shredded, one half cup
- » Pomegranate seeds, one half cup
- » Grapes, one cup
- » Apples, three, cored and cubed
- » Creamy Dressing
- » Cinnamon, one teaspoon
- » Lemon juice, one tablespoon
- » Almond yogurt, one half cup

1. Mix all of the listed Ingredients for the dressing.
2. In a large-sized bowl, toss the dressing with the shredded raw pumpkin, pomegranate seeds, apples, and the dressing. Serve immediately.

Calories: 161 Protein: 3g Fat: 1g Carbs: 40g

- » Balsamic vinegar, two teaspoons
- » Lemon juice, two tablespoons
- » Mint, fresh chopped, one tablespoon
- » Blueberries, one cup
- » Peaches, fresh, three, peeled and sliced thin
- » Strawberries, one pound, cleaned and sliced thin

1. Mix in a medium-sized serving bowl the basil, blueberries, peaches, and strawberries. In a small-sized bowl, mix the balsamic vinegar and the lemon juice.
2. Pour the liquid dressing over the mixed fruit and toss gently to coat all of the fruit pieces with the dressing.
3. Serve immediately or keep the salad covered in the refrigerator for no longer than two days.

Calories: 91 Protein: 1g Fat: 6g Carbs: 22g

- » Lemon juice, three tablespoons
- » Cardamom, one quarter teaspoon
- » Cinnamon, one half teaspoon
- » Mint, fresh, three tablespoons
- » Blackberries, one cup
- » Blueberries, one cup
- » Raspberries, one cup
- » Cherries, seeded, cut in half, one cup
- » Strawberries, cleaned, two cups quartered

1. In a small-sized bowl, mix the spices and the lemon juice well. In a medium-sized bowl, mix the fruits with the lemon juice and mint mixture.
2. Toss the fruits gently but thoroughly to coat all of the pieces. This will store well in the refrigerator for two to three days.

Calories: 113 Protein: 1g Fat: 1g Carbs: 27g

- » Salad
- » Mint, fresh chopped, one cup
- » Lime juice, two tablespoons
- » Kiwi, five, peeled and sliced
- » Mangoes, two, peeled and chopped
- » Green grapes, one cup cut in half
- » Blackberries, one cup
- » Blueberries, one cup
- » Strawberries, one cup sliced
- » Sweet Lime Dressing
- » Powdered sugar, two tablespoons
- » Lime juice, two tablespoons

1. Mix until smooth in a small-sized bowl the powdered sugar and the lime juice.
2. Mix in a large-sized bowl the fruits, then pour on the dressing and gently toss all of the fruits together well to coat all of the pieces.
3. This will stay good in the refrigerator for no more than one day.

Calories: 50 Protein: 1g Fat: 1g Carbs: 12g

- » Passion fruit, one-half cup (about six of the fruit)
- » Papaya, one chopped
- » Pineapple, one cup chunked
- » Oranges, two separated into segments
- » Star fruit, three sliced thin
- » Mangoes, two large, peeled and chunked
- » Mint, fresh, one-third cup chopped coarse
- » Lime juice, one third cup
- » Lime zest, one tablespoon
- » Ginger, ground, one tablespoon
- » Vanilla extract, one tablespoon
- » Brown sugar, one half cup
- » Water, four cups

1. Mix the water and the sugar in a medium-sized saucepan and put it over a medium to high heat until the sugar is dissolved.
2. Let this simmer for five minutes over a very low heat, so the sugar does not burn. Add in the vanilla extract and the ginger and stir well.
3. Let this cook for ten more minutes. Let the mix cool off the heat until it is room temperature, and then add in the mint, juice, and zest.
4. During the time the sauce is cooling mix together the remainder of the Ingredients in a large-sized bowl.
5. Pour the syrup mixture over the fruit in the bowl and mix gently to coat all pieces with the sauce.
6. Put the bowl in the refrigerator until the fruit is cold then serve.
7. Serve immediately or keep the salad covered in the refrigerator for no longer than two days.

Calories: 220 Protein: 3g Fat: 1g Carbs: 56g

- » Mint, fresh, one half cup
- » Orange juice, one half cup
- » Pineapple, one cup cut into small pieces
- » Strawberries, one cup cut into quarters
- » Blueberries, one cup
- » Blackberries, one cup
- » Kiwi, three peeled and sliced

1. In a large-sized bowl, mix all of the fruits and then top with the orange juice and the fresh mint.
2. Toss gently together all of the fruit until they are well mixed.

Calories: 215 Protein: 3g Fat: 1g Carbs: 49g

- » Basil, chopped, one tablespoon
- » Lime juice, two tablespoons
- » Mango, diced, one cup
- » Blueberries, one cup
- » Blackberries, one cup
- » Strawberries, sliced, one and one half cup
- » Quinoa, cooked, one cup

1. In a large-sized bowl, mix the fruits with the cooked quinoa and mix well.
2. Drizzle on the lime juice and add the chopped basil and mix the fruit gently but thoroughly to coat all of the pieces.

Calories: 246 Protein: 7g Fat: 1g Carbs: 44g

CONCLUSION

I hope you have enjoyed this book and all the green recipes here included. I also hope that by reading this book and trying as many of these recipes as possible, you will feel more energized and motivated to improve or maintain your healthy lifestyle.

Once you start a plant-based diet (particularly one that is low in fat and processed or prepared sugars), you will probably start seeing beneficial effects on your weight, especially if the diet will be supported with some good and regular physical exercise (a short 30 mins a day would do). Weight reduction (if that is what you need) can typically happen when you consume more fiber, vitamins, and minerals than animal fats and proteins. Most people can easily shed five pounds without going hungry or feeling denied in a few days of a plant-based diet.

A few studies indicate that organic products may also help slow the aging process, prevent psychological diseases and Alzheimer's illness in more seasoned grown-ups. Therefore, by embracing a plant-based lifestyle, you will live a healthier, happier, and longer life!

No need to say - without commitment, it will be impossible for you to achieve your set goals. Develop a practical plan that will help you transition smoothly into a plant-based lifestyle. While doing this, you will also need your environment to support and focus on your diet plan. Your efforts should be directed towards learning more about this diet. For instance, you should subscribe to YouTube channels to watch and enjoy other vegans' videos as they delve into their experiences.

When making a leap from other diets to plant-based diets, anything can happen along the way. Of course, there are instances where you might fall off the wagon and turn to animal-based diets or processed foods. However, what you should understand is that it is normal to fall and regress occasionally. The transformation is not easy; therefore, forgive yourself for making mistakes here and there. Concentrate on the bigger picture of living a blissful life where you are at a lower risk of cancer, diabetes, and other ailments. More importantly, keep yourself inspired by connecting with like-minded people. Do not overlook their importance in the transition, as they are also going through the challenge you are facing. Hence, they should advise you from time to time on what to do when you feel stuck. Happy, healthy eating!

RECIPES INDEX

BREAKFAST

1. Gingerbread Waffles — 33
2. Blueberry French Toast Breakfast Muffins — 33
3. Greek Garbanzo Beans on Toast — 34
4. Fluffy Garbanzo Bean Omelet — 34
5. Easy Hummus Toast — 35
6. No-Bake Chewy Granola Bars — 35
7. Tasty Oatmeal and Carrot Cake — 35
8. Almond Butter Banana Overnight Oats — 36
9. Peach & Chia Seed Breakfast Parfait — 36
10. Avocado Toast with White Beans — 36
11. Oatmeal & Peanut Butter Breakfast Bar — 37
12. Chocolate Chip Banana Pancake — 37
13. Avocado and 'Sausage' Breakfast Sandwich — 37
14. Cinnamon Rolls with Cashew Frosting — 38
15. Vegan Variety Poppy Seed Scones — 38
16. Sweet Pomegranate Porridge — 39
17. Apple Oatmeal — 39
18. Breakfast Cookies — 39
19. Vegan Breakfast Biscuits — 40
20. Orange French Toast — 40
21. Chocolate Chip Coconut Pancakes — 40
22. Chickpea Omelet — 41
23. Apple-Lemon Bowl — 41
24. Breakfast Scramble — 41
25. Black Bean and Sweet Potato Hash — 42
26. Apple-Walnut Breakfast Bread — 42
27. Vegan Salmon Bagel — 42
28. Mint Chocolate Green Protein Smoothie — 43
29. Dairy-Free Coconut Yogurt — 43
30. Vegan Green Avocado Smoothie — 43
31. Sun-Butter Baked Oatmeal Cups — 43
32. Chocolate Peanut Butter Shake — 44
33. Berries and Banana Smoothie Bowl — 44
34. Kale and Peanut Butter Smoothie — 44
35. Mint Chocolate Protein Smoothie — 45
36. Berry Breakfast Smoothie — 45
37. Sunrise Smoothie — 45
38. Sunshine Orange Smoothie — 46
39. Chocolate and Hazelnut Smoothie — 46
40. Blueberry Oatmeal Smoothie — 46
41. Cookie Dough Smoothie — 47
42. Coffee Smoothie — 47
43. Breakfast Muesli — 47
44. Banana Cream Pie and Chia Pudding — 48
45. Brown Rice Breakfast Pudding — 48
46. Oats with Chia — 48
47. Carrot Cake Oats — 49
48. Toast with Avocado and Berries — 49
49. Chocolate Chip and Coconut Pancakes — 50

SMOOTHIES AND FRESH JUICES

50. Max Power Smoothie — 53
51. Chai Chia Smoothie — 53
52. Trope-Kale Breeze — 53
53. Hydration Station — 54
54. Mango Madness — 54

55. Chocolate PB Smoothie	54	89. Mango, Pineapple and Banana Smoothie	65
56. TPink Panther Smoothie	55	90. Blueberry and Banana Smoothie	65
57. Banana Nut Smoothie	55	91. Chard, Lettuce and Ginger Smoothie	65
58. Overnight Oats On the Go	55	92. Red Beet, Pear and Apple Smoothie	66
59. Oatmeal Breakfast Cookies	56	93. Berry and Yogurt Smoothie	66
60. Sunshine Muffins	56	94. Chocolate and Cherry Smoothie	66
61. Applesauce Crumble Muffins	57	95. Strawberry and Chocolate Milkshake	66
62. Baked Banana French Toast with Raspberry Syrup	57	96. Zobo Drink	67
63. Kale Smoothie	58	97. Basil Lime Green Tea	67
64. Hot Tropical Smoothie	58	98. Turmeric Coconut Milk	67
65. Berry Smoothie	58	99. Berry Lemonade Tea	68
66. Cranberry and Banana Smoothie	58	100. Swedish Glögg	68

GRAINS

67. Pumpkin Smoothie	59		
68. Super Smoothie	59		
69. Kiwi and Strawberry Smoothie	59		
70. Banana and Chai Chia Smoothie	60	101. Veggie Barley Bowl	71
71. Chocolate and Peanut Butter Smoothie	60	102. Indian Lentil Dahl	71
72. Golden Milk	60	103. Kale and Sweet Potato Quinoa	72
73. Mango Agua Fresca	61	104. Brown Rice with Mushrooms	72
74. Light Ginger Tea	61	105. Veggie Paella	73
75. Classic Switchel	61	106. Vegetable and Wild Rice Pilaf	73
76. Lime and Cucumber Electrolyte Drink	61	52. Trope-Kale Breeze	74
77. Easy and Fresh Mango Madness	62	107. Brown Rice with Spiced Vegetables	74
78. Simple Date Shake	62	108. Spiced Tomato Brown Rice	75
79. Beet and Clementine Protein Smoothie	62	109. Noodle and Rice Pilaf	75
80. Matcha Limeade	63	110. Easy Millet Loaf	75
81. Fruit Infused Water	63	111. Walnut-Oat Burgers	76
82. Hazelnut and Chocolate Milk	63	112. Spicy Beans and Rice	76
83. Banana Milk	63	113. Black-Eyed Peas and Corn Salad	76
84. Apple, Carrot, Celery and Kale Juice	64	114. Indian Tomato and Garbanzo Stew	77
85. Sweet and Sour Juice	64	115. Simple Baked Navy Beans	77
86. Green Lemonade	64	116. Vinegary Black Beans	78
87. Pineapple and Spinach Juice	64	117. Spiced Lentil Burgers	78
88. Strawberry, Blueberry and Banana Smoothie	65	118. Pecan-Maple Granola	79

119. Bean and Summer Squash Sauté — 79
120. Peppery Black Beans — 79
121. Walnut, Coconut, and Oat Granola — 80
122. Ritzy Fava Bean Ratatouille — 80
123. Peppers and Black Beans with Brown Rice — 81
124. Black-Eyed Pea, Beet, and Carrot Stew — 81
125. Koshari — 82
126. Black Bean & Sweet Potato Hash — 82
127. Sweet and Salty Pineapple Fried Rice — 83
128. Rice & Veggie Bowl Rice — 83
129. Red Beans and Rice Rice — 84
130. Raw Noodles with Avocado 'N Nuts — 84
131. Rice & Bean Burritos — 85
132. Barbecued Greens & Grits — 85
133. Chickpea and Spinach Cutlets — 86
134. Flavorful Refried Beans — 86
135. Smoky Red Beans and Rice — 87
136. Savory Spanish Rice — 87
137. Delightful Coconut Vegetarian Curry — 88
138. Comforting Chickpea Tagine — 88
139. Black Bean Stuffed Sweet Potatoes — 89
140. Black Bean and Quinoa Salad — 89
141. Coconut Chickpea Curry — 90
142. Sweet Potato and White Bean Skillet — 90
143. Veggie Kabobs — 91
144. Pilaf with Garbanzos and Dried Apricots — 91
145. Spaghetti with Chickpeas Meatballs — 92
146. Black Bean Wrap with Hummus — 92

PASTA & NOODLES

147. Stir Fry Noodles — 95
148. Spicy Sweet Chili Veggie Noodles — 95
149. Creamy Vegan Mushroom Pasta — 96
150. Vegan Chinese Noodles — 96
151. Vegetable Penne Pasta — 97
152. Spaghetti in Spicy Tomato Sauce — 97
153. 20 Minutes Vegetarian Pasta — 98
154. Creamy Vegan Pumpkin Pasta — 98
155. Loaded Creamy Vegan Pesto Pasta — 99
156. Creamy Vegan Spinach Pasta — 99
157. Vegan Bake Pasta with Bolognese Sauce and Cashew Cream — 100
158. 5 Ingredients Pasta — 100
159. Traditional Indian Rajma Dal — 103

LEGUMES

160. Red Kidney Bean Salad — 103
161. Anasazi Bean and Vegetable Stew — 104
162. Easy and Hearty Shakshuka — 104
163. Old-Fashioned Chili — 105
164. Easy Red Lentil Salad — 105
165. Mediterranean-Style Chickpea Salad — 106
166. Traditional Tuscan Bean Stew (Ribollita) — 106
167. Beluga Lentil and Vegetable Mélange — 107
168. Mexican Chickpea Taco Bowls — 107
169. Indian Dal Makhani — 108
170. Mexican-Style Bean Bowl — 108
171. Classic Italian Minestrone — 109
172. Green Lentil Stew

with Collard Greens 109
173. Chickpea Garden Vegetable Medley 110
174. Hot Bean Dipping Sauce 110
175. Chinese-Style Soybean Salad 111
176. Old-Fashioned Lentil and Vegetable Stew 111
177. Indian Chana Masala 112
178. Red Kidney Bean Pâté 112
179. Brown Lentil Bowl 113
180. Hot and Spicy Anasazi Bean Soup 113
181. Black-Eyed Pea Salad (Ñebbe) 114
182. Mom's Famous Chili 114
183. Creamed Chickpea Salad with Pine Nuts 115
184. Black Bean Buda Bowl 115
185. Middle Eastern Chickpea Stew 116
186. Lentil and Tomato Dip 116
187. Creamed Green Pea Salad 117
188. Middle Eastern Za'atar Hummus 117

SOUPS AND STEWS

189. Tomato Gazpacho 119
190. Tomato Pumpkin Soup 119
191. Creamy Garlic Onion Soup 120
192. Avocado Broccoli Soup 120
193. Green Spinach Kale Soup 120
194. Cauliflower Asparagus Soup 121
195. African Pineapple Peanut Stew 121
193. Green Spinach Kale Soup 121
196. Cabbage & Beet Stew 122
197. Basil Tomato Soup 122
198. Mushroom & Broccoli Soup 122
199. Creamy Cauliflower Pakora Soup 123
200. Garden Vegetable and Herb Soup 123
201. The Mediterranean Delight with Fresh Vinaigrette 124
202. Vegetable Broth Sans Sodium 124
203. Amazing Chickpea and Noodle Soup 125
204. Lentil Soup the Vegan Way 125
205. Beet and Kale Salad 126
206. Kale and Cauliflower Salad 126
207. Asian Delight with Crunchy Dressing 127
208. Broccoli Salad the Thai Way 127
209. Sweet Potato, Corn and Jalapeno Bisque 128
210. Creamy Pea Soup with Olive Pesto 128
211. Spinach Soup with Dill and Basil 129
212. Coconut Watercress Soup 129
213. Roasted Red Pepper and Butternut Squash Soup 130
214. Cauliflower Spinach Soup 130
215. Avocado Mint Soup 131
216. Creamy Squash Soup 131
217. Zucchini Soup 131
218. Creamy Celery Soup 132
219. Avocado Cucumber Soup 132
220. Garden Vegetable Stew 132
221. Moroccan Vermicelli Vegetable Soup 133
222. Moroccan Vegetable Stew 133
223. Basic Recipe for Vegetable Broth 134
224. Cucumber Dill Gazpacho 134
225. Red Lentil Soup 135
226. Spinach and Kale Soup 135
227. Coconut and Grilled Vegetable Soup 136
228. Celery Dill Soup 136
229. Broccoli Fennel Soup 137
230. Tofu Goulash Soup 137
231. Pesto Pea Soup 138
232. Tofu and Mushroom Soup 138

SALADS AND SIDES DISHES

233. Cashew Siam Salad — 141
234. Cucumber Edamame Salad — 141
235. Spinach and Mashed Tofu Salad — 142
236. Super Summer Salad — 142
237. Roasted Almond Protein Salad — 143
238. Lentil, Lemon & Mushroom Salad — 143
239. Sweet Potato & Black Bean Protein Salad — 144
240. Lentil Radish Salad — 144
241. Jicama and Spinach Salad — 145
243. Southwest Style Salad — 145
244. Shaved Brussel Sprout Salad — 146
245. Colorful Protein Power Salad — 146
246. Edamame & Ginger Citrus Salad — 147
247. Taco Tempeh Salad — 147
248. Lebanese Potato Salad — 148
249. Chickpea and Spinach Salad — 148
250. Tempeh "Chicken" Salad — 149
251. Spinach & Dill Pasta Salad — 149
252. Italian Veggie Salad — 150
253. Glazed Carrots — 150
254. Broccoli Puree — 151
255. Lemon Cauliflower — 151
256. Lemongrass Rice — 152
257. Chives Couscous — 152
258. Coconut Cauliflower Mix — 153
259. Peppers Bowl — 153
261. Potato Mash — 154
262. Red Cabbage and Carrots — 154
263. Spaghetti Squash and Leeks — 155
264. Paprika Sweet Potato — 155
265. Cinnamon Carrots — 156
266. Wild Rice and Corn — 156
267. Kale Polenta — 157
268. Broccoli Salad — 157
269. Potato Carrot Salad — 158
270. Pea Salad — 158
271. Snap Pea Salad — 159
272. Cucumber Tomato Chopped Salad — 159
273. Zucchini Pasta Salad — 160
274. Egg Avocado Salad — 160
275. Pepper Tomato Salad — 161
276. Penne with Veggies — 161
277. Marinated Veggie Salad — 162
278. Arugula Salad — 162
279. Mediterranean Salad — 163
280. Potato Tuna Salad — 163
281. Shrimp Veggie Pasta Salad — 164
282. Sautéed Cabbage — 164

SNACKS AND SIDES

283. Black Bean Lime Dip — 167
284. Beetroot Hummus — 167
285. Zucchini Hummus — 168
286. Chipotle and Lime Tortilla Chips — 168
287. Carrot and Sweet Potato Fritters — 169
288. Buffalo Quinoa Bites — 169
289. Tomato and Pesto Toast — 170
290. Avocado and Sprout Toast — 170
291. Apple and Honey Toast — 170
292. Thai Snack Mix — 171
293. Zucchini Fritters — 171
294. Zucchini Chips — 171
295. Rosemary Beet Chips — 172
296. Quinoa Broccoli Tots — 172
297. Spicy Roasted Chickpeas — 172
298. Cinnamon Baked Apple Chips — 173
299. Acorn Squash with Mango Chutney — 173
300. Healthy Carrot Chips — 173
301. Hearty Brussels and Pistachio — 174
302. Buffalo Cashews Chutney — 174
303. Morning Peach — 174
304. Sticky Mango Rice — 175
305. Pecan and Blueberry Crumble — 175
306. Healthy Rice Pudding — 175

307. Oatmeal Cookies	176
308. Apple Slices	176
309. Easy Portobello Mushrooms	176
310. The Garbanzo Bean Extravaganza	177
311. Roasted Onions and Green Beans	177
312. Lemony Sprouts	177
313. Sausage Rolls	178
314. Onion Rings	178
315. Avocado Pudding	179
316. Almond Butter Brownies	179
317. Raspberry Chia Pudding	179
318. Chocolate fudge	180
319. Carrot Energy Balls	180
320. Crunchy Sweet Potato Bites	180
321. Roasted Glazed Baby Carrots	181
322. Oven-Baked Kale Chips	181
323. Cheesy Cashew Dip	181
324. peppery Hummus Dip	182
325. Traditional Lebanese Mutabal	182
326. Indian-Style Roasted Chickpeas	182
327. Avocado with Tahini Sauce	183
328. Sweet Potato Tater Tots	183

WRAPS AND SANDWICHES

329. Tofu Salad Sandwiches	185
330. Chickpea Salad Sandwiches	185
331. Seitan Shawarma	186
332. Chipotle Seitan Taquitos	186
333. Mediterranean Chickpea Wraps	187
334. Barbecue Chickpea Burgers with Slaw	187
335. Basic Hummus and Vegetable Sandwich	188
336. Green Pesto Sandwich	188
337. Chickpea Salad Sandwich	189
338. Avocado and White Bean Sandwich	189
339. Sweet Potato and Kale Sandwich Sandwich	190
340. Hummus and Quinoa Wrap	190
341. Mediterranean Veggie Wrap	191
342. Quick Lentil Wrap	191
343. Thai Vegetable and Tofu Wrap Sandwich	192
344. Plant-based Buffalo Wrap	192
345. Colorful Veggie Wrap	193
346. BBQ Chickpea Wrap	193
347. Chickpea and Mango Wraps	194
344. Plant-based Buffalo Wrap	194
348. Tofu and Pineapple in Lettuce	195
349. Quinoa and Black Bean Lettuce Wraps	195

SAUCES, DRESSINGS, AND DIPS

350. Satay Sauce	197
351. Tahini BBQ Sauce	197
352. Tamari Vinegar Sauce	198
353. Sweet and Tangy Ketchup	198
354. Homemade Tzatziki Sauce	199
355. Tangy Cashew Mustard Dressing	199
356. Avocado-dill Dressing	200
357. Easy Lemon Tahini Dressing	200
358. Sweet Mango and Orange Dressing	201
359. Creamy Avocado Cilantro Lime Dressing	201
360. Maple Dijon Dressing	201
361. Avocado Hummus	202
362. Avocado-chickpea Dip	202
363. Beer "Cheese" Dip	202
364. Creamy Black Bean Dip	203
365. Spicy and Tangy Black Bean Salsa	203
366. Homemade Chimichurri	203
367. Cilantro Coconut Pesto	204
368. Fresh Mango Salsa	204
369. Pineapple Mint Salsa	204
370. Asparagus Spanakopita	205
371. Black Bean and Corn	

Salsa from Red Gold ... 205
372. Avocado Bean Dip ... 205
373. Crunchy Peanut Butter Apple Dip ... 206
374. Herb Pockets ... 206
375. Creamy Cucumber Yogurt Dip ... 206
376. Chunky Cucumber Salsa ... 207
377. Healthier Guacamole ... 207
378. Garlic White Bean Dip ... 207
379. Fruit Skewers ... 208
380. Low-Fat: Stuffed Mushrooms ... 208
381. Marinated Mushrooms ... 208
382. Pumpkin Spice Spread ... 209
383. Maple Bagel Spread ... 209
384. Italian Stuffed Artichokes ... 209
385. Enchilada sauce ... 210
386. Keto Salsa Verde ... 210
387. Chimichurri ... 210
388. Keto Vegan Raw Cashew Cheese Sauce ... 211
389. Spicy Avocado Mayonnaise ... 211
390. Green Coconut Butter ... 211
391. Spiced Almond Butter Sauce ... 212
392. Keto Strawberry Jam ... 212
390. Green Coconut Butter ... 212
393. Chocolate Coconut Butter Sauce ... 213
394. Orange Dill Butter ... 213
395. Keto Caramel Sauce ... 213
396. Pecan Butter ... 214
397. Keto Vegan Ranch Dressing ... 214
398. Cauliflower Hummus ... 214
399. White Beans Dip ... 215
400. Edamame Hummus ... 215
401. Beans Mayonnaise ... 215
402. Cashew Cream ... 216
403. Lemon Tahini ... 216
404. Keto-Vegan Ketchup ... 216
405. Guacamole ... 217
406. Keto-Vegan Mayo ... 217
407. Peanut Sauce ... 217
408. Pistachio Dip ... 218
409. Smokey Tomato Jam ... 218
410. Tasty Ranch Dressing/Dip ... 218

VEGETABLES RECIPES

411. Steamed Cauliflower ... 221
412. Cajun Sweet Potatoes ... 221
413. Smoky Coleslaw ... 221
414. Mediterranean Hummus Pizza ... 222
415. Baked Brussels Sprouts ... 222
416. Basic Baked Potatoes ... 222
417. Miso Spaghetti Squash ... 223
418. Garlic and Herb Noodles ... 223
419. Thai Roasted Broccoli ... 223
420. Coconut Curry Noodle ... 224
421. Collard Green Pasta ... 224
422. Jalapeno Rice Noodles ... 225
423. Rainbow Soba Noodles ... 225
424. Spicy Pad Thai Pasta ... 226
425. Linguine with Wine Sauce ... 226
426. Cheesy Macaroni with Broccoli ... 227
427. Soba Noodles with Tofu ... 227
428. Plant Based Keto Lo Mein ... 228
429. Vegetarian Chow Mein ... 228
430. Veggie Noodles ... 229
431. Minutes Vegetarian Pasta ... 229
432. Asian Veggie Noodles ... 230
433. Cauliflower Latke ... 230
434. Roasted Brussels Sprouts ... 231
435. Brussels Sprouts & Cranberries ... 231
436. Potato Latke ... 231
437. Broccoli Rabe ... 232
438. Whipped Potatoes ... 232
439. Quinoa Avocado Salad ... 232
440. Roasted Sweet Potatoes ... 233
441. Cauliflower Salad ... 233
442. Garlic Mashed Potatoes & Turnips ... 233
443. Green Beans ... 234
444. Coconut Brussels Sprouts ... 234
445. Creamy Polenta ... 234
446. Skillet Quinoa ... 235

447. Green Beans with Balsamic Sauce — 235
448. Green Beans Gremolata — 235
449. Minted Peas — 236
450. Sweet and Spicy Brussels Sprout Hash — 236
451. Glazed Curried Carrots — 236
452. Pepper Medley — 237
453. Garlicky Red Wine Mushrooms — 237
454. Sautéed Citrus Spinach — 237
455. Lemon Broccoli Rabe — 238
456. Spicy Swiss Chard — 238
457. Red Peppers and Kale — 238
458. Mashed Cauliflower with Roasted Garlic — 239
459. Steamed Broccoli with Walnut Pesto — 239
460. Roasted Asparagus with Balsamic Reduction — 239
461. Sweet and Sour Tempeh — 240
462. Fried Seitan Fingers — 240
463. Vegetable Pie — 240
464. Collard Green Wrap — 241
465. Zucchini Garlic Fries — 241
466. Mashed Cauliflower — 241
467. Stir-Fried Eggplant — 242
468. Sautéed Garlic Mushrooms — 242
469. Stir-Fried Asparagus and Bell Pepper — 242
470. Wild Rice with Spicy Chickpeas — 243
471. Cashew Pesto & Parsley with veggies — 243
472. Spicy Chickpeas with Roasted Vegetables — 243
473. Special Vegetable Kitchree — 244
474. Mashed Sweet Potato Burritos — 244
475. Zucchini & Pepper Lasagna — 244
476. Toasted Cumin Crunch — 245
477. Spicy Vegetable Burgers — 245
478. Ratatouille Pasta shells — 246
479. Light Mushroom Risotto — 246

APPETIZERS AND SNACKS

480. Almond Vanilla Popcorn — 249
481. Carrot Hotdogs with Red Cabbage — 249
482. Broccoli Slaw Stir-fry with Tofu — 250
483. Eggplant and Sesame Stir-Fry — 250
484. Vegetable Teriyaki Stir-fry — 251
485. Chickpea Burgers — 251
486. Chickpea Crust Pizza with Veggie Topping — 252
487. Dark Chocolate Hazelnut Popcorn — 252
488. Greek Pizza — 253
489. Mexican Pizza — 253
490. Plant Based Crispy Falafel — 254
491. Cinnamon Roll Popcorn — 254
492. Pumpkin Flavored Popcorn — 255
493. Quinoa Tacos — 255
494. Vegan Caramel Popcorn — 256
495. Zucchini Nuggets — 256
496. Sunflower Seed Bites — 257
497. Sweet Nut Bars — 257
498. Peanut Butter Crunch Rice Cakes — 258
499. Spicy Edamame — 258
500. Sweet Pistachio Bites — 258
501. Bagel Popcorn — 258
502. Crispy Chickpeas — 259
503. Fruit and Nut Bars — 259
504. Creamy Log Boats — 260
505. Veggie Sticks and Dip — 260
506. Trail Mix — 260
507. Veggie Crisps — 261
508. Vegan Cheese Squares — 261
509. Tamari Almonds — 261
510. Sweet Tiffin — 262
511. Black Bean Balls — 262
512. Chia Soy Pudding — 262
513. Blueberry Ice Cream — 263

514. Chickpea Choco Slices 263
515. Sweet Green Cookies 263
516. Chocolate Orange Mousse 264
517. Easy Mango Tofu Custard 264
518. Chickpea Cookie Dough 264
519. Cacao Thin Mints 265
520. Banana Bars 265
521. Pumpkin Pudding 265
522. Sweet Hummus 266
523. Lentil Balls 266
524. Homemade Granola 266
525. Peanut Butter Quinoa Cups 267

DESSERTS

526. Apple Crumble 269
527. Cashew-Chocolate Truffles 269
528. Banana Chocolate Cupcakes 270
529. Minty Fruit Salad 270
530. Mango Coconut Cream Pie 271
531. Cherry-Vanilla Rice Pudding (Pressure cooker) 271
532. Lime in the Coconut Chia Pudding 272
533. Mint Chocolate Chip Sorbet 272
534. Peach-Mango Crumble (Pressure cooker) 273
535. Zesty Orange-Cranberry Energy Bites 273
536. Almond-Date Energy Bites 274
537. Pumpkin Pie Cups (Pressure cooker) 274
538. Coconut and Almond Truffles 275
539. Fudgy Brownies (Pressure cooker) 275
540. Chocolate Macaroons 276
541. Chocolate Pudding 276
542. Lime and Watermelon Granita 277
543. Coconut-Banana Pudding 277
544. Spiced Apple Chia Pudding 278
545. Caramelized Pears with Balsamic Glaze 278
546. Salted Coconut-Almond Fudge 279
547. Caramelized Bananas 279
548. Mixed Berries and Cream 280
549. "Rugged" Coconut BallsGlaze 280
550. Almond - Choco Cake 281
551. Banana-Almond Cake 281
552. Banana-Coconut Ice Cream 282
553. Coconut Butter Clouds Cookies 282
554. Chocomint Hazelnut Bars 283
555. Coco-Cinnamon Balls 283
556. Waffles with Almond Flour 284
557. Simple Banana Fritters 284
558. Coconut and Blueberries Ice Cream 285
559. Peach Crockpot Pudding 285
560. Raspberries & Cream Ice Cream 285
561. Healthy Chocolate Mousse 286
562. Fruits, Pine Nuts and Mint Salad 286
563. Vegan Mini Gingerbread Loaves 286
564. Vegan Chocolate Turron 287
565. Vegan Chocolate Orange Truffles 287
566. Gluten-Free Chocolate Orange Vegan Cake 287
567. Coconut Snowballs 288
568. Champagne Jelly with Fruits and Berries 288
569. Oranges with Cinnamon and Honey 288
570. Green Buckwheat Coffee Cake 289
571. Sweet Chocolate Hummus 289
572. Fruits and Berries in Orange Juice Salad 289
573. Tropical Fruits Salad 290
574. Peanut Paste (Halva) 290
575. Black Bean Orange Mousse 290
576. Cashew Pudding 291
577. Vanilla Mug Cake 291

578. Fruits and Sprouts Buckwheat Salad	291
579. Just Apple Slices	292
580. The Classic Rice Pudding	292
581. Cinnamon and Pumpkin Fudge	292
582. Blueberry and Pecan Bake	293
583. fantastic Sticky Mango Rice	293
584. Sesame Cookies	293
585. Cool Avocado Pudding	294
586. The No-Bake Faux Cheesecake	294
587. Berry Popsicles	294
588. Gingerbread Muffins	295
589. Bake-Free Fudge	295
590. Tasty Zucchini Brownies	295
591. Great Chia and Blackberry Pudding	296

592. Ambrosia with Pineapple	299
593. Tropical Fruit Salad	299
594. Fall Fruit with Creamy Dressing	299
595. Summertime Fruit Salad	300
596. Cherry Berry Salad	300
597. Fruit Salad with Sweet Lime Dressing	300
598. Asian Fruit Salad	301
599. Mimosa Salad	301
600. Honey Lime Quinoa Fruit Salad	301